Long-Term Outcomes of Epilepsy Surgery in Adults and Children

Kristina Malmgren • Sallie Baxendale
J. Helen Cross
Editors

Long-Term Outcomes of Epilepsy Surgery in Adults and Children

Springer

Editors
Kristina Malmgren
Sahlgrenska University Hospital and
Institute of Neuroscience and Physiology
Department of Clinical Neuroscience and
Rehabilitation Sahlgrenska Academy at
Gothenburg University
Gothenburg
Sweden

J. Helen Cross
UCL-Institute of Child Health
Great Ormond Street Hospital for
Children London and Young Epilepsy
Lingfield Surrey
UK

Sallie Baxendale
Department of Clinical
and Experimental Epilepsy
National Hospital for Neurology
and Neurosurgery
London
UK

ISBN 978-3-319-17782-3 ISBN 978-3-319-17783-0 (eBook)
DOI 10.1007/978-3-319-17783-0

Library of Congress Control Number: 2015941279

Springer Cham Heidelberg New York Dordrecht London

Printed on acid-free paper

Springer International Publishing AG Switzerland is part of Springer Science+Business Media (www.springer.com)

Contents

Contributors

Torsten Baldeweg, MD Cognitive Neuroscience and Neuropsychiatry Section, Developmental Neurosciences Division, Institute of Child Health, University College London, London, UK

Section of Cognitive Neuroscience and Neuropsychiatry, Great Ormond Street Hospital NHS Trust, London, UK

Sallie Baxendale, PhD, C.Psychol, AFBPsS Department of Clinical and Experimental Epilepsy, National Hospital for Neurology and Neurosurgery, London, UK

Ettore Beghi, MD Laboratorio di Malattie Neurologiche, Department of Neuroscienze, IRCCS-Istituto di Ricerche Farmacologiche "Mario Negri", Milan, Italy

Honor Coleman Melbourne School of Psychological Sciences, The University of Melbourne, Melbourne, VIC, Australia

J. Helen Cross, MB ChB, PhD, FRCP, FRCPCH Section of Clinical Neuroscience, UCL-Institute of Child Health, Great Ormond Street Hospital & Young Epilepsy, London, UK

Michael Duchowny, MD Comprehensive Epilepsy Program, Neurology and the Brain Institute, Miami Children's Hospital, Miami, FL, USA

John S. Duncan, MA, DM, FRCP, FMedSci Department of Epilepsy, National Hospital for Neurology and Neurosurgery, London, UK

Anna Edelvik, MD Department of Clinical Neuroscience and Rehabilitation, Institute of Neuroscience and Physiology, Sahlgrenska Academy, Gothenburg University, Gothenburg, Sweden

Department of Neurology, Sahlgrenska University Hospital, Gothenburg, Sweden

Siobhan Hannan, RN, RSCN, MSc, INP Paediatric Neurology, Chelsea and Westminster Hospital NHS Foundation Trust, London, UK

Melissa Hanson, BS Department of Neurology, University of Wisconsin School of Medicine and Public Health, Madison, WI, USA

George M. Ibrahim, MD, PhD Division of Neurosurgery, Department of Surgery, University of Toronto, Toronto, ON, Canada

Institute of Medical Science, University of Toronto, Toronto, ON, Canada

Division of Neurosurgery, The Hospital for Sick Children, Toronto, ON, Canada

Nathalie Jetté, MD, MSc Department of Clinical Neurosciences, Foothills Medical Centre, University of Calgary, Calgary, AB, Canada

Jana E. Jones, PhD Department of Neurology, University of Wisconsin School of Medicine and Public Health, Madison, WI, USA

Andres M. Kanner, MD, FANA Department of Neurology, Miller School of Medicine, University of Miami, Miami, FL, USA

Evan Cole Lewis, MD, FRCPC Department of Neurology, Miami Children's Hospital, Miami, FL, USA

Kristina Malmgren, MD, PhD Department of Clinical Neuroscience and Rehabilitation, Institute of Neuroscience and Physiology, Sahlgrenska Academy, Gothenburg University, Gothenburg, Sweden

Department of Neurology, Sahlgrenska University Hospital, Gothenburg, Sweden

Ailsa McLellan, MBChB, FRCP, FRCPCH Paediatric Neurosciences, Royal Hospital for Sick Children, Edinburgh, Scotland, UK

Ying Meng, BASc, MD Division of Neurosurgery, Department of Surgery, Toronto Western Hospital, University of Toronto, Toronto, ON, Canada

Anneli Ozanne, PhD Institute of Health Care Sciences, The Sahlgrenska Academy, University of Gothenburg, Gothenburg, Sweden

Klajdi Puka, HBSc Department of Psychology, The Hospital for Sick Children, Toronto, ON, Canada

Philippe Ryvlin, MD, PhD Department of Clinical Neurosciences, Centre Hospitalo-Universitaire Vaudois, Lausanne, Switzerland

Caroline Skirrow, PhD Cognitive Neuroscience and Neuropsychiatry Section, Developmental Neurosciences Division, Institute of Child Health, University College London, London, UK

Section of Cognitive Neuroscience and Neuropsychiatry, Great Ormond Street Hospital NHS Trust, London, UK

Mary Lou Smith, PhD Department of Psychology, The University of Toronto, Toronto, ON, Canada

Neurosciences and Mental Health Program, The Hospital for Sick Children, Toronto, ON, Canada

Department of Psychology, The Hospital for Sick Children, Toronto, ON, Canada

Torbjörn Tomson, MD, PhD Department of Clinical Neuroscience, Karolinska Institutet, Stockholm, Sweden

Department of Neurology, Karolinska University Hospital, Stockholm, Sweden

Samuel Wiebe, MD, MSc Department of Clinical Neurosciences, Foothills Medical Centre, University of Calgary, Calgary, AB, Canada

Sarah J. Wilson, PhD Melbourne School of Psychological Sciences, The University of Melbourne, Melbourne, VIC, Australia

Comprehensive Epilepsy Program, Austin Health, Melbourne, VIC, Australia

Chapter 1
Why a Volume on Long-Term Outcomes of Epilepsy Surgery?

Kristina Malmgren, Sallie Baxendale, and J. Helen Cross

Abstract Epilepsy surgery is a recognized option in the management of adults and children with drug-resistant epilepsy. Magnetic resonance imaging has increased the number of candidates by determining focal structural brain abnormalities not previously apparent. Advances in other techniques have widened the spectrum of surgical candidates both in adults and children. In the short term, rates of seizure freedom are relatively high, but seizure recurrence can still occur in the long term. There are methodological hurdles to overcome when assessing longer-term outcome. There are also the outcomes beyond seizures – cognition, neurodevelopment, academic and vocational outcomes, and quality of life – which are of importance when determining whether a treatment is beneficial. The aim of this volume is to focus on longer-term outcomes from epilepsy surgery in both adults and children.

Keywords Epilepsy surgery • Outcomes • Long term • Adults • Children

K. Malmgren, MD, PhD (✉)
Department of Clinical Neuroscience and Rehabilitation,
Institute of Neuroscience and Physiology, Sahlgrenska Academy,
Gothenburg University, Gothenburg, Sweden

Department of Neurology, Sahlgrenska University Hospital, Gothenburg, Sweden
e-mail: Kristina.malmgren@neuro.gu.se

S. Baxendale, PhD, C.Psychol, AFBPsS
Department of Clinical and Experimental Epilepsy,
National Hospital for Neurology and Neurosurgery, London, UK

J.H. Cross, MB ChB, PhD, FRCP, FRCPCH
Section of Clinical Neuroscience, UCL-Institute of Child Health, Great Ormond Street Hospital & Young Epilepsy 4/5 Long Yard, WC1N 3LU London, UK

Young Epilepsy, Lingfield Surrey, UK

K. Malmgren et al. (eds.), *Long-Term Outcomes of Epilepsy Surgery in Adults and Children*, DOI 10.1007/978-3-319-17783-0_1

Epilepsy surgery is now a recognized option in the management of carefully selected adults and children with drug-resistant epilepsy. It was Victor Horsley at the National Hospital for Neurology and Neurosurgery in London who performed the first recorded operation for epileptic seizures in 1886, reporting on three operations that "cured epilepsy." These were very much based on the knowledge acquired of brain function from motor stimulation in animals; therefore, localization was based on motor semiology and associated lesions found at surgery. Further, this was at a time when little in the way of medical treatment was available. With the development of EEG, providing greater information on localization, Wilder Penfield later established the technique of temporal lobe resection in adults. Hemispherectomy was initially performed on children with congenital hemiplegia, for the treatment of epilepsy and behavior disorder. Although short-term results were excellent, it was this group where long-term complications became evident with hydrocephalus from hemosiderosis, the result of the technique used, highlighting the importance of following patients in the longer term. In 1953, a young motor winder named Henry Molaison underwent a bilateral temporal lobe resection in Montreal. He became profoundly amnesic as a result and remained that way until his death in 2008. Detailed follow-up examination of previous patients who had undergone similar procedures revealed profound deficits in their memory function too. Recognition of the devastating cognitive outcomes that could be associated with epilepsy surgery led both to a prohibition on bilateral temporal procedures, and the recognition that cognitive evaluation must form an integral part of postoperative follow-up.

Murray Falconer, the pioneer of epilepsy surgery in the UK, first recognized that many of the adults who came to temporal lobe surgery for hippocampal sclerosis had experienced seizures since childhood, and that earlier surgery may have prevented some of the long-term consequences of chronic epilepsy. However, the evidence base for this premise has been limited.

Magnetic resonance imaging developed in the early 1980s greatly increased the number of possible candidates by determining focal structural brain abnormalities not previously apparent. Advances in other neurophysiological, neuroimaging, neurosurgical, and neuroanesthetic techniques have subsequently widened the spectrum of surgical candidates both in adults and children. Short-term outcomes have been widely reported, and a randomized controlled trial has definitively demonstrated efficacy of surgery over and above ongoing medical treatment in temporal lobe epilepsy. However, many studies report outcome assessed retrospectively, in selected groups of individuals, and many, specifically focus on seizure outcome. Further, there is a high degree of variability in duration of follow-up, with no standard practice. This can lead to selection and center bias. In the short term, rates of seizure freedom can appear relatively high but seizure recurrence can be reported as long as 10 years postoperatively. When epilepsy surgery was first advocated, particularly in children, attainment of seizure freedom was presumed to avoid the consequences of ongoing seizures in the longer term. A premise for early surgery is the longer-term benefits on neurodevelopment and cognition but few studies focus on such benefits, particularly those beyond seizures. Such may differ considerably across adult and pediatric populations.

There are, of course, methodological hurdles to overcome when assessing longer-term outcome. The first question is what may be considered "long term." Many studies report on 12 month, 3 year, or "last follow-up" – studies involving the latter having a wide range often from <12 months to 5 years in one study, reporting on the collective outcome. There is also often no indication of medication withdrawal. This aside, there are also the outcomes beyond seizures – cognition, neurodevelopment, academic and vocational outcomes, as well as quality of life, assessment of which may be latent in the shorter term but are of obvious importance in determining whether a treatment is overall beneficial.

A premise to pediatric surgery is to improve cognitive and psychosocial outcome – have we the evidence that this is achieved, and consequently are we counseling candidates appropriately with regard to expectations? Most adult candidates associate the possibility of postoperative seizure control with wide-ranging changes in many aspects of their lives. Long-term follow-up studies are needed to ensure they consider surgery with both a realistic scope and time frame for these changes.

The routine follow-up allowed within a healthcare system will vary considerably across geographical regions; ranging from 6 months to 2 years. For any longer-term follow-up, research funds are likely to be required. Moreover, funds required particularly to assess outcomes beyond seizures are likely to be substantial. The spectrum of epilepsy surgery across adults and children differs, and outcomes to be measured in the longer term not necessarily the same. The aims and expectations in different age groups, across differing pathologies and procedures are likely to differ and require different measures of outcome. Cross-sectional studies, therefore, may only give limited information. Individuals may be at differing points postoperatively, at differing starting points preoperatively and there will consequently be no information on the overall natural history following surgery. A long-term perspective is particularly important with respect to cognitive outcome where postoperative changes are not static, but interact with normal age-related changes and seizure control.

The aim of this text is to focus on longer-term outcomes from epilepsy surgery in both adults and children. We wished to address outcomes beyond seizure control, and beyond at least a 5-year time period following surgery.

In planning this volume, we wanted to highlight the methodological demands on long-term observational outcome studies. Chapter 2 is therefore devoted to addressing the methodological limitations of observational studies as well as the demands on future studies. In order to provide valid data, studies need to have a prospective design, representative study populations, a complete follow-up, and clear definitions of outcome measures. Many of the studies published to date do not fulfill all these demands but the Appendix tables at the end of the chapters summarize the characteristics and results of the studies and will hopefully make it easier for the reader to assess the quality of the literature.

An aspect that is not specifically addressed in this volume is the issue of the complications of epilepsy surgery. We know that around 3 % of patients suffer a surgical or neurological complication leading to permanent morbidity, while another 5–10 % have a complication with transient symptoms. Complications are reported shortly after surgery with follow-ups typically 3–6 months after surgery. However, the effects of complications may have a long-lasting impact especially on patients' quality of life and subjective experiences of epilepsy and these effects will therefore be reflected in the chapters covering these topics.

We acknowledge that in some areas data are few, but in addition to summarizing data available at present and so provide a baseline for discussion, both among ourselves and with our patients, we hope this volume highlights where further research is required.

Chapter 2
Methodological Demands on Observational Studies of Outcomes After Epilepsy Surgery

Ettore Beghi

Abstract The short- and long-term outcome of epilepsy surgery has been mostly assessed by observational studies because experimental designs in surgical patients are often unfeasible and have ethical implications. However, observational studies have methodological limitations, which include the retrospective design, the use of referral populations, the small sample size, the enrolment of patients at differing inception points, the use of differing inclusion criteria, differing definitions of prognostic predictors and outcome measures, the unmasked assessment of outcome, the short follow-up, the changing technologies and surgical procedures, and the inadequate statistical methods. These limitations are incorporated in systematic reviews of epilepsy surgery studies and cannot replace well-conducted prognostic studies. Key features of these studies should include representative populations at risk, well-defined inception cohorts, satisfactory and complete follow-up, prospective design, and standard definition of prognostic factors.

Keywords Epilepsy • Surgery • Design • Methodology

Resective surgery is a valuable option for the treatment of drug-resistant epilepsy. However, the short and long-term outcome of epilepsy surgery has been mostly assessed in observational reports. Despite the undisputed contribution of many of these studies in providing evidence of efficacy over time of epilepsy surgery, a number of concerns arise when the results are critically appraised. The methodological issues inherent in the design of such studies must be carefully inspected to put the results in a correct perspective, to separate valuable from less valuable findings, to assess the risk:benefit ratio of surgical approach, and to indicate where to move to improve future research in this field. The following points will be specifically discussed: (1) the impact of surgery on the outcome of seizures with reference to the various types of studies and the natural history of the disease; (2) the strengths and

E. Beghi, MD
Laboratory of Neurological Disorders, Department of Neuroscience, IRCCS-Institute for Pharmacological Research "Mario Negri", Via G. La Masa, 19, Milan, Italy
e-mail: ettore.beghi@marionegri.it

K. Malmgren et al. (eds.), *Long-Term Outcomes of Epilepsy Surgery in Adults and Children*, DOI 10.1007/978-3-319-17783-0_2

the limitations of the existing study designs; (3) a critical appraisal of prognostic indicators; (4) the effects of epilepsy surgery beyond seizure control; (5) the technical requirements of studies on the prognosis of epilepsy surgery and the prognostic indicators; (6) the issues to be considered when combining data in meta-analyses of epilepsy surgery; and (7) future perspectives.

The Impact of Surgery on the Outcome of Epilepsy with Reference to the Various Types of Studies and the Natural History of the Disease

The randomized clinical trial is the leading instrument to assess the impact of any therapeutic intervention, including surgery, on the natural history of a disease. The structure of the randomized trial implies the use of concurrent controls represented by patients with similar baseline characteristics receiving a treatment other than the investigational treatment. The few randomized trials so far published have provided undisputed evidence of greater efficacy of epilepsy surgery than pharmacological treatment over a short period of time. In one such trial, patients with temporal lobe epilepsy with seizures poorly controlled by medications were randomized to receive immediate surgery or to wait for 1 year before surgery [1]. At 1 year, the cumulative proportion of patients who were free from seizures impairing awareness was 58 % in the surgical group and 8 % in the medical group. Another randomized trial compared pharmacotherapy to surgery plus pharmacotherapy after failure of two antiepileptic drugs [2]. During a 2-year follow-up, 0/23 participants in the medical group and 11/15 in the surgical group were seizure free. However, given the technical constraints and the ethical and practical implications of randomized trials, the long-term outcome of epilepsy in patients randomized to the surgical and control groups cannot be assessed. For this reason, the long-term effects of surgical interventions mostly rely on the results of observational studies.

Even with the limitations of the uncontrolled setting (see below), observational studies are of value in assessing the efficacy and safety of a surgical intervention. In these studies, several pieces of evidence support the efficacy of epilepsy surgery. First of all, the significant number of cases with seizure remission after surgery (estimated in about 55–70 % of temporal lobe and 30–50 % of frontal lobe resections) [3] is per se evidence of efficacy, provided that virtually 100 % of patients have uncontrolled seizures before operation. These observations have been confirmed in a systematic review and meta-analysis of published reports by Schmidt and Stavem [4] who found that in appropriately selected patients with drug-resistant temporal lobe epilepsy, the combination of surgery with medical treatment is four times as likely as medical treatment alone to achieve freedom from seizures. Second, the consistency of results across studies carried out in different populations, centers and time periods, and with differing designs, is per se evidence of efficacy. In a systematic review and meta-analysis of 83 observational studies with a mean follow-up exceeding five years, Tellez-Zenteno and co-workers [5] found a median weighted pooled proportion of seizure-free patients of 66 % with temporal lobe resections, 46 % with occipital and parietal resections, and 27 % with frontal lobe resections. In this review, only 8/40 studies on temporal lobe surgery and 6/25 studies grouping temporal and extra-temporal surgery reported seizure freedom below the 25th percentile. Third, the efficacy is maintained at least in part in long-term studies. In their systematic review, Tellez-Zenteno et al. [5] found that the long-term seizure-free rate following temporal lobe surgery was similar to that of short-term controlled trials but consistently lower after extra-temporal and palliative surgery.

Although, based on the above findings, no one would object on the impact of surgery on the natural history of drug-resistant epilepsy, the long-term effects of surgical approach (and the indicators of successful surgery) are still ill-defined. In the absence of concurrent control groups (represented by patients with comparable baseline characteristics and receiving only pharmacological treatment), the possibility cannot be excluded that long-term seizure outcome could be (at least in part) independent from surgery itself. Long-term studies done in patients with newly diagnosed epilepsy from well-defined populations [6, 7] found that epilepsy presents differing prognostic patterns and drug resistance is a dynamic rather than a static process. In keeping with this, a prospective follow-up of patients with drug-resistant epilepsy in clinical series [8–10] show seizure remission in up to 33 % of cases. These findings support the view that long-term remission of seizures after epilepsy surgery can be obtained as part of the natural history of the disease in some patients regardless of the effects of surgical intervention.

In summary, patients with intractable focal epilepsy have a higher probability to achieve seizure freedom following resective (and to a lesser extent palliative) surgery than continued medication alone. However, the available data mostly address temporal lobe surgery and provide limited information on the long-term outcome of epilepsy, for which the effects of surgery, assessed by observational reports, cannot be disentangled from the natural history of the disease. The methodological limitations of these studies are summarized below along with the recommendations for improvement.

Study Designs with Strengths and Limitations

There are three main types of observational studies: the cohort studies, the case-control studies, and the cross-sectional studies. Studies on the outcome of epilepsy surgery mostly belong to the first and third type. In cohort studies, whether retrospective or prospective, the investigators enroll patients undergoing surgery (the cohort) and follow them over time. They obtain information on the baseline characteristics of the study population (eventually including the diagnostic investigations and the technical aspects of the surgical approach), and assess the occurrence of outcomes. When assessing the prognostic indicators of surgery, investigators commonly contrast individuals who are exposed to those who are not exposed (i.e., with and without a given baseline characteristic or among groups of individuals with different categories of exposure (i.e., with shorter or longer disease duration or with extended vs. limited resection). In case-control studies, investigators compare exposures between people with a particular disease outcome (cases) and people without that outcome (controls). The cases may be represented by patients in whom seizures persisted despite surgery and the controls by patients achieving seizure remission; the exposures are all variables that could impact on seizure outcome. In cross-sectional studies, investigators assess all individuals in a sample at the same point in time. Several investigations on the outcome of epilepsy surgery are cross-sectional studies and aim to quantify potential causal associations between exposures (surgery) and disease outcome (seizure reduction or remission).

These three study designs have common and design-specific limitations. These limitations include a retrospective design, a selected inception cohort, the lack of predefined definitions of the prognostic predictors and outcome measures, a small sample size, the unmasked assessment of outcome, a short follow-up period, the changing technologies and procedures, the uncontrolled use of antiepileptic drugs, and the use of incorrect statistical tests (Table 2.1).

A *retrospective design* may bias the study results for the lack of standardized data collection. The data collected in retrospective studies are generally retrieved from medical records and rely on the quality and completeness of the available information. In the absence of prespecified definitions, several baseline variables may reflect the accuracy of the caring physicians in filling the medical records and the differing interpretations given to each variable.

The *representativeness of the inception cohort* is another source of bias, more evident in (but not restricted to) retrospective studies, because "prevalent" cases (i.e., those still being followed at the time of the study) rather than "incident" cases (i.e., those included at the time of surgery) are preferably included. "Prevalent" and "incident" cases tend to differ in that the former are most likely represented by survivors, by patients with persisting seizures or with other epilepsy-related problems,

Table 2.1 Limitations of the design of observational studies on the outcome of epilepsy surgery

Retrospective design
Ill-defined study cohort
Subjective outcome measures
Poorly defined prognostic predictors
Follow-up of variable duration across patients
Small sample size
Absence of masking
Changing technologies and procedures
Inadequate control of confounding variables
Inappropriate statistical analyses

or perhaps by individuals better satisfied with the center's quality of care. In contrast, "incident" cases are represented by all patients enrolled at the time of surgery and as such include both patients who will achieve seizure remission and those who will continue to experience epilepsy-related problems.

In the *absence of precise definitions of the outcome measures and the prognostic predictors,* these variables are subjected to differing interpretations. The Engel classification of seizure outcome [11], still the most widely used, has been criticized for including patients' (and physicians') subjective opinions and for using terms like "disabling seizures" or "rare" which are open to widely different interpretations. The alternative use of quantitative measures to replace this terminology, as done in the ILAE Commission on Neurosurgery report [12], represents only a modest improvement because a 50 % reduction of baseline seizure frequency, as a measure of disease outcome, is strongly dependent on each individual's baseline seizures.

The *duration of follow-up* varies across patients depending on the timing of enrolment. As the prognosis of a disease is a time dependent variable, studies with long-term follow-up and high drop-out rate may be biased towards more positive results. Patients lost to follow-up might have discontinued their visits because of seizure-related problems and in general for the outcome of the disease. On the contrary, patients with short-term follow-up may have insufficient time to show the (lack of) benefits of surgery. Assessing the outcome of surgery by counting seizure-free patients at last follow-up does not take into account the length of follow-up and the drop-out rate and, as such, may be a source of biased results. Minimum follow-up periods should be allowed and appropriate statistical tests (see below) should be used to adjust for the length of follow-up.

The majority of surgical series are based on *small numbers of patients.* Small sample size may lead to imprecise estimates (as confirmed by the wide confidence intervals) in the proportions of patients meeting predefined outcome measures and is a source of sampling bias.

In the *absence of masking*, outcome measures (i.e., seizure counts) may reflect subjective interpretations, which vary across patients and investigators. In the absence of a prospective design and planning, the way the patients keep track of their seizures may lead to under-ascertainment, which is most likely to occur at the presence of minor events ("auras"). As well, the caring physicians and the investigators may give differing interpretations of events likely to be recorded as seizures. In an open setting, these events may be less likely to be diagnosed as seizures in patients who received surgery than in patients treated conservatively.

The *change of the technological and procedural approaches* may explain the increasing proportions of surgical successes over time, which may in turn prevent comparisons of studies done in different epochs.

A correct interpretation of the results of a study on the outcome of a disease in relation to a given intervention (in this case, surgery of epilepsy) should rely on an adequate control of the most important sources of bias, which are particularly relevant in an uncontrolled setting like that of observational studies. In most studies, an adequate *control of the confounding variables* was not included at the planning stage to become part of the study design. In studies where the control of confounders at the planning stage was unfeasible (which is mostly the case of retrospective studies), a correct statistical analysis, including use of multivariate analysis models, was infrequently planned. In addition, despite the differing periods of observation after surgery, appropriate statistical methods have been rarely used to adjust for the different length of follow-up across patients.

In their practice parameter on temporal lobe and localized neocortical resections, Engel [13] identified several major methodological deficiencies in the published studies, which included, among others, the retrospective design, the scarcity of data on preoperative seizures, and the absence of masking in seizure outcome assessment.

Data Pooling and Meta-analyses and a Critical Appraisal of Prognostic Indicators

The heterogeneity of the study populations and outcome measures and, most of all, the pitfalls in the study designs (see previous section) have a strong influence on data pooling. In a comprehensive review of the literature on seizure outcome after temporal lobectomy, McIntosh et al. [14] reported that good surgical outcome could be predicted by hippocampal sclerosis or abnormal MRI, prolonged febrile seizures, anterior temporal localization of interictal epileptiform activity on scalp EEG, extent of mesial resection, absence of perioperative generalized seizures, and absence of acute postoperative seizures. However, the authors identified several sources of variability across studies which prevented data pooling for the risk of biased results. These included, among others, the differing settings and the variability of the definitions used for the prognostic predictors.

A meta-analysis of 47 articles was also performed by Tonini et al. [15] who used strict inclusion and exclusion criteria to minimize the heterogeneity of the study designs. Febrile seizures, mesial temporal sclerosis, abnormal MRI, EEG/MRI concordance, and extensive surgical resection were the strongest prognostic indicators of seizure remission (positive predictors), whereas postoperative discharges and the use of intracranial monitoring predicted an unfavorable prognosis (negative predictors). Firm conclusions could not be drawn for extent of resection, EEG/MRI concordance, and postoperative discharges for the heterogeneity of study results. Neuromigrational defects, CNS infections, vascular lesions, interictal spikes, and side of resection did not affect the chance of seizure remission after surgery. However, limitations were indicated by the authors in the interpretation of the results. The first major limitation was intrinsic to all studies based on data pooling and meta-analysis. Data were extracted from studies using different criteria for seizure outcome. A second limitation was the variable length of the follow-up across studies. The authors limited the review to studies with an expected follow-up of at least 1 year (actually, duration of follow-up was less than 12 months in few patients). Although this interval can be considered crucial for the prediction of surgical outcome, the chance of seizure remission after surgery could be significantly affected by the differing duration of an extended follow-up (i.e., more than 12 months). A third limitation was inherent to the forced dichotomization of each putative prognostic predictor, which means that each factor could be contrasted to a variety of other factors or could include a number of different conditions, each of which associated with differing clinical outcomes. A fourth limitation was that any variable was examined without considering the role of other (known or unknown) confounders, which might have been the true prognostic predictors. This limitation refers to factors like the use of intracranial recording and febrile seizures. Last, the changing techniques and operative procedures might have affected seizure outcome preventing comparisons of studies done in different epochs.

The Effects of Epilepsy Surgery Beyond Seizure Control

To provide a comprehensive counseling to surgical candidates and their families, the impact of surgery should be assessed beyond seizure control and should include the effects of treatment on cognitive, psychosocial and behavioral functions, quality of life, mortality, and costs. All these outcome variables have been assessed by Spencer and Huh [16] in a comprehensive review of epilepsy surgery. The authors found that up to 4 % of adults with anterior mesial temporal lobectomy and up to 10 % of children with focal resection had neurological complications. Mortality related to surgery and late postoperative deaths were estimated at 0–2 % and were higher in children than in adults. Most studies described significant decline in verbal memory, mostly after dominant temporal resections. The methods and timing of neuropsychological assessments documenting these changes were, however, heterogeneous. Some studies reported improvements in verbal memory and full-scale IQ after resection of the non-dominant temporal lobe; however, the degree of contribution of the retest effect and the longevity of these findings was unclear. Between 40 and 50 % of children with epilepsy had high rates of comorbid learning disabilities, developmental delay, psychiatric and behavioral difficulties, and psychosocial problems. After surgery, 4–30 % of patients developed new affective disorders. 1–5 % developed psychosis, although reports from the past decade showed lower incidences than earlier studies. Most studies trying to define the effects of surgery on psychiatric disturbances and the risk factors for sequelae did not include presurgical and postsurgical assessments. Most studies of developmental and cognitive results of medial temporal resections in children suggested a lack of significant change in IQ or verbal memory. Seizure-free outcome was not always clearly related to cognitive outcome.

Although studies provide valuable information on the improvement of quality of life after surgery and indicate seizure freedom as the strongest and most consistent predictor for quality of life improvement, the lack of preoperative comparisons and absence of true control populations in most studies limits the validity of the results. The review by Spencer and Huh (2008) [16] did not compare surgical to medical outcomes. A number of studies have, however, compared surgical to medical therapy in terms of seizure control, cognitive status, psychosocial complications, quality of life, and mortality. These studies were carefully examined by Perry and Duchowny [17] who concluded that, based on limited evidence, successful epilepsy surgery, defined by complete seizure freedom, has the potential to improve cognitive functions, quality of life, and mortality, and may even prove cost-effective. However, the authors acknowledged that in these studies surgical and medical groups were significantly different at baseline (the latter being often unsuitable surgical candidates), the findings were frequently inconsistent, and the purported benefits of surgery on cognitive and psychosocial functions and on quality of life were mostly mediated by seizure freedom and reduction of the pharmacological burden.

One must also consider the use of different outcome measures. A critical appraisal of the quality of evidence on neuropsychological outcomes after epilepsy surgery has been recently published [18] and can be summarized here. The authors examined 147 articles and verified the application of 45 items used as measures of neuropsychological outcome of surgery. Among the socio-demographic characteristics of the patients, education was reported only by 54 % of studies and ethnicity and employment in rare instances. Only 16 % of studies reported on presurgical and 14 % on postsurgical drug treatment. Blinding of clinicians and/or assessors was almost never performed and an independent blind outcome assessment was never performed. Reasons for loss to follow-up were given in only 31 % of studies. Postsurgical deficits were indicated in only 25 % of reports. Quantitative measures of changes were applied in only 64 % of studies. Validated measures of change were used in 26 % of studies. The study results could be generalized in only 23 % of cases. Randomization of treatment was rare and a predefined sample size calculation was almost never performed. A quality assessment of psychosocial outcome measures was not performed.

In summary, assessment of surgical outcome in epilepsy beyond seizure control has received little attention in terms of rating of the quality of evidence using the principles of evidence-based medicine. A correct determination of the neuropsychological outcomes after surgery is relevant in helping the identification of patients at risk for postoperative cognitive decline.

Requirements of Studies on Prognosis of Epilepsy Surgery and Prognostic Indicators

Observational studies are a useful complement to the results of randomized trials and, if well-designed, can identify clinically important differences among therapeutic options (including surgery) and are the only ways to provide long-term data on the risk:benefit ratio of epilepsy surgery. However, in order to improve the quality of the information from observational studies, precise recommendations must be imparted to increase the external validity of published reports. An international group of methodologists, researchers, and journal editors developed a set of guidelines to improve the reports of observational studies. These recommendations are summarized in the Strengthening the Reporting of Observational Studies in Epidemiology (STROBE) [19, 20]. The checklist of items included in the STROBE statement is reported in Table 2.2. The recommendations refer to the reporting of observational studies and to the three main study designs. They can be usefully applied to studies on the outcome of epilepsy surgery.

The design of an ideal study on the prognosis of epilepsy surgery should have the following prerequisites: (1) well-defined criteria for the inclusion of patients; (2) standard (homogeneous) definitions of the prognostic predictors and outcome measures; and (3) adequate duration of follow-up and proper statistical methods to adjust for drop-outs and limited periods of observation. The criteria for the inclusion

Table 2.2 The STROBE Statement—Checklist of items to be addressed in reports of observational studies

Title and abstract Indicate the study's design with a commonly used term in the title or the abstract; provide in the abstract an informative and balanced summary of what was done and what was found
Introduction *Background and rationale*: Explain the scientific background and rationale for the investigation being reported *Objectives*: State specific objectives, including any prespecified hypotheses
Methods *Study design*: Present key elements of study design early in the paper *Setting:* Describe the setting, locations, and relevant dates, including periods of recruitment, exposure, follow-up, and data collection *Patients*: (a) Cohort study—Give the eligibility criteria, and the sources and methods of selection of participants. Describe methods of follow-up. (b) Case-control study—Give the eligibility criteria, and the sources and methods of case ascertainment and control selection. Give the rationale for the choice of cases and controls. (c) Cross-sectional study—Give the eligibility criteria, and the sources and methods of selection of participants *Controls*: (a) Cohort study—For matched studies, give matching criteria and number of exposed and unexposed. (b) Case-control study—For matched studies, give matching criteria and the number of controls per case *Variables*: Clearly define all outcomes, exposures, predictors, potential confounders, and effect modifiers. Give diagnostic criteria, if applicable *Data sources and measurement*: For each variable of interest, give sources of data and details of methods of assessment (measurement). Describe comparability of assessment methods if there is more than one group *Bias:* Describe any efforts to address potential sources of bias *Study size*: Explain how the study size was arrived at *Quantitative variables*: Explain how quantitative variables were handled in the analyses. If applicable, describe which groupings were chosen, and why *Statistical methods*: (a) Describe all statistical methods, including those used to control for confounding. (b) Describe any methods used to examine subgroups and interactions; (c) Explain how missing data were addressed. (d) Cohort study—If applicable, explain how loss to follow-up was addressed. Case-control study—If applicable, explain how matching of cases and controls was addressed. Cross-sectional study—If applicable, describe analytical methods taking account of sampling strategy. (e) Describe any sensitivity analyses

(continued)

Table 2.2 (continued)

Results *Participants*: (a) Report the numbers of individuals at each stage of the study—e.g., numbers potentially eligible, examined for eligibility, confirmed eligible, included in the study, completing follow-up, and analyzed. (b) Give reasons for non-participation at each stage. (c) Consider use of a flow diagram *Descriptive data*: (a) Give characteristics of study participants (e.g., demographic, clinical, social) and information on exposures and potential confounders. (b) Indicate the number of participants with missing data for each variable of interest. (c) Cohort study—Summarize follow-up time (e.g., average and total amount) *Outcome data*: Cohort study—Report numbers of outcome events or summary measures over time. Case-control study—Report numbers in each exposure category, or summary measures of exposure. Cross-sectional study—Report numbers of outcome events or summary measures *Main results*: (a) Give unadjusted estimates and, if applicable, confounder-adjusted estimates and their precision (e.g., 95 % confidence intervals) Make clear which confounders were adjusted for and why they were included. (b) Report category boundaries when continuous variables were categorized (c) If relevant, consider translating estimates of relative risk into absolute risk for a meaningful time period *Other analyses*: Report other analyses done—e.g., analyses of subgroups and interactions, and sensitivity analyses
Discussion *Key results*: Summarize key results with reference to study objectives *Limitations*: Discuss limitations of the study, taking into account sources of potential bias or imprecision. Discuss both direction and magnitude of any potential bias *Interpretation*: Give a cautious overall interpretation of results considering objectives, limitations, multiplicity of analyses, results from similar studies, and other relevant evidence *Generalizability*: Discuss the generalizability (external validity) of the study results
Other information *Funding*: Give the source of funding and the role of the funders for the present study and, if applicable, for the original study on which the article is based

Reprinted from: Vandenbroucke et al. [20]. Creative Commons Attribution (CC BY) license

of the patients should be in keeping with the requirement that patients must be representative of the underlying surgical candidates. The authors should provide a clear description of the stage of disease at which patients entered the study and describe the source of their patients, to minimize referral and selection bias. The use of homogeneous (preferably standard) definitions for the commonest prognostic indicators is encouraged. Details should be also given of all putative prognostic predictors, to provide a comprehensive overview of the prognosis of the disease in question and give the best explanation of the results after controlling for the known prognostic indicators. Prolonged follow-up is required with an attempt to obtain information on the surgical outcome in all patients. In order to adjust for the duration of follow-up, survival tables and curves should be used in order to censor patients who did not achieve a predefined outcome measure (e.g., seizure relapse over time) at the time of the last observation.

Outcome measures should be clearly defined and, if possible, reliable. Proper statistical methods should be employed to assess the independent role of each prognostic predictor. Multivariate analysis models are encouraged.

Table 2.3 American academy of neurology evidence classification scheme for a therapeutic article

Class I: Prospective, randomized, controlled clinical trial with masked outcome assessment, in a representative population
The following are required: (a) primary outcome(s) is/are clearly defined; (b) exclusion/inclusion criteria are clearly defined; (c) adequate accounting for drop-outs and crossovers with numbers sufficiently low to have minimal potential for bias; (d) relevant baseline characteristics are presented and substantially equivalent among treatment groups or there is appropriate statistical adjustment for differences
Class II: Prospective matched group cohort study in a representative population with masked outcome assessment that meets a–d above OR a randomized, controlled trial in a representative population that lacks one criteria a–d
Class III: All other controlled trials (including well-defined natural history controls or patients serving as own controls) in a representative population, where outcome assessment is independent of patient treatment
Class IV: Evidence from uncontrolled studies, case series, case reports, or expert opinion

With permission: Engel et al. [21], Table 1. Wolters Kluwer

These recommendations are consistent with the evidence classification scheme of the American Academy of Neurology (AAN) for a therapeutic article [21]. Based on the quality of evidence, the AAN identified four classes, Class I being represented by prospective, randomized, controlled clinical trials with masked outcome assessment in representative populations, and (at the other extreme) Class IV by uncontrolled studies, case series, case reports, or expert opinions (Table 2.3).

Issues to Be Considered When Combining Data in Meta-analyses of Epilepsy Surgery

As previously indicated, a meta-analysis incorporates all the defects of the original studied. For this reason, attempts should be made to minimize all sources of heterogeneity and pool the data only from studies with similar design and methods. The strategy of a systematic review should be first outlined in an ad hoc study protocol in which the methods of assessment of the eligible studies are clarified, any effort should be made to include fairly large (sub)populations at risk, reliable outcome measures, and clear (and homogeneous) definitions of the variables to be selected as prognostic predictors of epilepsy surgery. Selection bias is a relevant source of erroneous inferences in open studies, particularly from surgical series. This is even greater when small samples of patients are being considered. Homogeneity of diagnostic findings and surgical procedures should be also assured because a systematic review of published studies tends to cover a prolonged time span, during which diagnostic and surgical procedures may vary significantly. For these reasons, the neuroimaging techniques used should be clearly reported and data pooling should be limited to studies employing the same (hopefully the most updated) diagnostic aids. However, as the reliability of these diagnostic procedures is suboptimal, one should always consider the possibility of inter-rater disagreement when comparing data from different centers (even in the same study). This is particularly important when dealing with some imaging findings, like mesial temporal sclerosis or cortical dysplasia. Patients with and without underlying epileptogenic lesions should be identified and assessed separately and each putative lesion should tentatively undergo separate analysis. Other prognostic predictors (like febrile seizures, CNS infections or other neurological disorders occurred in the patient's past history) require proper predefinition as they mostly rely on history, in the absence of imaging or pathologic findings. In each study, details should be given of age at onset of seizures, family history of epilepsy, history of febrile seizures, etiology, disease severity (i.e., seizure frequency), preoperative EEG, imaging and (where available) pathological findings, disease duration, age at surgery, surgical factors (type and extent of surgery) including resection volume, and postoperative clinical (i.e., seizure frequency) and EEG findings. The outcome of seizures after epilepsy surgery must be assessed using valid, reliable and standard criteria. In the large majority of the surgical series, the Engel's four categories were used [13]. The reliability of this classification still needs verification. Another important issue is the duration of the follow-up, which is strongly correlated to seizure outcome. In that sense, prolonged observation and the use of actuarial methods (survival tables and curves) are strongly encouraged to provide meaningful findings. Multivariate analysis models should be used to assess seizure outcome and all the above prognostic indicators should be included to assess the independent predictors and control for confounding and interactions. Finally, each study's results must be assessed for heterogeneity, which must be low before drawing conclusions based on the meta-analysis.

Future Perspectives

An increasing number of surgical options have been used in the last decades. These include, among others, vagus nerve stimulation and deep brain stimulation. Along with classical resective and palliative surgery, these techniques require long-term outcome assessment. As indicated above, future studies on the prognosis of epilepsy surgery should have minimum evidence-based requirements to provide acceptable results. These include a prospective design, the inclusion of representative study populations and well-defined inception cohorts, a prolonged and complete follow-up, and a standard definition of prognostic factors and outcome measures. Multicenter studies are a valuable alternative to increase sample size and to compare different countries, institutions, and technical approaches. As with meta-analyses, pooling data from different sources implies the use of study protocols fulfilling all the previously discussed requirements and the accomplishment of the recommendations of evidence-based medicine.

References

1. Wiebe S, Blume WT, Girvin JP, Eliasziw M, Effectiveness and Efficiency of Surgery for Temporal Lobe Epilepsy Study Group. A randomized, controlled trial of surgery for temporal lobe epilepsy. N Engl J Med. 2001;345:311–8.
2. Engel Jr J, McDermott MP, Wiebe S, Langfitt JT, Stern JM, Dewar S, Sperling M, Gardiner I, Erba G, Fried I, Jacobs M, Vinters HV, Mintzer S, Kieburtz K. Early surgical therapy for drug-resistant temporal lobe epilepsy. JAMA. 2012;307:922–30.
3. National Institutes of Health Consensus Conference. Surgery for epilepsy. JAMA. 1990;264:729–33.
4. Schmidt D, Stavem K. Long-term seizure outcome of surgery versus no surgery for drug-resistant partial epilepsy: a review of controlled studies. Epilepsia. 2009;50:1301–9.
5. Tellez-Zenteno JF, Dhar R, Wiebe S. Long-term seizure outcomes following epilepsy surgery: a systematic review and meta-analysis. Brain. 2005;128:1188–98.
6. Sillanpaa M, Schmidt D. Natural history of treated childhood-onset epilepsy: prospective, long-term population-based study. Brain. 2006;129:617–24.
7. Shorvon SD, Goodridge DMG. Longitudinal cohort studies of the prognosis of epilepsy: contribution of the National General Practice Study of Epilepsy and other studies. Brain. 2013;136:3497–510.
8. Luciano A, Shorvon SD. Results of treatment changes in patients with apparently drug-resistant chronic epilepsy. Ann Neurol. 2007;62:375–81.
9. Callaghan B, Schlesinger M, Rodemer W, Pollard J, Hesdorffer D, Hauser WA, French J. Remission and relapse in a drug-resistant epilepsy population followed prospectively. Epilepsia. 2011;52:619–26.
10. Neligan A, Bell GS, Sander JW, Shorvon SD. How refractory is refractory epilepsy? patterns of relapse and remission in people with refractory epilepsy. Epilepsy Res. 2011;96:225–30.
11. Engel Jr J, Van Ness PC, Rasmussen TB, Ojemann LM. Surgical treatment of the epilepsies outcome with respect to epileptic seizures. In: Engel Jr J, editor. Surgical treatment of the epilepsies. 2nd ed. New York: Raven; 1993. p. 609–21.
12. Wieser HG, Blume WT, Fish D, Goldensohn E, Hufnagel A, King D, et al. ILAE commission report. Proposal for a new classification of outcome with respect to epileptic seizures following epilepsy surgery. Epilepsia. 2001;42:282–6.
13. Engel Jr J. Approaches to localization of the epileptogenic lesion. In: Engel Jr J, editor. Surgical treatment of the epilepsies. New York: Raven; 1987. p. 75–96.
14. McIntosh AM, Wilson S, Berkovic SF. Seizure outcome after temporal lobectomy: current research practice and findings. Epilepsia. 2001;42:1288–307.
15. Tonini C, Beghi E, Berg AT, Bogliun G, Giordano L, Newton RW, Tetto A, Vitelli E, Vitezic D, Wiebe S. Predictors of epilepsy surgery outcome: a meta-analysis. Epilepsy Res. 2004;62:75–87.
16. Spencer S, Huh L. Outcomes of epilepsy surgery in adults and children. Lancet Neurol. 2008;7:525–37.
17. Perry MS, Duchowny M. Surgical versus medical treatment for refractory epilepsy: outcomes beyond seizure control. Epilepsia. 2013;54:2060–70.
18. Hrabok M, Dykeman J, Sherman EMS, Wiebe S. An evidence-based checklist to assess neuropsychological outcomes of epilepsy surgery: how good is the evidence? Epilepsy Behav. 2013;29:443–8.
19. von Elm E, Altman DG, Egger M, Gøtzsche PC, Pocock SJ, Vandenbroucke JP, STROBE Initiative. The Strengthening the Reporting of Observational Studies in Epidemiology (STROBE) statement: guidelines for reporting observational studies. PLoS Med. 2007;4:e296.
20. Vandenbroucke JP, von Elm E, Altman DG, Gøtzsche PC, Mulrow CD, Pocock SJ, Poole C, Schlesselman JJ, Egger M, STROBE Initiative. Strengthening the Reporting of Observational Studies in Epidemiology (STROBE): explanation and elaboration. PLoS Med. 2007;4:e297.

21. Engel Jr J, Wiebe S, French J, Sperling M, Williamson P, Spencer D, Gumnit R, Zahn C, Westbrook E, Enos B, Quality Standards Subcommittee of the American Academy of Neurology; American Epilepsy Society; American Association of Neurological Surgeons. Practice parameter: temporal lobe and localized neocortical resections for epilepsy: report of the Quality Standards Subcommittee of the American Academy of Neurology, in association with the American Epilepsy Society and the American Association of Neurological Surgeons. Neurology. 2003;60:538–47.

Chapter 3
Long-Term Seizure and Antiepileptic Drug Outcomes After Epilepsy Surgery in Adults

Kristina Malmgren, Anna Edelvik, and John S. Duncan

Abstract Epilepsy surgery is an efficacious treatment for selected persons with drug-resistant focal epilepsy, rendering many seizure-free and others significantly improved. There is Class I evidence for short-term efficacy of epilepsy surgery from two randomized controlled studies of temporal lobe resection. In order for patients to make an informed decision about the treatment option of epilepsy surgery, they also need data on the probability of long-term remission or improvement. Long-term longitudinal observational studies are necessary in order to obtain valid outcome data. From a number of such studies, the proportion of patients who have been continuously free from seizures with impairment of consciousness since resective surgery seems to be 40–50 % after 10 years, while a higher proportion have been seizure-free at least a year at each time-point assessed. The best longitudinal data are in patients who have undergone temporal lobe resection and in whom the histopathology was mesial sclerosis, and in these patients the majority of relapses occur within 5 years. Whether this course is applicable to other resection types and pathologies is not clear. There is much less information on the longitudinal course in patients who have undergone other resection types and have other causes. For many resection types, the number of patients in single-center long-term follow-ups is limited and for almost all studies there is a lack of controls. Multicenter observational studies following both operated and nonoperated patients are needed in order to obtain more robust data.

Keywords Epilepsy surgery • Seizure outcome • Long term • Predictors • Antiepileptic drugs

K. Malmgren, MD, PhD (✉) • A. Edelvik, MD
Department of Clinical Neuroscience and Rehabilitation, Institute of Neuroscience and Physiology, Sahlgrenska Academy, Gothenburg University, Gothenburg, Sweden

Department of Neurology, Sahlgrenska University Hospital, Gothenburg, Sweden
e-mail: Kristina.Malmgren@neuro.gu.se

J.S. Duncan, MA, DM, FRCP, FMedSci
Department of Epilepsy, National Hospital for Neurology and Neurosurgery, London, UK

K. Malmgren et al. (eds.), *Long-Term Outcomes of Epilepsy Surgery in Adults and Children*, DOI 10.1007/978-3-319-17783-0_3

Introduction

Surgical treatment for epilepsy has long been recognized as a valuable treatment option for carefully selected patients with drug-resistant focal epilepsy. In adults, most operations are temporal lobe resections (TLR), with smaller numbers of patients having frontal lobe resections (FLR) or other extratemporal resections. Very few adults undergo multilobar resections or hemispherectomies. In some patients in whom resective surgery is not possible, palliative procedures such as callosotomy or other dissociative procedures may be indicated. Until recently, the knowledge about seizure outcomes after different epilepsy surgery procedures has been based on 1–2-year follow-ups. Epilepsy surgery candidates, however, are mainly young adults and along with information about the short-term chances of seizure control versus risks (complications as well as expected adverse effects), they need detailed advice about likely long-term seizure outcome before deciding to undergo brain surgery. Many patients also have expectations to withdraw antiepileptic drugs (AEDs) after successful surgery [1] since side effects of AEDs contribute to poor quality of life [2]. Realistic expectations concerning long-term seizure and AED outcomes are part of the information they need to consider (see also Chap. 17 of this volume).

There are no randomized controlled trials (RCTs) for long-term follow-up and for obvious reasons such trials would be practically and ethically difficult to implement. In the absence of RCTs, observational cohort studies are important. In order to compare data from different observational studies, defined quality criteria are needed. A number of requirements for well-conducted studies on the prognosis after epilepsy surgery have been suggested: representative study populations, well-defined inception cohorts, satisfactory and complete follow-up, prospective design, and standard definition of prognostic factors as discussed in Chap. 2 of this volume [3].

Reporting of Seizure Outcomes

One problem when assessing the literature on seizure outcomes after epilepsy surgery is how seizure outcome and especially seizure freedom is defined. The most commonly used scheme is the Engel classification; another is the International League Against Epilepsy (ILAE) outcome scale [4, 5]. While the Engel classification assesses the seizure outcome taking account of the whole postoperative period, the ILAE classification refers to the seizure outcome the last year of follow-up and the seizure outcome class should be determined for each year at annual intervals after surgery. However, both classifications make it possible to identify those patients who have been completely seizure-free without auras since the operation (Engel class I A, and ILAE class 1a). In the Engel classification class I B identifies those patients who have had auras only but no seizures with impairment of consciousness since surgery (Engel class I B) but this is not possible in the ILAE classification. Both classifications exclude early postoperative seizures.

Most studies report seizure outcome the last year of follow-up and do not distinguish patients with sustained seizure freedom since surgery, although this is the most important patient group to identify in order to advise surgical candidates about their chances of good outcome. Seizure freedom is most often defined as freedom from seizures with impairment of consciousness, or Engel I (which also includes patients who have had some seizures with impairment of consciousness after surgery but then been seizure-free at least 2 years and patients who have had secondary generalized tonic-clonic seizures (SGTCS) on antiepileptic drug (AED) withdrawal). Some studies differentiate into completely seizure-free (Engel I A or ILAE Class 1a) or include patients with auras only in the category of seizure-free (Engel I A and B or ILAE Class 1a and 2). In the following, we will therefore as far as possible state how seizure freedom is defined in the studies reviewed. Although both scales include a possibility to note worsening of seizure frequency postoperatively, this is seldom reported.

Seizure outcome after epilepsy surgery is not only a question of having sustained seizure freedom or relapse of seizures. More recently, different patterns of remission have also been described, which will be further commented on.

Class I Evidence for Short-Term Seizure Outcomes

There is Class I evidence for short-term efficacy of epilepsy surgery from two randomized controlled studies (RCTs) of TLR [6, 7]. In the Canadian intention to treat RCT 58 % of the 40 patients who were randomized to presurgical evaluation (64 % of those operated) were free from seizures with impairment of consciousness after 12 months compared with 8 % of the 40 patients randomized to optimized medical treatment [6]. These results were shown in the American Academy of Neurology practice parameter to be practically identical to those from 24 class IV series of TLR, which led a recommendation of epilepsy surgery as the treatment of choice for drug-resistant temporal lobe epilepsy (TLE) [8]. Other systematic reviews have shown similar short-term outcomes.

Late referral for epilepsy surgery remains a major problem [9–11] and the ERSET (Early Randomized Surgical Epilepsy Trial) study including 16 US epilepsy surgery centers was therefore designed to determine whether surgery soon after failure of two AEDs in people with drug-resistant mesial temporal lobe epilepsy is superior to continued medical treatment in controlling seizures. Even though this study was prematurely terminated due to slow accrual, the benefits of early surgery were demonstrated: none of the 23 patients in the medically treated group versus 11/15 in the surgical group were free from seizures with impairment of consciousness during the 2 years of follow-up [7].

The limitations of these RCTs are that they only concern TLR and are therefore not generalizable to other resective procedures.

Worsening of seizures was not reported in the Canadian study [6], while in the ERSET study the seizure frequency during the 2-year study period was tabulated for each patient, showing that none of the 15 operated patients had a worsening in seizure frequency compared to 3/23 in the medical group [7]. In studies without control groups, it is difficult to interpret an increase in seizure frequency, since this could represent variation over time without any causal relationship with the resection. Some patients, however, do not only continue to have their habitual seizures but also have new-onset SGTCS after surgery. In a retrospective study from the Cleveland Clinic investigating seizure worsening in 276 patients with postoperative seizure recurrence, 1.4 % of the patients had new-onset SGTCS after surgery [12].

Long-Term Seizure Outcomes

During the last decade, an increasing number of epilepsy surgery centers have reported long-term outcomes in cohorts of patients following a variety of surgical interventions. The studies which best fulfill the requirements for well-conducted studies as outlined in Chap. 2 have been summarized in Table 3.1. A summary table of all the referenced studies of long-term outcomes after resective epilepsy surgery in adults can be found after the chapter (Appendix).

Long-term outcome after resective epilepsy surgery is often reported cross-sectionally, which makes it difficult to discern temporal trends. In a meta-analysis from 2005 based on 78 studies, 66 % of TLR patients, 46 % of patients who had parietal or occipital resections (P/OLR) and 27 % of FLR patients were seizure-free at follow-up ≥5 years postsurgery, but the authors point out that few studies reported sustained seizure freedom from surgery; most report seizure status last year of follow-up. Almost all studies described patient cohorts without controls [13].

Several recent studies with prospectively collected long-term data on seizure outcome have provided better information about the chances of sustained seizure freedom. In the largest of these, which is a single-center study of 1,160 patients (adults and children) with a cross-sectional follow-up of at least 2 years (mean follow-up 5.4 years, range 2.0–20.5 years), 50.5 % were continuously seizure-free without auras [9]. In another single-center longitudinal follow-up of 615 adults, 52 % of all patients remained free from seizures with impairment of consciousness from the time of surgery (using an outcome classification which equals Engel I A and B) 5 years after surgery and 47 % at 10 years [14]. In a population based national study of 278 patients who had 5 or 10 year follow-up 190 were adults [15]. This study had a control group of 80 adults who had been presurgically evaluated but not had surgery. At long-term 41 % of the operated adults had sustained seizure freedom (Engel I A and B) since surgery, compared to none of the controls.

Table 3.1 Characteristics of well-conducted long-term seizure outcome studies in adults

Author, year	Study design	Number in study group	Type of surgery	Lesion type (histology)	Outcome measure	2 year outcome %	5 year outcome %	10 year outcome %
Asztely, 2007	P S X	65	RES, T+XT	All	ILAE 1+2	54		58
Aull-Watschinger, 2008	P S L	72	RES, T	HS	ILAE 1a ILAE 1+2	56 71	46 79	
de Tisi, 2011	R S L	234 at 5 years, 122 at 10 years	All (only 7 NRES)	All	ILAE 1+2 sustained		52	47
Edelvik, 2013	P N L	190	RES, T+XT	All	ILAE 1+2 sustained ILAE 1+2	50 59	41 62	
Elsharkawy, 2008	R S L	66 at 5 years, 31 at 10 years	RES, F	All	Engel I A Engel I	41 49	35 47	35 42
Elsharkawy, 2009	R S L	419 at 5 years, 366 at 10 years	RES, T	All	Engel I	72	71	71
Jeha, 2007	R S L	22 at 5 years	RES, F	All	Engel I	55	27	
Luyken, 2003	R S X	180 at 5 years, 67 at 10 years	RES, T+XT	Tumors	Engel I	82	81	81
McIntosh, 2004	R S L	138 at 5 years, 56 at 10 years	RES, T	All	Engel I A+B+D	55	48	41
McIntosh, 2012	R S L	81	RES, XT	All	Engel I A+B ILAE 1+2		14 37	
Paglioli, 2004	P S L	135, 69 at 5 years	RES, T	HS	Engel I A Engel I	76 89	75 91	
Spencer, 2005	P M X	339	RES, T+XT	All	At least 2 years seizure remission, allowing auras		69	
Sperling, 1996	R S L	89	RES, T	All	At least 1 year seizure remission, allowing auras		70	

Abbreviations:
Study design: *P* prospective, *R* retrospective, *S* single center, *N* national (population based), *X* cross-sectional, *L* longitudinal
Type of surgery: *RES* resective surgery, *NRES* nonresective surgery, *T* temporal lobe, *XT* extratemporal lobes
Outcome measure: Sustained: continuous seizure freedom since surgery

Long-Term Seizure Outcome After Temporal Lobe Resections

A number of recent longitudinal long-term outcome studies report sustained seizure freedom after TLR. Most are retrospective single-center series, only a few are prospective. Sustained seizure freedom is reported as Engel I [4, 16, 17], Engel I A [18, 19], or Engel I A and B [20], and in a few studies as ILAE class 1 and 2 [14, 21]. The proportion of patients with sustained seizure freedom around 5 years postoperatively varies between 44 and 55 % [14, 15, 17, 18, 21] and 60–80 % [16, 19, 20, 22]. Among the studies with more moderate rates of sustained seizure freedom three of five are prospective [14, 15, 21]. All studies reporting higher rates of sustained seizure freedom were retrospective.

A few studies report longitudinal follow-up until 10 years. In one retrospective single-center study in 325 patients (adults and children), 48 % were continuously seizure-free (defined as Engel I A, B and D) after 5 years and 41 % after 10 years [17]. In the earlier mentioned study of 615 adults, 497 had TLR and 55 % of them were seizure-free (without or with auras) after 5 years and 49 % after 10 years [14].

TLR constitute the majority of resective epilepsy surgery procedures in adults. It is therefore not surprising that most of the long-term outcome studies and especially those presenting longitudinal outcome data using survival methods concern TLR. It is possible to study the long-term prognosis in this more homogenous group of patients. Many factors may influence seizure outcomes, for example, referral bias, epilepsy center experience and resources, time period, and histopathology. In Fig. 3.1, we present a Kaplan-Meier analysis of time to first seizure (defined as seizures with impairment of consciousness) in adult patients (18 and older) who have undergone any variety of TLR and in whom the main histopathology was mesial sclerosis. The analysis includes data from three large epilepsy centers from three continents and with data partly from different time periods. The patients from Austin Health, Melbourne, Australia were enrolled 1979–1998 (courtesy for sharing these data to Drs Anne McIntosh and Sam Berkovic), those from Jefferson Comprehensive Epilepsy Center, Philadelphia, USA, were included 1987–2014 (courtesy for sharing these data to Drs Ali Asadi-Pooya and Michael Sperling), and the patients from UCL, London, UK 1990–2008.

As seen in Fig. 3.1, the curves are remarkably similar, with most relapses in the first 5 years and then some flattening of the gradient. The similarity between the curves from three large single-center series from three continents indicates that although factors such as referral or selection bias and differences in presurgical evaluation or surgical procedures may influence outcomes, there are in these patient populations common underlying risks for relapse.

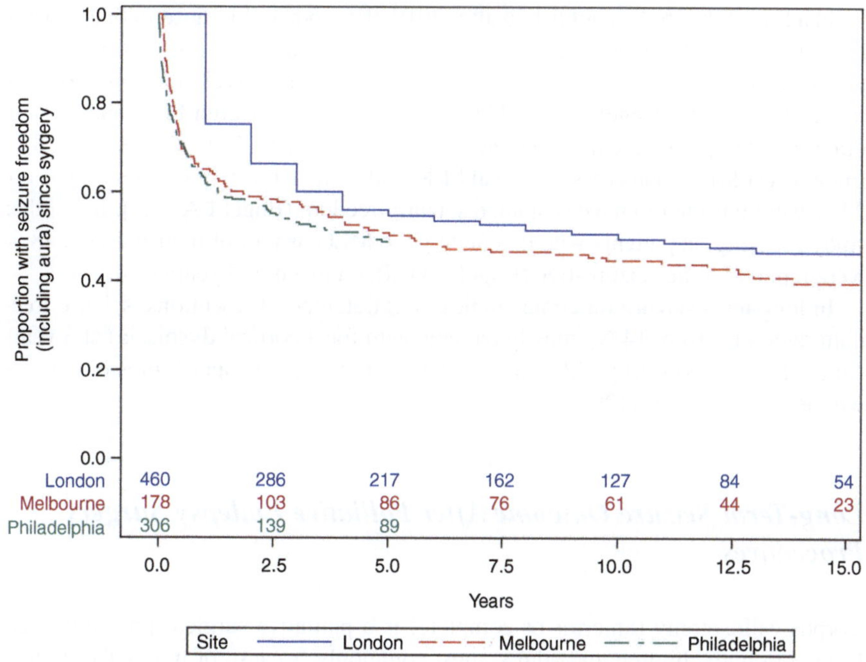

Fig. 3.1 Kaplan-Meier curve for continuous seizure freedom (allowing auras) after temporal lobe resection for hippocampal sclerosis. Data from three large epilepsy surgery centers: Austin Health, Melbourne, Australia (Courtesy of Drs A. McIntosh and S. Berkovic), Jefferson Comprehensive Epilepsy Center, Philadelphia, USA (Courtesy of Drs A. Asadi-Pooya and M. Sperling), and UCL, London, UK. The data from UCL were collected at each anniversary after surgery, hence the step-wise appearance of the curve

Long-Term Seizure Outcome After Frontal Lobe and Other Extratemporal Resections

In a recent systematic review of long-term outcomes after FLR, the authors identified 21 articles from 1991 to 2010 containing data from 1,199 patients (adults and children) with a mean or median follow-up of at least 4 years [23]. All studies were retrospective or prospective single-center series and the seizure-free rates at long term varied from 20 to 78 % across individual studies with no significant trend towards better outcomes over time. The overall rate of postoperative seizure freedom reported as Engel I was 45 %. The seizure outcome at 5 years defined as Engel I in the two studies that provided longitudinal data were 47 % and 27 %, respectively [24, 25].

In a few of the studies published after 2010, the reports of long-term outcomes in patients after FLR or other extratemporal resections include information on sustained seizure freedom since surgery. Five years postoperatively these proportions range from 14.7 % (Engel I) [26], 27 % (Engel I) [25], 35 % after FLR, and 33 % in other extratemporal resections (Engel I A and B) [15] to 47 % (Engel I, 34.8 % Engel I A) [24]. In one cross-sectional FLR study with a mean of 6 years follow-up, 24 % were reported to have sustained seizure freedom (Engel I A) [27]. In another study focusing on patients who had undergone MEG as part of their workup, 48 % were reported to be seizure-free (Engel I A) after a mean of 5 years [28].

In long-term seizure outcome studies of extratemporal resections, seizure freedom rates vary from 14 % (mostly patients with focal cortical dysplasia) at 5 years (Engel I A and B) [26] to 52 % at 5 and also at 10 years (Engel I, mostly patients with lesional etiology) [29].

Long-Term Seizure Outcome After Palliative Epilepsy Surgery Procedures

Corpus callosotomy (anterior or complete) is a palliative surgical procedure performed in both children and adults, most commonly because of traumatizing drop attacks (tonic or atonic). Most follow-up studies are single-center, retrospective, and report outcome cross-sectionally with different outcome measures making comparisons difficult. Series including both children and adults have outcomes comparable to the purely pediatric series [30]. In the only purely adult series comprising 15 adults with a mean follow-up of 2.6 years (range 0.6–10.2 years), 5 patients (33 %) reported >60 % reduction in all seizures while 7 (47 %) reported >60 % reduction in drop attacks [31]. One long-term outcome study of 95 patients, children and adults, with a minimum follow-up of 5 years reported improvement in GTCS in 77.3 % and in drop attacks in 77.2 % [32]. In another long-term study of 78 patients (27 adults) with a median follow-up of 8 years, 61/73 patients with drop attacks were reported free from these at follow-up (84 %) [33]. A recent long-term follow-up, which is population-based, multicenter, and prospective [34], also included both children and adults ($N=31$). In this study, there was a sustained reduction in seizure frequency at long term, which even improved over time. At the long-term follow-up (5 or 10 years), 10 of the 18 patients with preoperative drop attacks were free of these attacks.

Surgical treatment of patients with hypothalamic hamartomas is another mainly palliative procedure that can be performed as open surgery, radiosurgery, or as a disconnective procedure. As for callosotomies, series are often single-center and retrospective with limited sample sizes. In a series of 24 children and adults who underwent interstitial radiosurgery 46% had an Engel I or II outcome after a mean follow-up of 2 years [35]. In a recent study of 40 adults who underwent gamma knife treatment, 29 % were reported to be seizure-free in the long term (mean 4.8 years) [36].

Predictors of Remission and Relapse at Long-Term After Resective Epilepsy Surgery

Predictors for seizure freedom (positive) or seizure recurrence (negative) at long term (at least 4 years) have been sought by several investigators. While some found no remaining predictors in multivariate analysis [18, 21, 27], others have identified a number of predictors. Commonly identified predictors for seizure freedom or "good outcome" are positive MRI and histopathology (varying depending on types of pathology included in analysis) [14–17, 25, 26, 37, 38]. Positive predictors in patients at least 4 years after FLR were lesional epilepsy, abnormal MRI, localized resection as opposed to more extensive frontal or multilobar resections [23]. In lesional cases, gross-total resection (as opposed to subtotal resection) led to better seizure outcome. In the study evaluating the predictive value of MEG, monofocal MEG and nondominant side resections were predictive of seizure freedom [28].

Several factors have been identified as predictors negatively related with long-term seizure freedom: SGTCS at baseline [17, 39, 40], long epilepsy duration [9, 15, 38, 41–43], higher age at surgery [14, 29, 40], high baseline seizure frequency [15, 44], postoperative interictal epileptiform discharges [37, 41, 45], and early postoperative seizures [25, 26, 46].

The one predictive factor that is tractable – epilepsy duration before undertaking presurgical investigation – has repeatedly been shown not to have shortened significantly over the years [7, 9, 47]. These results from long-term outcome studies underline the importance of earlier identification of good candidates for resective epilepsy surgery.

The duration of epilepsy in adults referred for presurgical evaluation is still 15–20 years [48], a time period that for many of the young adults referred is more than half of their lives. Earlier epilepsy surgery has the important potential to decrease or even prevent many of the disabling psychological and social consequences of epilepsy.

Patterns of Remission and Relapse

Although seizure outcome is often reported as a static measure (seizure-free or not at a certain time-point), seizure outcomes after epilepsy surgery are more complicated. Several studies have pointed out the changing pattern of seizure control over time that complicates the process of evaluating surgical outcomes. In a retrospective study of 175 patients who had been seizure-free for 1 year after resective epilepsy surgery, 63 % never relapsed during a mean follow-up of 8.3 years. The likelihood of remaining seizure-free declined to 56 % over 10 years, but half of the patients who relapsed had at most one seizure per year [49].

In a US multicenter follow-up of 223 patients who at some point during follow-up (2–7 years) had entered a 2-year remission, 25 % relapsed later. Patients who entered a 2-year remission immediately after surgery were less likely to relapse later than those who had a 2-year remission at a later time [39]. In another study of 285 patients who had 1 year of postoperative seizure freedom, 18 % had relapsed by 5 years and 33 % by 10 years, but at last follow-up (after a mean of 8 years), only 13 % were not seizure-free [40].

In the UCL long-term follow-up of 615 adults, 68–73 % of patients had been seizure-free (or had only aura) the previous year at any time during follow-up. Most patients were stable, but 3–15 % changed seizure status. Patients who were seizure-free 2 years after surgery, had an 80 % chance of still being seizure-free after another 5 years, and those who were continuously seizure-free 5 years postoperatively had an 89 % chance of still being seizure-free after another 5 years. So the longer the preceding seizure-free period was, the less likely it was that the patients would relapse, even if they would never be completely free of risk for recurrence [14]. Of those who were not seizure-free in the first 2 years after surgery, 24 % were seizure-free for the next 5 years. Of those who were not seizure-free in the first 5 years after surgery, 20 % were seizure-free for the next 5 years.

Long-Term Outcomes of Antiepileptic Drug Treatment

There are no systematic studies of the optimal timing of postoperative drug withdrawal in adults. The proportion of seizure-free adults (and children) in whom AEDs have been withdrawn after successful epilepsy surgery varies widely across studies. In a meta-analysis from 2007, nine studies were identified and a pooled analysis showed that 27 % of seizure-free children and 19 % of seizure-free adults had discontinued AEDs at a mean follow-up of 7 years [50]. However, in an Indian study, AED withdrawal was systematically planned for all seizure-free patients after TLR and was successful in 63 % of 258 patients who were followed for at least 5 years [37].

In a cross-sectional follow-up study after neocortical resections, 61/223 (27 %) had stopped AEDs after a mean of 7 years [51], which is the same proportion as in the UCL study where 104 of 365 (28 %) seizure-free individuals were off AEDs at the latest follow-up (median 8 years) [14].

In a study of outcomes in 106 patients after extratemporal (mainly lesional) resections in adults and children, 59 % were seizure-free without aura (ILAE 1) during the last year of follow-up. Twenty-five percent had stopped AEDs (and had been off AEDs for at least 1 year) after a mean of 4.6 years, and another 40 % had reduced the number of AEDs [41].

In the prospective-population-based Swedish long-term follow-up study, 43 % of the adults who were seizure-free 10 years postsurgery had stopped AED treatment [15]. Figure 3.2 illustrates the proportion of patients who are off AEDs 10 years after surgery but also the numbers of seizure-free patients who had reduced polytherapy 10 years after epilepsy surgery [52].

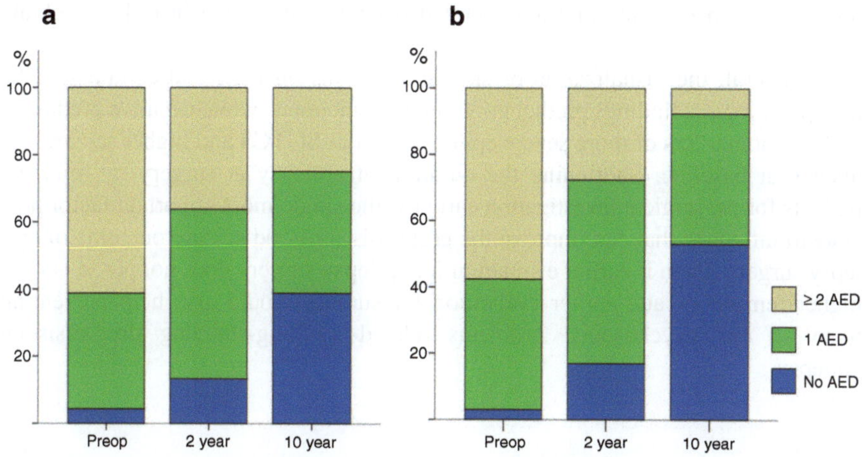

Fig. 3.2 (**a, b**) Number of antiepileptic drugs at the start of preoperative investigations, and 2 and 10 years after surgery. Panel **a**: Adult patients who were seizure-free at least the year before the 10-year follow-up ($n=116$). Panel **b**: Adult patients with sustained seizure freedom since surgery at the 10-year follow-up ($n=66$). *AED* antiepileptic drug

Conclusions and Future Directions

Epilepsy surgery is an efficacious treatment for selected persons with drug-resistant focal epilepsy, rendering many seizure-free and others significantly improved. For many years, follow-up data were limited to a few years after surgery. However, most adults who undergo epilepsy surgery are young and in order for them to make an informed decision about the treatment option of neurosurgery, they need not only short-term data but also data on the probability of long-term remission or improvement. In order to make their own risk-benefit assessment, they also need information on many other outcome aspects, many of which are discussed in other chapters of this volume.

Long-term longitudinal observational studies are necessary in order to obtain valid outcome data. From a number of such studies, the proportion of patients who have been continuously free from seizures with impairment of consciousness since resective epilepsy surgery seems to be 40–50 % after 10 years, while a higher proportion have been seizure-free at least a year at each time-point assessed. The best longitudinal data are in patients who have undergone TLR and in whom the histopathology was mesial sclerosis, and from these data (Fig. 3.1) it seems that the majority of relapses occur within 5 years, and after that there is a lesser relapse rate. Whether this course is applicable to other resection types and pathologies is not clear.

There is much less information on the longitudinal course in patients who have undergone other resection types and have other causes. For many resection types, the number of patients in single-center long-term follow-ups is limited and for almost all studies there is a lack of controls. Multicenter observational studies following both operated and nonoperated patients are needed in order to obtain more robust data.

In general, the visualization of structural lesions on MRI and certain specific histopathological findings predict good seizure outcomes, while negative predictors include biomarkers of more severe epilepsy such as SGTCS and higher seizure frequency at baseline. Shortening the duration of epilepsy at surgery by referring patients for presurgical investigation earlier is the single most important factor possible to influence that can improve the prognosis for good seizure outcome of epilepsy surgery. Even if earlier evaluation for epilepsy surgery does not per se carry a higher remission rate, earlier evaluation for surgery would also help preventing many of the psychosocial problems related to long-standing drug-resistant epilepsy.

Appendix. Summary of Study Characteristics and Results from Long-Term Studies of Seizure Outcome in Adults

Author, year	Study design	Type of surgery	Pathology	Operated patients *N*	Dropouts *N*	Number in study group	Follow-up, years mean (min-max)	Males %	Age at surgery mean (min-max)	Prognostic indicators studied	Outcome measures	Good outcome	Statistical methods
Asztely, 2007	P S X	RES T+XT	All	70	5	65	12.4 (8.6–16.2)	51	35 (19–58)	None	ILAE 1&2	58 % ILAE 1&2	MW
Aull-Watschinger, 2008	P S L	RES T	HS	135	3	72 at 5 years	5	45	35 (15–52)	A B D E G	ILAE 1&2	46 % ILAE 1a, 79 % ILAE 1&2	LogReg
Bien, 2001	R S X	RES T	All	NS	NS	148	4.8 (2–10)	45	31.5 (9–64)	None	Engel I, ILAE 1	44 % Engel IA, 62 % ILAE 1	MW
Bien, 2006	R S X	RES T+XT	All	175 identified	44	131	6.9 (SD 2.7)	53	31.1 (SD 10.6)	None	Not defined	52 % seizure-free last year	t-test, Ch, MW, ANCOVA
Bien, 2012	R S X	RES T+XT	All	1,721	NS	1,160	5.4 (2–20.5)	52	31 (0–74)	None	Engel IA, ILAE 1	50 % Engel IA, 63 % ILAE 1	MW
Cohen-Gadol, 2006	R S X+L	RES T+XT	Non-lesional (incl HS)	399	14	156 at 5 years 73 at 10 years	6.2 (0.6-15.7)	46	32 (3–69)	A D G H *Histopathology, sex, lobe, previous surgery* (unclear if multivariate analysis)*	Engel I	74 % at 5 years 72 % at 10 years	KM, CPH

(continued)

Author, year	Study design	Type of surgery	Pathology	Operated patients *N*	Dropouts *N*	Number in study group	Follow-up years mean (min-max)	Males %	Age at surgery mean (min-max)	Prognostic indicators studied	Outcome measures	Good outcome	Statistical methods
de Tisi, 2011	R S L	All	All	649	34	615; 234 at 5 years 122 at 10 years	8 (1–19)	47	(16–63)	A D G H *Age, type of surgery, histopathology, postop auras*	ILAE 1&2, sustained seizure freedom	Sust SF incl aura: 52 % at 5 years, 47 % at 10 years. 68–73 % ILAE 1&2 at each year	KM, CPH
Di Gennaro, 2014	R S X+L	RES T	HS	113 identified	6	107	8.3 (5–12)	61	35 (11–62)	A C D E *Postop IED**	Engel IA, ILAE 1	62 % Engel IA, 81 % ILAE 1	LR, Ch, LogReg
Dunlea, 2010	R N X+L	RES T+XT	All	329 identified	130	199	7 (1–24)	48	26.3 (1–61)	None	Engel I (not consistent)	43 % Engel I after mean 7 years. 41 % SF at 5 years, 44 % at 10 years, 25 % at 15 years	NS
Dupont, 2006	R S X	RES T	HS	183	73	110	7 (1–17)	51	35 (SD 10)	None	Engel	43 % Engel IA, 71 % Engel I after mean 7 years. KM-estimates: Engel IA 59 % at 5 years, 43 % at 10 years	Ch, Fi, KM
Edelvik, 2013	P N X+L	RES T+XT	All	219	29	190	7.6 (5 and 10 years)	46	37.7 (19–67)	A D F G H *Duration, seizure frequency, MRI*	ILAE 1&2	41 % sust SF incl aura, 62 % ILAE 1&2 at mean 7 years	Ch, Fi, LogReg

Elsharkawy, 2008	R S X+L	RES F	All	134	37	97; 66 at 5 years 31 at 10 years	6.9 (2–14)	59	28.5 (16–69)	A D E F G *MRI lesion, postop aura**	Engel IA, Engel I	35 % Engel IA and 47 % Engel I at 5 years. 35 % Engel IA and 42 % Engel I at 10 years	KM, CPH, LogReg
Elsharkawy, 2008 [2]	R S X+L	RES XT	All	NS	NS	154	8.8 (1–14)	59	~29 (16–59)	A B D E G *invasive EEG, single operation, early surgery, auditory aura*, GTCS* (only univariate testing)*	Engel I	52 % at 5 and 10 years	KM, CPH
Elsharkawy, 2009	R S X+L	RES T	All	483	49	434; 419 at 5 years 366 at 10 years 147 at 16 years	NS (0.5–16)	51	NS	A D E F H *hippocampal atrophy, family history of ep, bilateral IED*, versive seizures**	Engel I	71 % at 5 years 71 % at 10 years 69 % at 16 years	KM, CPH, LogReg
Ferrier, 1999	R S X	RES F	All	42	5	37	5.9 (1–19)	49	16.8 (1–38)	A B D E F β *Contralateral head version*, MRI lesion*	Engel I	32 % Engel I	MW, Ch, Fi, LogReg
Foldvary, 2000	R S X	RES T	All	NS	17	79	14 (2–34)	57	24 (SD 9)	A B D G *Seizure frequency (only univariate testing)*	Engel I	35 % Engel IA and 65 % Engel I at mean 14 years. 52 % Engel I at 5 years, 45 % at 10 years	KM, logrank

(continued)

Author, year	Study design	Type of surgery	Pathology	Operated patients *N*	Dropouts *N*	Number in study group	Follow-up, years mean (min-max)	Males %	Age at surgery mean (min-max)	Prognostic indicators studied	Outcome measures	Good outcome	Statistical methods
Hanakova, 2014	R S L	RES XT	All	77	4	73	6 (1–15)	63	28.3 (1–51)	A F H *MRI, histopathology (only univariate testing)*	Engel I	51 % Engel I after mean 6 years. 55 % Engel I at 5 years	ANOVA, Ch, KM
Jeha, 2006	R S X	RES T	All	497	126	371	5.5 (1–14)	NS	NS, "adults"	A D E F G H *ECoG, histopathology (only univariate testing)*	Not defined	Seizure relapse in 37 %	Multiphase hazard modeling
Jeha, 2007	R S X	RES F	All	NS	NS	70; 22 at 5 years	4.1 (1–11)	57	22 (1–57)	A B D E F G H *Predictors for recurrence: MRI-negativity, extrafrontal MRI-finding, non-localizing EEG, APOS, incomplete resection*	Engel	44 % Engel IA + B after mean 4 years. KM-estimate: 27 % at 5 years (6/22)	W, Ch, Fi, CPH, KM
Jobst, 2000	R S X	RES F	All	25 identified	0	25	4.3 (1–7)	58	27 (11–44)	None	Engel I	64 % Engel I	NS
Kelley, 2005	R S X	RES T	All	56 identified	11	45	29.9 (SD 4.9)	NS	NS	A C E G *Seizures first postop year*, invasive EEG**	SF last 20 years	50 % SF 30 years after surgery	Ch, KM, LogReg
Kim, 2010	R S X	RES F	All	NS	NS	76	6.8 (SD 2.9)	62	28.5 (SD 9.3)	A B C D E F G H K *MRI*	Engel I	55 % Engel I	MW, Ch KM, CPH
Lazow, 2012	R S X	RES F	All	58 identified	0	58	6.6 (1–17)	55	30 (9–58)	C E F H K	Engel, ILAE	24 % Engel IA 57 % Engel I 50 % ILAE	Ch, Fi, LogReg, KM

Luyken, 2003	R S X+L	RES T+XT	Tumors	214	7	207	8 (2–14)	50	28 (5–67)	A B D E G H *Duration, unifocal EEG, type of tumor, dual pathology*, extent of resection, surgical approach*	Engel I	81 % Engel I at 5 years, 81 % Engel I at 10 years	Ch, Fi, KM, MW, LogReg
McIntosh, 2004	R S X+L	RES T	All	360	35	325 138 at 5 years 56 at 10 years	9.6 (0.7–23)	NS	NS (6.7–59)	A D H K *Histopathology, GTCS**	Engel IA+B+D	48 % SF at 5 years 41 % SF at 10 years	Ch, Fi, LogReg, KM
McIntosh, 2012	R S X+L	RES XT	All	87	6	81	10.3 (1–17.7)	47	27.5 (4–60)	A D E G H *Histopathology, early seizures**	Engel IA+B, ILAE 1&2	At 5 years: Engel IA+B 14 %, ILAE 1&2 38 %	KM, CPH
Menon, 2012	R SX	RES XT	All	NS	NS	106	4.6 (2–11)	69	19.7 (3–45)	A D E G H *Duration, postop IED**	Engel IA, ILAE 1	38 % Engel IA 59 % ILAE 1	MW, Ch, Fi, KM, LogReg
Mihara, 2004	R S X	RES T+XT	All	488	131	282 T 75 XT	6 (2–16) T 5 (2–13) XT	NS	~24 (2–55)	None	Engel I	78 % Engel I (T) 64 % Engel I (XT)	None
Mohammed, 2012	R S X	All	All	361	244	117	26.5 (21–42)	62	20 (2–51)	A B D G H	Engel I	48 % Engel I	Ch, Fi

(continued)

Author, year	Study design	Type of surgery	Pathology	Operated patients *N*	Dropouts *N*	Number in study group	Follow-up, years mean (min-max)	Males %	Age at surgery mean (min-max)	Prognostic indicators studied	Outcome measures	Good outcome	Statistical methods
Mosewich, 2000	R S X	RES F	All	68	0	68	~4.0 (SD 2.5)	66	30.1 (4–51)	A C D E F G *MRI, febrile seizures*, (only univariate testing)*	SF or nondisabling seizures	59 % "excellent outcome" (not completely SF)	Ch, Fi, W, LogReg
Mu, 2014	R S X	RES F	All	NS	NS	46	5.0 (0.5–17)	61	30.4 (10–58)	A B G K *Monofocal MEG, side*	Engel IA	48 % Engel IA	W, Ch, Fi, KM, CPH
Murphy, 2010	R S X	RES T	HS	21	0	21	9.5 (SD 2 4)	33	54.9 (50–72)	A B C F G	"Modified" Engel	81 % Engel I	Fi, MW, LogReg
Paglioli, 2004	P S L	RES T	HS	135	1	134; 69 at 5 years	5.5 (2–11)	NS	31.6 (8–62)	A E F G H	Engel I	At 5 years: 91 % Engel I 75 % Engel IA	KM, Ch, Fi
Paillas, 1983	R S X	All	All	NS	NS	44	NS (11–26)	NS	NS	None	NS	Study of patients who have been SF beyond 10 years. 32/44 (73 %) continued SF up to 26 years after surgery	None
Park, 2010	R S X	RES neocortical	All	283 identified	60	223	7 (2–12)	NS	NS	NS	NS	54 % SF	Ch, Fi, CPH, KM
Phi, 2009	R S X+L	RES T	Tumors	87 identified	0	87	4.5 (1–10.7)	56	22	A B D E G H *Duration, non-concordant EEG*, extent of resection*	NS	79 % SF at 5 years	KM, CPH

Ramesha, 2011	R S L	RES T	All	513	21	492	5.2 (2–11)	56	29 (1–60)	A B D G H *Early relapse*, seizure type at relapse (CPS/GTCS)**	ILAE 1	If no relapse during first year, 90 % SF at 5 years; if relapse during first year, 63 % SF at 5 years	Fi, KM, CPH
Rathore, 2011	R S L	RES T	HS, non-lesional	327	17	310	8.0 (SD 2.0)	55	27.1 (SD 9.2)	A D E F H *HS, postop IED**	ILAE	82 % ILAE 1 45 % ILAE 1a	KM, Fi, Ch, LogReg
Schwartz, 2006	R M X+L	All	All but vascular and neocortical tumors	NS	NS	285 with 1 year seizure freedom	7.9 (SD 3.1)	NS	33.4 (SD 9.6)	A D E G H K *Age, GTCS**	Not defined	After 1 year of seizure freedom 28 % will relapse; Risk estimation: 18 % after 5 years, 33 % after 10 years	KM, CPH
Spencer, 2005	P M X+L	RES T+XT	All	396	57	339	4.6 (2–7)	NS	NS, over age 12	A B C D E F G H *GTCS*, HS*	SF ≥ 2 years incl aura	66 % SF at mean 4.6 years. 69 % SF at 5 years	Ch, CPH, KM
Sperling, 1996	R S L	RES T	All	93	4	89	5	51	32 (10–60)	A D E K No multivariate analysis	SF last year incl aura	70 % SF at 5 years	Ch, Fi, t-test, ANOVA
Tanriverdi, 2008	R S L	RES T	All	63	15	48	12	49	34 (SD 11)	None	Engel IA	71 % Engel IA at 12 years	MW, Ch
Vickrey, 1995	R S X	RES T+XT	All	202	5	197	5.8	48	27.0	None	ILAE 1	31 % ILAE 1	t-test, Ch, Fi, W, MW

(continued)

Author, year	Study design	Type of surgery	Pathology	Operated patients *N*	Dropouts *N*	Number in study group	Follow-up, years mean (min-max)	Males %	Age at surgery mean (min-max)	Prognostic indicators studied	Outcome measures	Good outcome	Statistical methods
Wieser, 2003	R S L	RES SelAH	HS, lesions	464	95	369 234 at 5 years 125 at 10 years	7.2 (1–24)	58	~32 (SD ~12)	None	Engel ILAE (only in diagrams)	~65 % Engel I, ~55 % ILAE 1 at 5 and 10 years; ILAE 1a: ~38 % at 5 and ~34 % at 10 years	Fi, MW

Abbreviations:
General: *NS* not specified, *SD* standard deviation
Study design: *P* prospective, *R* retrospective, *S* single center, *N* national (population based), *X* cross-sectional, *L* longitudinal
Type of surgery: *RES* resective surgery, *NRES* nonresective surgery *T* temporal lobe, *XT* extratemporal lobes, *F* frontal lobe, *SelAH* selective amygdalohippocampectomy
Pathology: *HS* hippocampal sclerosis
Prognostic indicators studied: *A* age-related factors (age at onset, epilepsy duration, age at surgery, age at epileptogenic event), *B* sex or race, *C* coexisting conditions (mental retardation, preop psychiatric history, head trauma, comorbidities), *D* seizure-related factors (seizure frequency, history of GTCS, history of status epilepticus, history of febrile seizures, head version, ictal dystonic posturing, seizure types preop/at relapse, acute postop seizures (APOS), seizure freedom 1 year postop, early postop seizures, postop auras), *E* EEG (localization or unilateral interictal epileptiform discharges (IED), postop IED, invasive EEG, subdural grids, preop electrocorticography (ECoG)), *F* MRI (MRI finding, hippocampal volumetry), *G* surgical factors (type of resection (lobe), side of resection, size of resection, bilateral surgery, previous surgery, surgical approach), *H* histopathology (histopathology, dual pathology), *K* other (SPECT, MEG, PET, WADA scores, postop cessation of AEDs, era of surgery)
Significant predictors in multivariate analysis in italics. Prediction of seizure freedom for most studies. Prediction for seizure relapse is marked with *. Prediction for "favorable outcome" = Engel I + II was analyzed in one study marked with β
Outcome measures: Engel classification, ILAE classification (Wieser 2001), SF ≥ 2 years incl aura: seizure-free at least 2 years allowing auras
Good outcome: *SF* seizure-free according to outcome measure, *Sust SF incl aura* sustained seizure freedom since surgery allowing auras (equivalent to Engel 1A + B)
Statistical methods: *MW* Mann-Whitney U-test, *LR* likelihood ratio, *LogReg* logistic regression, *Fi* Fisher's exact test, *Ch* Chi2, *KM* Kaplan-Meier, *CPH* Cox proportional hazard, *W* Wilcoxon rank-sum

References

1. Wilson SJ, Saling MM, Kincade P, Bladin PF. Patient expectations of temporal lobe surgery. Epilepsia. 1998;39(2):167–74.
2. Luoni C, Bisulli F, Canevini MP, De Sarro G, Fattore C, Galimberti CA, et al. Determinants of health-related quality of life in pharmacoresistant epilepsy: results from a large multicenter study of consecutively enrolled patients using validated quantitative assessments. Epilepsia. 2011;52(12):2181–91.
3. Beghi E, Tonini C. Surgery for epilepsy: assessing evidence from observational studies. Epilepsy Res. 2006;70(2–3):97–102.
4. Engel J. Surgical treatment of the epilepsies. New York: Raven Press; 1987.
5. Wieser HG, Blume WT, Fish D, Goldensohn E, Hufnagel A, King D, et al. ILAE Commission Report. Proposal for a new classification of outcome with respect to epileptic seizures following epilepsy surgery. Epilepsia. 2001;42(2):282–6.
6. Wiebe S, Blume WT, Girvin JP, Eliasziw M. A randomized, controlled trial of surgery for temporal-lobe epilepsy. N Engl J Med. 2001;345(5):311–8.
7. Engel Jr J, McDermott MP, Wiebe S, Langfitt JT, Stern JM, Dewar S, et al. Early surgical therapy for drug-resistant temporal lobe epilepsy: a randomized trial. JAMA. 2012;307(9):922–30.
8. Engel Jr J, Wiebe S, French J, Sperling M, Williamson P, Spencer D, et al. Practice parameter: temporal lobe and localized neocortical resections for epilepsy. Epilepsia. 2003;44(6):741–51.
9. Bien CG, Raabe AL, Schramm J, Becker A, Urbach H, Elger CE. Trends in presurgical evaluation and surgical treatment of epilepsy at one centre from 1988–2009. J Neurol Neurosurg Psychiatry. 2013;84(1):54–61.
10. Choi H, Carlino R, Heiman G, Hauser WA, Gilliam FG. Evaluation of duration of epilepsy prior to temporal lobe epilepsy surgery during the past two decades. Epilepsy Res. 2009;86(2–3):224–7.
11. Haneef Z, Stern J, Dewar S, Engel Jr J. Referral pattern for epilepsy surgery after evidence-based recommendations: a retrospective study. Neurology. 2010;75(8):699–704.
12. Sarkis RA, Jehi L, Bingaman W, Najm IM. Seizure worsening and its predictors after epilepsy surgery. Epilepsia. 2012;53(10):1731–8.
13. Tellez-Zenteno JF, Dhar R, Wiebe S. Long-term seizure outcomes following epilepsy surgery: a systematic review and meta-analysis. Brain. 2005;128(Pt 5):1188–98.
14. de Tisi J, Bell GS, Peacock JL, McEvoy AW, Harkness WF, Sander JW, et al. The long-term outcome of adult epilepsy surgery, patterns of seizure remission, and relapse: a cohort study. Lancet. 2011;378(9800):1388–95.
15. Edelvik A, Rydenhag B, Olsson I, Flink R, Kumlien E, Kallen K, et al. Long-term outcomes of epilepsy surgery in Sweden: a national prospective and longitudinal study. Neurology. 2013;81(14):1244–51.
16. Cohen-Gadol AA, Wilhelmi BG, Collignon F, White JB, Britton JW, Cambier DM, et al. Long-term outcome of epilepsy surgery among 399 patients with nonlesional seizure foci including mesial temporal lobe sclerosis. J Neurosurg. 2006;104(4):513–24.
17. McIntosh AM, Kalnins RM, Mitchell LA, Fabinyi GC, Briellmann RS, Berkovic SF. Temporal lobectomy: long-term seizure outcome, late recurrence and risks for seizure recurrence. Brain. 2004;127(Pt 9):2018–30.
18. Dupont S, Tanguy ML, Clemenceau S, Adam C, Hazemann P, Baulac M. Long-term prognosis and psychosocial outcomes after surgery for MTLE. Epilepsia. 2006;47(12):2115–24.
19. Sindou M, Guenot M, Isnard J, Ryvlin P, Fischer C, Mauguiere F. Temporo-mesial epilepsy surgery: outcome and complications in 100 consecutive adult patients. Acta Neurochir. 2006;148(1):39–45.

20. Paglioli E, Palmini A, da Costa JC, Portuguez M, Martinez JV, Calcagnotto ME, et al. Survival analysis of the surgical outcome of temporal lobe epilepsy due to hippocampal sclerosis. Epilepsia. 2004;45(11):1383–91.
21. Aull-Watschinger S, Pataraia E, Czech T, Baumgartner C. Outcome predictors for surgical treatment of temporal lobe epilepsy with hippocampal sclerosis. Epilepsia. 2008;49(8):1308–16.
22. Jeha LE, Najm IM, Bingaman WE, Khandwala F, Widdess-Walsh P, Morris HH, et al. Predictors of outcome after temporal lobectomy for the treatment of intractable epilepsy. Neurology. 2006;66(12):1938–40.
23. Englot DJ, Wang DD, Rolston JD, Shih TT, Chang EF. Rates and predictors of long-term seizure freedom after frontal lobe epilepsy surgery: a systematic review and meta-analysis. J Neurosurg. 2012;116(5):1042–8.
24. Elsharkawy AE, Alabbasi AH, Pannek H, Schulz R, Hoppe M, Pahs G, et al. Outcome of frontal lobe epilepsy surgery in adults. Epilepsy Res. 2008;81(2–3):97–106.
25. Jeha LE, Najm I, Bingaman W, Dinner D, Widdess-Walsh P, Luders H. Surgical outcome and prognostic factors of frontal lobe epilepsy surgery. Brain. 2007;130(Pt 2):574–84.
26. McIntosh AM, Averill CA, Kalnins RM, Mitchell LA, Fabinyi GC, Jackson GD, et al. Long-term seizure outcome and risk factors for recurrence after extratemporal epilepsy surgery. Epilepsia. 2012;53(6):970–8.
27. Lazow SP, Thadani VM, Gilbert KL, Morse RP, Bujarski KA, Kulandaivel K, et al. Outcome of frontal lobe epilepsy surgery. Epilepsia. 2012;53(10):1746–55.
28. Mu J, Rampp S, Carrette E, Roessler K, Sommer B, Schmitt FC, et al. Clinical relevance of source location in frontal lobe epilepsy and prediction of postoperative long-term outcome. Seizure. 2014;23(7):553–9.
29. Elsharkawy AE, Behne F, Oppel F, Pannek H, Schulz R, Hoppe M, et al. Long-term outcome of extratemporal epilepsy surgery among 154 adult patients. J Neurosurg. 2008;108(4):676–86.
30. Asadi-Pooya AA, Sharan A, Nei M, Sperling MR. Corpus callosotomy. Epilepsy Behav. 2008;13(2):271–8.
31. Park MS, Nakagawa E, Schoenberg MR, Benbadis SR, Vale FL. Outcome of corpus callosotomy in adults. Epilepsy Behav. 2013;28(2):181–4.
32. Tanriverdi T, Olivier A, Poulin N, Andermann F, Dubeau F. Long-term seizure outcome after corpus callosotomy: a retrospective analysis of 95 patients. J Neurosurg. 2009;110(2):332–42.
33. Sunaga S, Shimizu H, Sugano H. Long-term follow-up of seizure outcomes after corpus callosotomy. Seizure. 2009;18(2):124–8.
34. Stigsdotter-Broman L, Olsson I, Flink R, Rydenhag B, Malmgren K. Long-term follow-up after callosotomy-a prospective, population based, observational study. Epilepsia. 2014;55(2):316–21.
35. Schulze-Bonhage A, Trippel M, Wagner K, Bast T, Deimling FV, Ebner A, et al. Outcome and predictors of interstitial radiosurgery in the treatment of gelastic epilepsy. Neurology. 2008;71(4):277–82.
36. Drees C, Chapman K, Prenger E, Baxter L, Maganti R, Rekate H, et al. Seizure outcome and complications following hypothalamic hamartoma treatment in adults: endoscopic, open, and Gamma Knife procedures. J Neurosurg. 2012;117(2):255–61.
37. Rathore C, Panda S, Sarma PS, Radhakrishnan K. How safe is it to withdraw antiepileptic drugs following successful surgery for mesial temporal lobe epilepsy? Epilepsia. 2011;52(3):627–35.
38. Luyken C, Blumcke I, Fimmers R, Urbach H, Elger CE, Wiestler OD, et al. The spectrum of long-term epilepsy-associated tumors: long-term seizure and tumor outcome and neurosurgical aspects. Epilepsia. 2003;44(6):822–30.
39. Spencer SS, Berg AT, Vickrey BG, Sperling MR, Bazil CW, Shinnar S, et al. Predicting long-term seizure outcome after resective epilepsy surgery: the multicenter study. Neurology. 2005;65(6):912–8.

40. Schwartz TH, Jeha L, Tanner A, Bingaman W, Sperling MR. Late seizures in patients initially seizure free after epilepsy surgery. Epilepsia. 2006;47(3):567–73.
41. Menon R, Rathore C, Sarma SP, Radhakrishnan K. Feasibility of antiepileptic drug withdrawal following extratemporal resective epilepsy surgery. Neurology. 2012;79(8):770–6.
42. Simasathien T, Vadera S, Najm I, Gupta A, Bingaman W, Jehi L. Improved outcomes with earlier surgery for intractable frontal lobe epilepsy. Ann Neurol. 2013;73:646–54.
43. Phi JH, Kim SK, Cho BK, Lee SY, Park SY, Park SJ, et al. Long-term surgical outcomes of temporal lobe epilepsy associated with low-grade brain tumors. Cancer. 2009;115(24):5771–9.
44. Foldvary N, Nashold B, Mascha E, Thompson EA, Lee N, McNamara JO, et al. Seizure outcome after temporal lobectomy for temporal lobe epilepsy: a Kaplan-Meier survival analysis. Neurology. 2000;54(3):630–4.
45. Di Gennaro G, Casciato S, D'Aniello A, De Risi M, Quarato PP, Mascia A, et al. Serial postoperative awake and sleep EEG and long-term seizure outcome after anterior temporal lobectomy for hippocampal sclerosis. Epilepsy Res. 2014;108(5):945–52.
46. Ramesha KN, Mooney T, Sarma PS, Radhakrishnan K. Long-term seizure outcome and its predictors in patients with recurrent seizures during the first year aftertemporal lobe resective epilepsy surgery. Epilepsia. 2011;52(5):917–24.
47. Rydenhag B, Flink R, Malmgren K. Surgical outcomes in patients with epileptogenic tumours and cavernomas in Sweden: good seizure control but late referrals. J Neurol Neurosurg Psychiatry. 2013;84(1):49–53.
48. Ryvlin P, Cross JH, Rheims S. Epilepsy surgery in children and adults. Lancet Neurol. 2014;13(11):1114–26.
49. Yoon HH, Kwon HL, Mattson RH, Spencer DD, Spencer SS. Long-term seizure outcome in patients initially seizure-free after resective epilepsy surgery. Neurology. 2003;61(4):445–50.
50. Tellez-Zenteno JF, Dhar R, Hernandez-Ronquillo L, Wiebe S. Long-term outcomes in epilepsy surgery: antiepileptic drugs, mortality, cognitive and psychosocial aspects. Brain. 2007;130(Pt 2):334–45.
51. Park KI, Lee SK, Chu K, Jung KH, Bae EK, Kim JS, et al. Withdrawal of antiepileptic drugs after neocortical epilepsy surgery. Ann Neurol. 2010;67(2):230–8.
52. Edelvik A, Rydenhag B, Flink R, Malmgren K. Seizure outcome ten years after resective epilepsy surgery – a population-based, prospective, longitudinal study. Abstracts from 10th European Congress on Epileptology in London 2012. Epilepsia. 2012;53 Suppl 5:11.

Chapter 4
Long-Term Seizure and Antiepileptic Drug Outcomes After Epilepsy Surgery in Children

Evan Cole Lewis and Michael Duchowny

Abstract Seizure outcomes in children are typically assessed using the Engel classification system. However, they may be reported at variable duration of follow-up, often a wide range in individual studies. Completeness of resection is the major predictor of seizure freedom for all epilepsy cases; otherwise, positive and negative predictors depend on specific presurgical, surgical, and postsurgical variables. Lobar seizure-free outcomes are variable: frontal (33.7–66 %), insular (about 80 %), occipital (30–69.2 %), parietal (40–82 %), and temporal (63.2–85 %) in the longer term from data available. Rates of seizure freedom in temporal lobe epilepsy (TLE) are better than for extratemporal lobe epilepsy (ETLE) and comparable to adult rates. Hemidisconnection outcomes range from 41 to 83 % which is better than for tailored multilobar approaches. For seizure foci not amenable to focal resection, corpus callosotomy (CC) remains a potential treatment option for children with atonic seizures. Early decisions should be made about weaning of medication to determine which children require antiepileptic drugs (AEDs) in the longer term.

Keywords Epilepsy surgery • Hemispherectomy • Corpus callosotomy • Drug-resistant epilepsy • Seizure outcome • Focal epilepsy • Pediatric epilepsy • Outcome assessment • Temporal lobe surgery

Introduction

Seizure freedom, or at the very least seizure reduction, remain the primary aims of epilepsy surgery in childhood, accepting secondary aims may include improvement in neurodevelopment, behavior, and quality of life. Data on long-term seizure outcomes from epilepsy surgery in childhood are limited; many studies report on

E.C. Lewis, MD, FRCPC
Department of Neurology, Miami Children's Hospital, Miami, FL, USA

M. Duchowny, MD (✉)
Comprehensive Epilepsy Program, Neurology and the Brain Institute,
Miami Children's Hospital, Miami, FL, USA
e-mail: michael.duchowny@mch.com

K. Malmgren et al. (eds.), *Long-Term Outcomes of Epilepsy Surgery in Adults and Children*, DOI 10.1007/978-3-319-17783-0_4

types of surgery or pathologies with a wide range of follow-up, as well as being inclusive of both adults and children. Late recurrence of seizures may be seen following surgery, although may be more likely in certain pathologies. There is also a wide variation as to how seizure outcome is reported, meaning comparison between studies is difficult. Determining longer-term outcomes beyond 3–5 years from surgery is important to appropriately counsel families with regard to expectation, follow-up, and medical contact. Further, informed decisions will need to be made about withdrawal of medication.

How Is Seizure Outcome Assessed?

Seizure freedom after surgery is assessed using either the Engel or International League Against Epilepsy (ILAE) classification system (Figs. 4.1 and 4.2). The Engel classification, developed in 1993 [1] is the most widely used but has been criticized for its interpretive ambiguity by utilizing terms such as "worthwhile" and "disabling," its inability to facilitate direct comparison with antiepileptic drug (AED) trials which commonly use 50 % seizure reduction as a primary outcome measure, and its lack of distinct categorizations for absolute seizure freedom and postsurgical worsening.

For these reasons, the ILAE proposed a classification system in 2001 [2] that addressed the shortcomings of the Engel system. Specifically, the introduction of "seizure days," referring to the incidence of at least one seizure in a 24-h period is

Engel Classification	
Class I: Free of Disabling Seizures	
A:	Seizure free since surgery
B:	Nondisabling simple partial seizures only since surgery
C:	Some disabling seizures after surgery, but free of disabling seizures for at least 2 years
Class II: Rare Disabling Seizures ("almost seizure free")	
A:	Initially free of disabling seizures but has rare seizure now
B:	Rare disabling seizures since surgery
C:	More than rare disabling seizures since surgery, but rare seizures for the last 2 years
D:	Nocturnal seizures only
Class III: Worthwhile Improvement	
A:	Worthwhile seizure reduction
B:	Prolonged seizure-free intervals amounting to greater than half the followed-up period, but not <2 years
Class IV: No Worthwhile Improvement	
A:	Significant seizure reduction
B:	No appreciable change
C:	Seizure worse

Fig. 4.1 Engel classification of postoperative seizure outcome

ILAE Classification	
Class 1:	Completely seizure free; no auras
Class 1a:	*Completely seizure free *since surgery*; no auras
Class 2:	Only auras; no other seizures
Class 3:	1-3 seizure days per year; ± auras
Class 4:	Four seizure days per year to 50 % reduction of baseline seizure days; ± auras
Class 5:	<50 % reduction of baseline seizure days to 100 % increase of baseline seizure days; ± auras
Class 6:	>100 % increase of baseline seizure days

***Differentiates from Class 1 which refers to seizure freedom within the last year of follow-up**

Fig. 4.2 ILAE classification system of postoperative seizure outcome. Seizure outcome class determined for each year at annual intervals after the date of surgery. *Differentiates from Class 1 which refers to seizure freedom within the last year of follow-up

thought to be more clinically meaningful and addresses patients who occasionally have clusters of seizures or episodes of status epilepticus.

To utilize the ILAE system correctly for surgical patients, baseline seizure days for the 12-month period prior to surgery must be known. This makes the ILAE system applicable to individuals and populations both on a year-by-year basis and cumulatively to the last documented outcome. However, ILAE outcome determination for retrospective studies is not possible if baseline data is unavailable. This latter point may explain why the Engel system continues to be popular in epilepsy surgery studies as most published series are retrospective and baseline data for the preceding 12-month period is often unknown. Further, there may be a relatively high frequency of seizures in young children in whom benefit may not be captured utilizing the ILAE scheme.

Only one published study has compared the ILAE and Engel classification systems [3]. Independent interpreters assessed a mixed cohort of 76 patients that included 25 children and both systems were found to have high inter-rater agreement.

There currently is no pediatric-specific outcome scale and reliance on either the Engel or ILAE classification systems is acceptable [4]. However, the Engel system is the most widely employed outcome measure and has adequate inter-rater reliability. The Engel system is, therefore, utilized throughout this chapter to maintain consistency across interpretation of data unless referenced studies specifically applied the ILAE classification system.

The Engel and ILAE classification systems address only seizure outcome and do not assess psychosocial, behavioral, cognitive, or vocational development, all vital to gauging the utility of epilepsy surgery [4, 5]. Discussion of these measures and their relationship to quality of life is beyond the scope of this chapter and are discussed in detail in other chapters. Further, the system does not specify or include duration of follow-up at the time of reporting, meaning direct comparison between studies is not possible.

Predictors of Seizure Outcome

Predicting seizure freedom after epilepsy surgery in childhood is imperative for guiding candidate selection and family counseling. This can be a challenging task as children have unique clinical, developmental, and pathological variables that make comparisons with adults difficult [6]. Furthermore, factors that influence surgical outcome in adults such as temporal lobe location and presence of a gross structural lesion are less important in childhood [6]. An understanding of both positive and negative predictors of seizure freedom greatly assists in candidate selection. Table 4.1 presents various clinical and peri-operative factors associated with seizure outcome.

Presurgical Predictors of Seizure Freedom

Patient Demographics

Most preoperative clinical features do not predict seizure freedom [6–9]. There is no reported association of sex, age at surgery, duration of epilepsy, seizure frequency, seizure type (partial or secondarily generalized) or presence of

Table 4.1 Factors that result in favorable and unfavorable outcomes or have no effect on postsurgical seizure freedom in all types of epilepsy in children

	Presurgical	Surgical	Postsurgical
Favorable outcome	Abnormal MRI Presence of MRI lesion Focal interictal discharges Regionalized ictal discharges MEG clusters within ictal onset zone	Completeness of resection Temporal resections	Focal cortical dysplasia
No effect on outcome	Sex Age at surgery Duration of epilepsy Seizure frequency Seizure type (partial or generalized) Cognitive impairment Normal/non-focal MRI PET SPECT		Tuberous sclerosis Low grade tumor
Unfavorable outcome	No MEG Clusters within ictal onset zone Multiple MEG clusters overlapping the ictal onset zone		Interictal discharges within/near resection cavity Interictal discharges lateralized to side of resection Nonspecific histopathology Postencephalitic histopathology

cognitive impairment with postsurgical seizure status [6–8]. In contrast, a single preoperative seizure semiology is an important predictor in MR-negative cases [8, 10] and the absence of generalized seizures also correlates with favorable outcome in TLE and ETLE [11, 12]. The effect of age at onset of epilepsy and subsequent postsurgical seizure freedom is often confounded by the underlying substrate. For instance, surgical success is less likely in patients who present in early life with focal cortical dysplasia possibly due to associated atypical widespread epileptogenic networks that are established prenatally or in early postnatal life [13, 14].

Presence of MRI Lesion

Data on investigative predictors of outcome are limited. The presence of a discrete lesion on MR imaging has been shown consistently to correlate with a favorable seizure outcome [11, 12, 15]. MR abnormalities provide anatomical landmarks for intracranial electrode placement, assist in determining resection margins and confirm localizing findings derived from other presurgical investigations. These factors all contribute to completeness of resection and surgical success [6]. Seizures associated with highly demarcated MRI lesions such as hamartomas, vascular malformations or developmental tumors are often alleviated by lesionectomy alone. In contrast, non-lesional or subtle pathological substrates such as infection, trauma, or degenerative disorders are typically associated with a more diffuse insult with potential secondary areas of epileptogenesis that may activate after initial resection [12].

Interictal Discharges

Focal interictal discharges on scalp and video EEG positively predict seizure freedom while ictal patterns more often only lateralize or regionalize the epileptogenic zone [16, 17]. In a mixed cohort of adult and pediatric patients (mean age 30.8 years; range, 8–57 years) with HS or non-lesional MTLE, seizure freedom correlated with regionalized ictal onset, the absence of contralateral propagation and lateralization of interictal discharges to the operated temporal lobe. When these features are present the likelihood of postoperative seizure freedom is increased [16].

Conversely, postoperative persistence of interictal discharges is linked to poor outcome with a 71 % negative-predictive value for seizure freedom [18]. Rathore and Radhakrishnan (2010) reviewed 1,345 adults and children from 20 studies and noted that postoperative interictal discharges were associated with unfavorable seizure outcome for all resections (odds ratio 3.3, 95 % CI: 2.5–4.5). Further classification by anatomical location showed that the odds of poor seizure outcome was more likely for extratemporal resections (odds ratio 5.6; 95 % CI: 3.9–9.3) compared to temporal resections (odds ratio 2.5; 95 % CI: 1.6–4.0) if postoperative interictal discharges were present [18].

Neurophysiological Findings

The predictive power of scalp interictal and ictal activity is in part related to their assistance with intracranial electrode placement to precisely delineate the epileptogenic zone [6, 17]. This is particularly relevant in MRI negative cases. Jayakar et al. (2008) examined 102 pediatric patients with normal or non-focal MRI scans and identified two variables predicting seizure freedom- convergent focal interictal spikes on scalp EEG and completeness of resection. The definition of completeness of resection included electrophysiologic delineation of the ictal onset zone by intracranial EEG findings consisting of focal transformations into rhythmic activity, bursts of high frequency discharges, repetitive spiking or electrodecremental patterns [17]. Abnormal intracranial EEG findings are more predictive of seizure freedom when they are concordant with anatomical abnormalities. In the pediatric cohort described by Paolicchi et al. (2000), completeness of resection of the abnormal anatomic and electrographic region was the only predictor of seizure freedom [6].

The overall utility of further neurophysiological investigations remains controversial and unclear. There are no outcome studies evaluating the role of EEG source localization in children. A meta-analysis of adult and pediatric studies of magnetoencephalography found insufficient evidence to support a positive relationship between MEG and seizure freedom [19], whereas subsequent reclassification produced the opposite finding [20].

Surgical Predictors of Seizure Freedom

Completeness of Resection

Completeness of resection is the primary determinant of postoperative seizure freedom [6–8, 21]. Most studies define completeness of resection as the complete removal of the epileptogenic zone defined by intraoperative or extraoperative subdural EEG and, in lesional patients, removal of the lesion based on the postoperative MRI.

Patients with incomplete resections can still do well [21]. Thus, children should not be excluded from surgical consideration based on the likelihood that surgery would result in an incomplete resection of either the ictal onset zone or the lesion. In most cases, proximity to eloquent cortex limits the resection boundaries and is responsible for residual tissue. For patients with incomplete resection, factors including unilobar procedures, temporal resection, and the finding of a contiguous lesion on MRI are associated with seizure freedom [21].

Site of Resection: Temporal Versus Extratemporal

Higher rates of seizure freedom are observed in children undergoing temporal compared to extratemporal resections, a finding consistent across all age groups [11, 12, 14, 15, 22–26]. Completeness of resection with diffuse lesions in extratemporal lobe epilepsy, compared to common focal lesions of the temporal lobe

Table 4.2 Positive and negative predictors of postsurgical seizure freedom in temporal lobe epilepsy in children [12, 22, 28]

Positive Predictors	Negative Predictors
Lesion on MR Lateralized interictal or ictal EEG abnormality (not necessarily localized to temporal lobe) At least one semiology sign of temporal lobe origin at onset of the habitual seizure	Sensory motor deficit Intellectual disability MRI abnormalities extending outside of temporal lobe History of generalized seizures Status epilepticus Unremarkable histology Acute postop seizures Ipsilateral epileptiform activity on postoperative EEG

such as hippocampal sclerosis, can be more difficult to achieve due to more complicated localization and surgical access issues. In addition, the anterior temporal lobe is more amenable to aggressive resections which increases the likelihood of completeness and contributes to the superior prognosis [10, 14]. Positive and negative predictors of seizure-free outcome in temporal lobe epilepsy are shown in Table 4.2

Postsurgical Predictors of Seizure Freedom

Histopathology

Histopathologic substrate is variably reported as a predictive outcome factor in large mixed cohorts of postoperative patients which makes it difficult to definitively define its role in seizure outcome in children. Two studies reported improved outcomes in pediatric patients with glial-neuronal tumors and focal cortical dysplasia while inflammation, polymicrogyria, and "normal tissue" correlated with diminished rates of seizure freedom [10, 14]. For temporal lobe epilepsy, children with HS and tumors fare better than all other reported substrates [12].

Other studies have generated conflicting findings. D'argenzio et al. (2012) created Cox proportional hazard model survival plots for seizure recurrence in relation to etiology in a cohort of 80 pediatric ETLE patients (Fig. 4.3) [27]. Nonspecific pathology (scar tissue, gliosis, atrophy, perinatal injury, and normal brain) was the only variable significantly associated with a higher risk of seizure recurrence compared to focal cortical dysplasia; whereas, the presence of a low-grade tumor or tuberous sclerosis complex revealed no comparative difference. Similar poor outcomes have been demonstrated in lesional TLE when the histopathology is unremarkable [28].

Postencephalitic epilepsy in children tends to be quite intractable and is associated with particularly poor outcomes despite localization of seizure foci with extensive presurgical evaluation and invasive monitoring [29–31]

The wide variation in seizure outcome in relation to histopathology suggests an indeterminate correlation and need for more data.

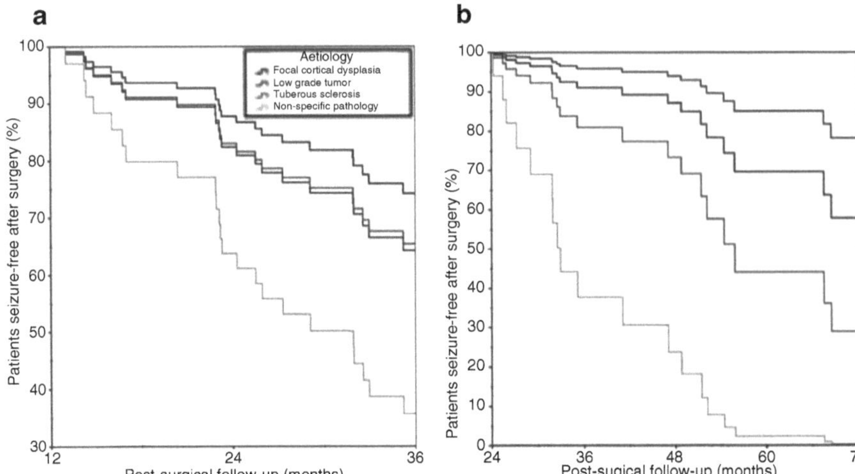

Number at risk	Year 0	Year 1	Year 2	Year 3	Year 4	Year 5	Year 6
Focal cortical dysplasia	37	34	23	13	11	9	6
Low-grade tumor	22	19	9	5	3	3	2
Tuberous sclerosis	9	9	8	7	6	2	2
Non-specific pathology	12	12	10	3	2	0	0
Total	80	74	50	28	22	14	10

Fig. 4.3 Cox proportional hazards model survival plots depicting seizure freedom with respect to histopathology. (**a**) Survival plot up to 36 months for the whole study population ($n=80$). (**b**) Survival plot from 24 to 72 months for patients with a follow-up of 2 years or more ($n=50$). The table shows the number of patients at risk of seizure relapse by year of observation and etiology (With Permission: John Wiley and Sons, D'Argenzio et al. [27], Fig. 2.1)

Type of Surgery

Hemispherectomy, Hemispherotomy, and Multilobar Surgery

Hemidisconnection procedures involve the surgical removal of a portion of one cerebral hemisphere or the disconnection of the lobes within that hemisphere. The classic anatomic hemispherectomy procedure has been modified in an effort to improve outcomes and reduce complications [32]. Typically, hemidisconnection is performed in patients with drug-resistant epilepsy arising from one cerebral hemisphere with evidence of concurrent hemiparesis and hemianopic visual field defect. For all patients under consideration for a hemidisconnection, the possibility of new neurologic deficits arising from the surgery is weighed against the potential neurodevelopmental benefits of seizure control [33].

The largest review to date reported seizure freedom or Engel Class Ia outcomes in 66 % (112/170) of patients at mean follow-up of 5.3 years [33]. Major improvement (>90 % reduction in seizures or greater) was obtained in 80 % of this cohort at 4.8 years median follow-up. This result is consistent with reported seizure-free outcomes ranging from 41 to 83 %.

Seizure freedom tends to be enduring in hemidisconnection patients. Moosa et al. (2013) used a Kaplan-Meier survival analysis to estimate seizure-free rates at 1, 2, and 5 years postsurgery at 76, 71, and 63 %. The majority of patients who fail hemidisconnection do so in 4–6 months, whereas, seizure freedom persists in patients who are seizure-free at 6 months postoperatively. Patients who are seizure-free at 6 months have a 98, 92, and 81 % chance of seizure freedom at 1, 2, and 5–10 years, respectively [33].

The relationship between substrate and seizure outcome in hemidisconnection patients is less clear as studies reveal contradictory results [34, 35]. Many studies separate substrates into developmental (e.g., hemimegelencephaly), acquired (e.g., encephalomalacia as a sequelae of stroke) and progressive (e.g., Rasmussen encephalitis).

Studies that have established a relationship between seizure freedom and substrate report poorer seizure outcomes for developmental lesions, especially hemimegalencephaly [36, 37], whereas, acquired and progressive substrates are associated with better seizure outcomes [35–37]. In the latter study, older age at surgery predicted seizure freedom but the authors recognized that older children were more likely to undergo hemidisconnection for acquired rather than developmental substrates. Seizures due to developmental substrates present earlier in life and are operated on at an earlier age, especially hemimegalencephaly, falsely indicating that older children fair better in terms of seizure outcomes [35]. Notable negative predictors of seizure outcome for hemidisconnection include bilateral PET abnormalities [33] and early postoperative seizures [33, 35]. Bilateral interictal and ictal EEG and bilateral MRI abnormalities do not correlate with seizure outcomes [33–35, 38].

Multilobar surgery is performed more often in childhood [6, 14, 39]. In three different large pediatric epilepsy surgery cohorts, reported seizure-free rates after multilobar resection were 15 % (64/425), 22 % (25/113), and 69 % (43/62 posterior cortex surgeries) [14, 40, 41] compared to 11.5 % (16/139) and as low as 3 % in other series reporting on mixed cohorts of adults and children [42, 43]. Long-term seizure freedom after childhood multilobar resections ranges from 55 to 68 % [14, 40] with resections within the posterior cortex resulting in better outcomes than in anterior locations [41]. Importantly, in a cohort of 63 pediatric and adult patients, Sarkis et al. (2012) showed that seizure freedom for multilobar resections typically decreased over time [43]. The likelihood of seizure freedom was 71 % at 6 months followed by 64, 52 and 41 % at 1, 5 and 10 years (Fig. 4.4).

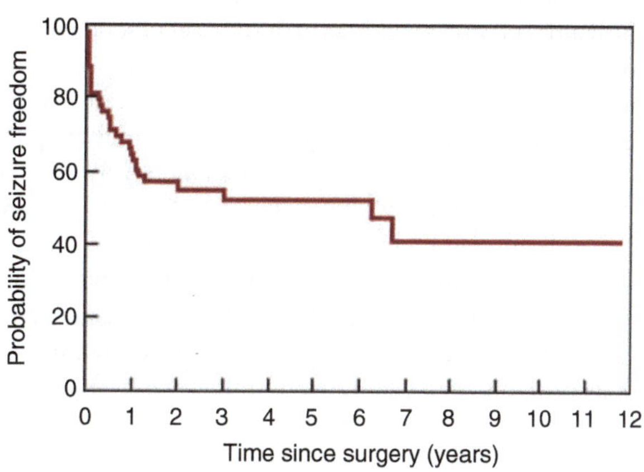

Fig. 4.4 Kaplan-Meier curve showing postoperative survival rates for multi-lobar resection at 6 months, 1 year, 5 years, and 10 years (With permission: John Wiley and Sons, Sarkis et al. [43], Fig. 3.2)

Table 4.3 Reported percent seizure-free outcomes by anatomical site

Lobe	Seizure-free outcomes (%)
Frontal	33.7–66
Cingulate	100
Insular	~80
Occipital	30–69.2
Parietal	40–82
Temporal	63.2–85

Cingulate = small case series and case reports
Insular = small mixed series
Occipital = mixed adult-pediatric cohorts
Parietal = mixed adult-pediatric cohorts

Epileptologists recommending hemidisconnection often consider more restricted multilobar resections to spare patient morbidity such as hemiparesis or visual field deficit. No studies have directly compared hemidisconnection to multilobar resection in the pediatric age group but Cossu et al. (2008) found that a tailored "wide multilobar" approach aiming to spare eloquent cortex resulted in relatively poor outcomes compared to hemispherectomy [14].

Focal Resections: Extratemporal and Temporal Lobes

A global summary of seizure-free outcomes by anatomical lobe of origin is given in Table 4.3 and a summary of outcomes of the major studies referenced in this chapter can be found in the Appendix.

Frontal Lobe

Reported rates of postoperative seizure freedom in frontal lobe epilepsy (FLE) in mixed adult-pediatric series are highly variable, ranging from 20 to 60 %. There is little information regarding FLE surgical outcomes in childhood populations and all existing data are derived from retrospective case series or uncontrolled meta-analyses. Rates of seizure freedom in the pediatric population range from 34 to 66 % at a mean age of 9–11 years; variable follow-up from a minimum of 1–2 years, and/or mean follow-up from 34 to 40 months [9–11, 44–46].

Predictors of FLE seizure freedom include the presence of a gross structural lesion, abnormal preoperative MRI, and localized ictal findings with total resection of the lesion being the most significant single predictor of seizure freedom [44, 45]. However, the presence of a lesion does not guarantee a better outcome [9] and non-lesional FLE surgery outcomes are poorer than non-lesional posterior cortex surgeries [10]. This difference may be related to the establishment of complex neuronal networks in the frontal lobe and the surgical constraints conferred by language and motor cortex. These factors also likely contribute to the poorer outcomes in lesional and non-lesional FLE in comparison to temporal lobe epilepsy (TLE) [9, 10].

Cingulate Epilepsy

Due to its deep anatomical location and various inter-neuronal connections, localization of ictal onset within the cingulate gyrus is challenging and associated with seizure outcomes in children that are likely underreported [47]. Data is limited to small series and individual case reports with consequently limited follow-up. In a large mixed adult-pediatric cohort [47] that included three anterior and two posterior cases, all cases were lesional and had mixed neoplastic and non-neoplastic pathology. All patients were seizure-free between 1 and 11 years postsurgery.

Insular Lobe

Reported seizure outcomes after insular resection are variable and based on small pediatric cohorts in long-term epilepsy surgery studies. More recent case reports describe good outcomes [48–50]. Von Lehe et al. (2009) reported six children in a mixed pediatric-adult sample with follow-up ranging from 12 to 164 months [51]. Four patients had lesions localized solely to the insula; five were seizure-free, and one achieved a 50 % seizure reduction.

Occipital Lobe

There is a paucity of studies in the adult and mixed adult-pediatric literature reporting occipital lobe epilepsy (OLE) surgery, and only one study explored surgical outcomes for OLE in a pure pediatric cohort [41]. All other reports describe either mixed adult-pediatric cohorts or mixed anatomical surgical locations (i.e., "posterior cortex" surgery) encompassing the parietal and occipital lobes or multilobar resections. The small number of studies is due to the low incidence of focal lesional, "pure" occipital lobe epilepsy, and the diminished reliability of standard investigations to localize occipital lobe ictal onset [52]. The incidence of occipital lobe epilepsy in children is unknown but believed to be rare with only one large case series, albeit an older study, showing an incidence of 8 % [53, 54]. Investigations including video EEG, SPECT, and MRI are unreliable predictors of occipital seizure onset [55].

Surgery for OLE is less successful than temporal lobe epilepsy surgery. Studies reporting outcomes in OLE are variable due to non-standardized inclusion criteria, mixed underlying substrates, and inconsistent use of seizure outcome scales [52]. The current literature suggests a range of seizure freedom from 50 to 69.2 % in mixed cohorts of adult and pediatric patients with OLE with follow-up ranging from 13 to 157 months [41, 52, 55–57].

Pediatric outcomes can be extracted from two studies [41, 56]. The first is a series of pediatric posterior cortex surgeries of which eight patients had surgery for "pure" OLE; all were seizure-free at follow-up [41]. Mean age of seizure onset was 8.5 years but specific duration of follow-up was not reported. The second study (Tandon et al., 2009) reported a mixed adult-pediatric sample with 11/21 patients under age 17 years [56]. This cohort was followed from 34 to 157 months with 55 % seizure-free at the last follow-up.

There is a trend in the adult and pediatric literature that particular clinical features can be associated with anatomical features of OLE. OLE is more likely to present with preoperative visual field deficits in comparison to parietal or multilobar occipital epilepsies but the deficit tends to be less clinically significant [52, 56]. Medial or lobar occipital lesions have a higher likelihood of preoperative visual field defects while lateral or basal occipital lesions are more likely to present with visual auras and concordant lateralized scalp EEG onset [57]. Jobst et al. (2010) found better outcomes in patients with inferior occipital lobe seizure onset [55].

Parietal Lobe

Outcomes of PLE surgery in children have been reported only rarely as a distinct cohort. Gleissner et al. (2008) described 15 children who underwent parietal lobe surgery for epilepsy of various pathological diagnoses [58]. At 1-year follow-up, 87 % (13/15) were seizure-free. Long-term follow-up with a mean interval of 4.4 years (range: 2–9 years) was available for 11 patients with seizure freedom of 82 %.

Temporal Lobe

The pediatric epilepsy surgery literature typically separates out temporal lobe epilepsy (TLE) and discusses extratemporal lobe epilepsy (ETLE) as a collective cohort although TLE accounts for only 15–20 % of epilepsy cases in children [12, 59]. Similarities and differences exist in presentation of TLE in young children, older children, and adults. Despite these differences, children have similar outcomes as adults and surgery for TLE in children has been proven to be safe and effective [23].

One consistently identified difference between children and adults is TLE etiology. Whereas, hippocampal sclerosis (HS) is the most common cause of intractable TLE in adults, TLE etiologies in children are more variable [12]. In a recent systematic review of TLE surgery, children with HS and tumors are more likely to experience long-term seizure freedom [12].

There are no published randomized control trials in pediatric TLE surgery and all published studies are either retrospective or prospective observational studies with the vast majority having a cross-sectional or longitudinal design with no control group. Skirrow et al. (2011) analyzed long-term TLE surgery outcomes against a

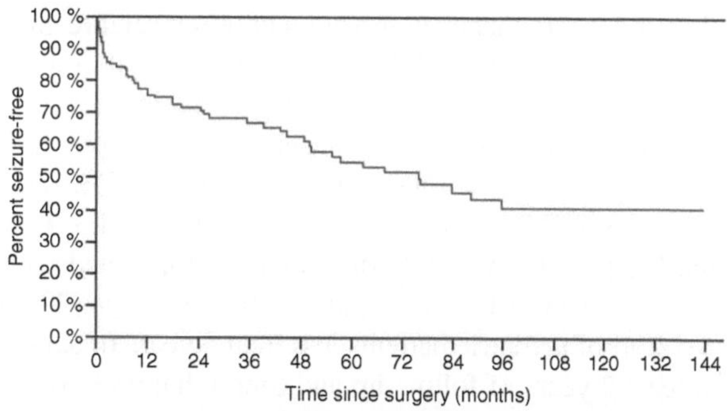

	1 year	2 years	5 years	12 years
% seizure-free (overall group)	76 %	72 %	54 %	41 %
N at risk	86	69	35	12

Fig. 4.5 Kaplan-Meier curve expressing seizure-free outcomes at 1, 2,5, and 12 years after temporal lobe resection in children with TLE ($n=130$; from 1996 to 2006) (With permission: Wolters Kluwer Health, Lopez-Gonzalez et al. [62], Fig. 5.6.1)

small nonsurgical control group ($n=11$) and found improved outcomes in the cohort of 42 patients comprising the surgical group (86 % vs. 36 %, respectively) at mean follow-up of 9 years [60].

Individual published cohorts of TLE surgery in children ranging from 19 to 130 patients with follow-up of 1–23 years reveal rates of seizure freedom between 63.2 and 85 % which are comparable to the published adult findings [23, 28, 59, 61–65]. A recent review by Englot et al. (2013), covering the period between 1993 and 2012, accumulated data on 1,318 pediatric patients from 36 studies and found that 76 % (1,002/1,318) were seizure-free at last postsurgical follow-up with a minimum follow-up of 1 year. Ages of the patients ranged from 0 to 19 years (mean [±SEM] 10.7 ± 0.3 years).

Lopez-Gonzalez et al. (2012) showed that seizure freedom rates typically decrease over time in children. This group used a Kaplan-Meier seizure-freedom curve to show that the rate of seizure freedom in their population was 76, 72, 54, and 41 % at 1, 2, 5, and 12 years postsurgery (Fig. 4.5). Although an explanation for this finding is not forthcoming, it is possible that secondary epileptogenesis or incomplete resection of the ictal onset zone was responsible.

Age of the pediatric patient is an essential factor to consider in TLE surgery evaluation and has been analyzed extensively [12, 28, 63, 65, 66]. It is important to acknowledge that cortical maturation likely plays a role in the presentation of TLE [66] and incorrect interpretation of semiology in young patients may impede surgical evaluation by falsely identifying a concordant semiology as a non-concordant one. Younger children tend to have fewer auras and dyscognitive features and more prominent motor manifestations; some have been reported to present with epileptic spasms [28, 63].

A recent systematic review of TLE surgery outcomes in children did not stratify outcomes by age, but this data can be found in some of the studies they included [12]. Developmental substrates, malignant tumors, and dual pathology (hippocampal plus extrahippocampal findings) tend to predominate in younger children and are all associated with less favorable seizure-free outcomes [12, 23, 63]. Despite this, it appears that even in young children seizure-free outcome rates still approximate those in older children and adults. Mittal et al. (2005) separated their cohort into children (<12 years old) and adolescents (13–18 years old) and found that, at the last follow-up, 84.8 % of children were seizure-free compared to 79.4 % of adolescents (median follow-up of 11.3 years). The rate of persistent seizures (Engel Class III or IV) was comparable at 13.0 and 14.3 %, respectively. The group from the Hospital for Sick Children in Toronto, Canada reported no differences in outcomes in 106 TLE surgery patients based on age [22]. Maton et al. (2008) analyzed a cohort of pediatric patients less than 5 years of age (mean age, = 26 months) with at least 2 years of follow-up and found that 65 % of patients were seizure-free and 15 % had >90 % seizure reduction.

Corpus Callosotomy

For patients with drug-resistant seizures that are not amenable to focal resection, corpus callosotomy (CC) can be a useful treatment option in appropriately selected patients whose predominant seizure type is drop attacks. Often there may be discussion about the merits of callosal section vs. vagal nerve stimulation (VNS); comparative studies suggest superiority of callosotomy over VNS for atonic seizures. VNS alternatively may result in improvement in a wider range of seizure types [67, 68]

CC is primarily indicated for atonic drop attacks but is also beneficial for complex partial seizures with rapid secondary generalization without a defined epileptogenic focus [69]. Disconnecting the corpus callosum blocks the interhemispheric spread of seizures; thus, the primary aim of callosal sectioning is to reduce seizure intensity and decrease seizure burden rather than eliminate seizures completely [70, 71].

Observational studies support the effectiveness of CC for drop attacks and GTC seizures [69–71]. A prospective mixed adult-pediatric cohort with a mean age at surgery of 13 years (range: 2–41 years), went from 190 drop attacks per month presurgery to 100 per month at 2 year follow-up and 20 per month between 5 and 10 years [69]. Seizure freedom was obtained in 10/18 patients and 3 of the remaining 8 patients achieved a >75 % seizure reduction.

Sunaga et al. (2009) reported that complete callosotomy increases seizure freedom for drop attacks in comparison to partial sectioning. In 78 patients (51 patients less than 18 years of age), 90 % who underwent complete callosotomy were free of drop attacks with a relapse rate of 7 % at 6 years in comparison to 54 % seizure freedom after partial callosotomy and a relapse rate of 31 % at 6 years. Twenty-one percent of patients developed new postural seizures.

GTC seizures improved after callosotomy in a retrospective review of 95 mixed adult-pediatric patients (mean age of 24 years) [70]. Forty-two percent were seizure-free at a mean follow-up of 17 years and 35 % were free from drop attacks over the same time period.

Antiepileptic Medications and Long-Term Seizure Freedom

Prior to undergoing epilepsy surgery, most studies report that pediatric patients are taking two or more antiepileptic drugs (AED) in keeping with the ILAE definition of drug-resistant epilepsy [72]. Eventual weaning of AEDs is a key objective for patient's who ultimately undergo epilepsy surgery; therefore, understanding the likelihood of achieving this is important to assist patients and their families in the decision making process.

Patients with substrates and clinical findings that require larger resections, such as multilobar procedures or hemidisconneciton, tend to be using a greater number of AEDs at baseline and surgery can have a meaningful impact on reducing this number [36]. In a cohort of 33 patients who underwent hemispherectomy, 16 were no longer taking AEDs at a median of 3.4 years follow-up and the remaining 17 patients significantly reduced the amount of AEDs they were using [36].

Regardless of type of surgery, most pediatric patients will require less AEDs over time [27, 33, 38, 40, 41]. Hemb et al. (2010) demonstrated this in their 22 year cohort in which the number of AEDs per patient decreases with increased time from surgery. In patients who underwent temporal lobectomy reported by Miserocchi et al. (2013), 35 % had been weaned with mean follow-up of 67.2 months, 43 % with mean follow-up of 31.2 months were tapering AEDs, and 22 % with mean follow-up of 22.3 months were maintaining their presurgical regimen. Other studies have shown this trend over long-term intervals following various types of resections. For example, discontinuation of AEDs has been reported in 37.5 % (15/40) of seizure-free children with extratemporal resections (median follow-up, 3 years), 77 % (41/53) of seizure-free children with lobar/multilobar posterior cortex resections (median follow-up, 6.92 years), and 57 % of seizure-free children with temporal lobe resections (mean follow-up, 9 years) [27, 41, 65].

There remains a risk for postsurgical seizure recurrence even with the use of AEDs. Lopez-Gonzalez et al. (2012) reported that over the 12-year follow-up period in their temporal lobectomy cohort, seizures recurred at one point in 54 patients (41 %) and only 33 % (18/54) of these were associated with an attempt to withdraw AEDs. By adjusting medication they were able to re-establish seizure freedom in half (27/54) of all the individuals. Because the risk of recurrence despite AED use is now well established, it is not surprising to see that proportionately higher AED use was observed in the first 2 years of follow-up in a cohort of patients from UCLA who underwent epilepsy surgery after 1997 compared to the group who received surgery prior to 1997 [40]. This probably reflects the more current shift in practice to maintain AEDs following surgery until patients have demonstrated long-term seizure freedom which is typically considered to be about 1–2 years. However, for both cohorts at 5 years follow-up, AED use was similar and, overall, 40 % of all patients were seizure-free and no longer required antiepileptic medication. However, the evidence regarding the risk of postsurgical seizure recurrence and timing of AED withdrawal is conflicting and there are no guidelines or standards of care in pediatric epilepsy surgery. For example, Kim et al. (2008) reported no recurrence of seizures due to antiepileptic medication withdrawal attempts in their large mixed cohort of 134 patients at a mean follow-up of 5.2 years [73]. One large multicenter retrospective European study found that 728 of 766 children who had undergone surgery and had initiated an AED reduction, after a mean postoperative follow-up of 61.6 months, were seizure-free for at least 12 months [74]. The time interval from surgery to the start of AED reduction and complete discontinuation was not related to seizure freedom, cure at final follow-up or the ability to regain seizure freedom after restarting treatment. The conclusion was that early AED withdrawal following surgery did not affect long-term outcome or cure but that it could unmask incomplete surgical success sooner.

Conclusions

Children undergoing epilepsy surgery make up a heterogeneous group. The underlying substrates for their epilepsy differ proportionately to what is observed in adults and they experience a range of different types of surgical procedures. There is little consistent longitudinal data with regard to seizure outcome. There is a suggestion that outcome at 12 months is in part an indicator of longer-term outcome but some attrition occurs over time, more so in nonspecific and gliotic pathologies than ischaemic lesions or cortical malformations. A key question is when and if medication can be withdrawn. Recent data indicate that earlier rather than later withdrawal should be considered in seizure-free patients; this is not likely to affect longer-term outcome but will unmask those in whom continued medication is likely to be required. Further prospective studies consisting of homogeneous cohorts are required for accurate data to be collected about long-term seizure outcome and its true relationship to other outcome measures.

Appendix. Longer term seizure outcome in series published to date, with analysis of predictors of outcome

Author, year	Study design	Operated patients *N*	Drop-outs *N*	Number in study group	Follow-up, years mean (min-max)	Males %	Age at surgery mean (min–max)	Type of surgery	Pathology	Prognostic indicators studied	Outcome measures	Good outcome	Statistical methods
Lopez-Gonzalez, 2012	R, L	130	0	130	NR (1–12)	48	12.3 years (1–18 years)	RES, T	All	A, B, D, F, G, H, K *Side of surgery, number of AEDs, type of surgery, presence of tumor*	Engel	SF: 76 % at 1 year, 72 % at 2 years, 54 % at 5 years and 41 % at 12 years	CPH, Fi, KM, W
Benifla, 2006	R, L	126	0	126	5.6 (2–13)	52	13.5 years (5 months–19.8 years)	RES, T	All	A, D, E, H	Engel	At mean of 5.6 years: 74 % Engel I 2 % Engel II 6 % Engel III 19 % Engel IV (20/126 did not have min. 2 years follow-up & were excluded from analysis of outcomes)	Fi, LogReg

(continued)

Appendix (continued)

Author, year	Study design	Operated patients *N*	Drop-outs *N*	Number in study group	Follow-up, years mean (min-max)	Males %	Age at surgery mean (min–max)	Type of surgery	Pathology	Prognostic indicators studied	Outcome measures	Good outcome	Statistical methods
Mittal, 2005	R, L	109	0	109	Median: 10.9 (5–20.2)	52.3	Median: 13.2 years (2 months–18.9 years)	RES, T	All	A, B, C, D, F, G, H	Engel	At median of 11.3 years: 81.7 % Engel I 4.6 % Engel II 13.7 Engel III & IV	Ch, Fi, LogReg
Maton, 2008	R, L	20	0	20	5.5 (2–23 years)	70	26.4 months (6 months–4.4 years)	RES, T	All	C, D, E, F, G, H	Engel	At mean of 5.5 years: 65 % Engel I 15 % Engel II 20 % Engel III & IV	NR
Skirrow, 2011	R, C, L	60	18	53 (11/53 were control group)	9 (5–15 years)	45	13.3 years	RES, T	HS DNET	D	Seizure Freedom	At mean of 9 years: 86 % of surgery patients SF 36 % of surgery patients SF	Ch, Fi, LogReg,
Kim, 2008	R, L	134	0	134	5.2 (1–14)	56	8.5 years (8 months–18 years)	RES, T, XT, FH, CAL, MST, DIS	All	E, F, G, H *Predictors for recurrence: MRI-negative, developmental lesions, bilateral or multifocal abnormal postop EEG, incomplete resection*	Engel	At mean of 5.2 years: 69 % Engel I 5 % Engel II 7 % Engel III 19 % Engel IV SF temporal: 88 % SF extratemporal: 55 %	Ch

Vadera, 2012	R, L	45	0	45	5 (4 months–12.3 years)	56	Median: 12 years	RES, T	HS HS + FCD	None	Engel	At mean of 5 years: 69 % Engel I 16 % Engel II 9 % Engel III 7 % Engel IV	None
Miserocchi, 2013	R, L	186	0	68	Minimum: 1 year	63	8.9±4.5 years (1–15 years)	RES, T	All	A, B, C, D, E, F, G, H *Predictors for recurrence (bivariate analysis): preop sensory-motor deficit, mental retardation, abnormal MRI beyond temporal lobe, history of generalized seizures or status epilepticus, unremarkable histology, postop seizures, ipsilateral postop epileptiform activity on EEG*	Engel	85 % Engel I 16 % Engel II 9 % Engel III 7 % Engel IV (Time period for outcome measure not reported)	Fi, KW (Bivariate analysis)

(continued)

Appendix (continued)

Author, year	Study design	Operated patients *N*	Drop-outs *N*	Number in study group	Follow-up, years mean (min-max)	Males %	Age at surgery mean (min–max)	Type of surgery	Pathology	Prognostic indicators studied	Outcome measures	Good outcome	Statistical methods
Lee, 2010	R, L	19	0	19	2.4 ± 0.7 years (1.2–3.5)	57.9	14.6 ± 2.8 years (9.3–18.0)	RES, T	All	A, B, D, E, G, H *Predictors for recurrence: secondary generalized seizures, wider resection with subtotal temporal lobectomy, malformation of cortical development*	Engel	At mean of 2.4 years: 63.2 % Engel I 26.3 % Engel II 10.5 % Engel III 0 % Engel IV	PPM, Ch, Fi
Smyth, 2007	R, N, L	49	0	49	2.2 (5 months–6.2 years)	57	9.1 year (1.3–13.9)	RES, T	All (Neoplasm excluded)	A, C, D, E, F, G, H, K *Predictors for recurrence: more than one seizure type, moderate to severe development delay*	Engel	At mean of 2.2 years: 63.3 % Engel I & II 36.7 % Engel III-IV	MW, Ch, Y
Vachhrajani, 2012	R, L	40	0	40	3.35 (0–13.4 years)	50	11.7 years (NR)	RES, F, MST	All	A, E, F, G, H *No predictors identified*	Engel	At mean of 3.35 years: 62.5 % Engel I 12.5 % Engel II 17.5 % Engel III 5 % Engel IV	STT, LogReg, Ch, Fi

Kral, 2001	R, L	32	0	32	2.9 years (1– 9.4 years)	69	10.8 years (1– 17 years)	RES, F, CAL	All	A, B, C, D, E, F *Significant predictors of SF: Lesional MRI, ECOG, Lesionectomy* (Univariate analysis unless significant predictor identified)	Engel	At mean of 2.9 years: 65.6 % Engel I 0 % Engel II 18.8 % Engel III 15.6 % Engel IV	Ch, Fi, W
D'Argenzio, 2012	R, L	102	22	80	Median: 3.08 years (8 months– 10.6 years)	52.5	Median: 9.08 years (3 months– 18.6 years)	RES, F, PR, O	All	A, C, D, G, K *Predictor of seizure recurrence: nonspecific lesion pathology*	Engel	At median of 3.08 years: 50 % Engel Ia 3 % Engel Ib 3 % Engel Ic 10 % Engel II 15 % Engel III 20 % Engel IV	Ch, Fi, STT, MW, CPH,
Kasasabeh, 2012	R, L	39	0	39	"Extended Follow-Up" defined as >24 months	51	12.2±4.8	RES, F	All	A, B, D, E, F, G, H *Early postoperative seizures correlated with poor short-term SF (<12 months) but was not significant for long-term SF (>24 months)*	Engel	At 1 year ($n=37$): 68 % Engel I 16 % Engel II 11 % Engel III 5 % Engel IV At extended F/U ($n=22$): 55 % Engel I 18 % Engel II 23 % Engel III 5 % Engel IV	W, Fi, Sp

(continued)

Appendix (continued)

Author, year	Study design	Operated patients *N*	Drop-outs *N*	Number in study group	Follow-up, years mean (min-max)	Males %	Age at surgery mean (min–max)	Type of surgery	Pathology	Prognostic indicators studied	Outcome measures	Good outcome	Statistical methods
Lehe, 2009	R, L	24	0	6 (Pediatric patients)	5.16 years (1–13.7 years)	50	7 years (1–17 years)	RES, INS, INS+F, INS+F+T	All	None	ILAE	At mean of 5.16 years: 83 % ILAE 1 17 % ILAE 4	Descri-ptive
Park, 2009	R, L	6	0	6	1.48 years (6 months–2.75 years)	50	4.16 years (2–7 years)	RES, INS	All	None	Engel	At mean of 1.48years: 83 % Engel I 17 % Engel II	Descri-ptive
Limbrick Jr, 2009	R,L	49	0	49	2.38 years (0.5 months –7.4 years)	63.3	0.2–20.5 years	FH, FIH	All	E, G, H, *No statistically significant predictors identified*	Engel	At mean of 2.38 years: 77.6 % Engel I 12.2 % Engel II 10.2 % Engel III 0 % Engel IV	W, Fi, Ch, KM, CAT
Liava, 2014	R, L	312	0	62 (Pediatric patients)	6.94 years (2–16)	61	7.9 years (1–16)	RES, P, O, P+O, O+T	All	A, D, E, F, G H *Bonferroni correction showed that there were no predictors of SF*	Engel	At mean of 6.94 years: 85.5 % Engel I 3 % Engel II 6.5 % Engel III 5 % Engel IV	Fi, STT, BON
Hemb, 2010	R, L, S (Comparison of two cohorts)	580	0	425 (resective surgery)	(0.5–5 years)	54	7.7±6.3 years	RES, H, ML, L	All	A, B, D, E, F, G, H, K *Predictor of SF: AED use at 2 years, hemispherectomy, temporal lobectomy, HS, tumor*	SF	SF at 2 years ($n=326$): 69 % SF at 5 years ($n=236$): 59 %	STT, Ch, LogReg

Cossu, 2008	R, L	113	0	113	4.59 years (2–9.58 years)	59	8.8 years (1–15 years)	RES, F, T, XT, ML	All	A, B, C, D, E, F, G, H *Predictor of decreased seizure recurrence (multivariate): unifocal MRI, older age at seizure onset, temporal unilobar resection, completeness of resection, glioneuronal tumor*	Engel	At mean of 4.59 years: 68 % Engel I 9 % Engel II 10 % Engel III 13 % Engel IV	KW, Fi, LogReg
Moosa, 2012	R, L	186	16	170	5.3 ± 3.3 years	60	7.02 ± 5.2 years	RES, H	All	A, B, C, D, E, F, G, H, K *Predictors of seizure recurrence (multivariate): bilateral PET abnormalities, acute postoperative seizures*	Engel	At mean of 5.3 years: 66 % SF (Engel 1a) 34 % Not-SF	W, Ch, Fi, CPH, KM

(continued)

Appendix (continued)

Author, year	Study design	Operated patients *N*	Drop-outs *N*	Number in study group	Follow-up, years mean (min-max)	Males %	Age at surgery mean (min–max)	Type of surgery	Pathology	Prognostic indicators studied	Outcome measures	Good outcome	Statistical methods
Devlin, 2003	R, L	33	0	33	Median: 3.4 years (1–8 years)	64	Median: 4.25 years (0.33–17 years)	RES, H	All	H Decreased chance of SF: developmental pathology	Modified Engel	At median of 3.4 years: 52 %, SF 9 %, rare seizures 30 %, >75 % reduction 9 %, <75 % reduction or no improvement	MW, KW

Abbreviations:
General: *NS* not specified, *SD* standard deviation, *NR* not reported
Study design: *P* prospective, *R* retrospective, *S* single center, *N* national (population based), *X* cross-sectional, *L* longitudinal, *SR* systematic review, *C* control group
Type of surgery: *RES* resective surgery, *T* temporal lobe, *XT* extratemporal lobes, *F* frontal lobe, *PR* parietal lobe, *OC* occipital lobe, *INS* insular cortex, *CNG* Cingulate gyrus, *H* hemispherectomy, *FH* functional hemispherectomy, *PIH* Peri-insular hemispherectomy, *ML* Multilobar, *L* lobar, *CAL* callosotomy, *MST* multiple subpial transection, *DIS* disconnection
Pathology: *HS* hippocampal sclerosis, *NL* non-lesional, *DNET* dysembryoplastic neuroepithelial tumor
Prognostic indicators studied: *A* age-related factors (age at onset, epilepsy duration, age at surgery, age at epileptogenic event), *B* sex or race, *C* coexisting conditions (mental retardation, preop psychiatric history, head trauma, comorbidities), *D* seizure-related factors (seizure frequency, history of GTCS, history of status epilepticus, history of febrile seizures, head version, ictal dystonic posturing, seizure types preop/at relapse, acute postop seizures (APOS), seizure freedom 1 year postop, early postop seizures, postop auras), *E* EEG (localization or unilateral interictal epileptiform discharges (IED), postop IED, invasive EEG, subdural grids, preop electrocorticography (ECoG)), *F* MRI (MRI finding, hippocampal volumetry), *G* surgical factors (type of resection (lobe), side of resection, size of resection, bilateral surgery, previous surgery, surgical approach), *H* histopathology (histopathology, dual pathology), *K* other (SPECT, MEG, PET, WADA scores, postop cessation of AEDs, era of surgery)
Significant predictors in multivariate analysis in italics. Prediction of seizure freedom for most studies
Outcome measures: Engel classification, ILAE classification (Wieser 2001), SF $\geq$ 2 years incl aura: seizure free at least 2 years allowing auras
Good outcome: *SF* seizure free according to outcome measure, *Sust SF incl aura* sustained seizure freedom since surgery allowing auras (equivalent to Engel1a+b)
Statistical methods: *MW* Mann–Whitney *U*-test, *LR* likelihood ratio, *LogReg* logistic regression, *Fi* Fisher's exact test, *Ch* Chi2, *KM* Kaplan-Meier, *CPH* Cox proportional hazard, *W* Wilcoxon rank-sum, *KW* Kruskal-Wallis rank-sum test, *PPM* Pearson's product–moment correlation test, *Y* Yates correction for continuity, *STT* Student *t*-test, *SP* Spearman correlation, *CAT* Cochrane Armitage test, *BON* Bonferroni correction

References

1. Engel J, Cascino GD, Ness P, Rasmussen T, Ojermann L. Outcome with respect to epileptic seizures. In: Engel J, editor. Surgical treatment of the epilepsies. New York: Raven Press; 1993.
2. Wieser HG, Blume WT, Fish D, Goldensohn E, Hufnagel A, King D, et al. ILAE Commission Report. Proposal for a new classification of outcome with respect to epileptic seizures following epilepsy surgery. Epilepsia. 2001;42(2):282–6.
3. Durnford AJ, Rodgers W, Kirkham FJ, Mullee MA, Whitney A, Prevett M, et al. Very good inter-rater reliability of Engel and ILAE epilepsy surgery outcome classifications in a series of 76 patients. Seizure. 2011;20(10):809–12.
4. Cross JH, Jayakar P, Nordli D, Delalande O, Duchowny M, Wieser HG, et al. Proposed criteria for referral and evaluation of children for epilepsy surgery: recommendations of the Subcommission for Pediatric Epilepsy Surgery. Epilepsia. 2006;47(6):952–9.
5. Perry MS, Duchowny M. Surgical versus medical treatment for refractory epilepsy: outcomes beyond seizure control. Epilepsia. 2013;54(12):2060–70.
6. Paolicchi JM, Jayakar P, Dean P, Yaylali I, Morrison G, Prats A, et al. Predictors of outcome in pediatric epilepsy surgery. Neurology. 2000;54(3):642–7.
7. Cross JH. Epilepsy surgery in childhood. Epilepsia. 2002;43 Suppl 3:65–70.
8. RamachandranNair R, Otsubo H, Shroff MM, Ochi A, Weiss SK, Rutka JT, et al. MEG predicts outcome following surgery for intractable epilepsy in children with normal or nonfocal MRI findings. Epilepsia. 2007;48(1):149–57.
9. Vachhrajani S, de Ribaupierre S, Otsubo H, Ochi A, Weiss SK, Donner EJ, et al. Neurosurgical management of frontal lobe epilepsy in children. J Neurosurg Pediatr. 2012;10(3):206–16.
10. Ansari SF, Maher CO, Tubbs RS, Terry CL, Cohen-Gadol AA. Surgery for extratemporal nonlesional epilepsy in children: a meta-analysis. Childs Nerv Syst. 2010;26(7):945–51.
11. Englot DJ, Breshears JD, Sun PP, Chang EF, Auguste KI. Seizure outcomes after resective surgery for extra-temporal lobe epilepsy in pediatric patients. J Neurosurg Pediatr. 2013;12(2):126–33.
12. Englot DJ, Rolston JD, Wang DD, Sun PP, Chang EF, Auguste KI. Seizure outcomes after temporal lobectomy in pediatric patients. J Neurosurg Pediatr. 2013;12(2):134–41.
13. Duchowny M, Jayakar P, Levin B. Aberrant neural circuits in malformations of cortical development and focal epilepsy. Neurology. 2000;55(3):423–8.
14. Cossu M, Lo Russo G, Francione S, Mai R, Nobili L, Sartori I, et al. Epilepsy surgery in children: results and predictors of outcome on seizures. Epilepsia. 2008;49(1):65–72.
15. Edelvik A, Rydenhag B, Olsson I, Flink R, Kumlien E, Kallen K, et al. Long-term outcomes of epilepsy surgery in Sweden: a national prospective and longitudinal study. Neurology. 2013;81(14):1244–51.
16. Schulz R, Luders HO, Hoppe M, Tuxhorn I, May T, Ebner A. Interictal EEG and ictal scalp EEG propagation are highly predictive of surgical outcome in mesial temporal lobe epilepsy. Epilepsia. 2000;41(5):564–70.
17. Jayakar P, Dunoyer C, Dean P, Ragheb J, Resnick T, Morrison G, et al. Epilepsy surgery in patients with normal or nonfocal MRI scans: integrative strategies offer long-term seizure relief. Epilepsia. 2008;49(5):758–64.
18. Rathore C, Radhakrishnan K. Prognostic significance of interictal epileptiform discharges after epilepsy surgery. J Clin Neurophysiol. 2010;27(4):255–62.
19. Lau M, Yam D, Burneo JG. A systematic review on MEG and its use in the presurgical evaluation of localization-related epilepsy. Epilepsy Res. 2008;79(2–3):97–104.
20. Lewine JD. Commentary on Lau et al., 2008. A systematic review on MEG and its use in the presurgical evaluation of localization-related epilepsy. Epilepsy Res. 2008;82(2–3):235–6; author reply 240–1.
21. Perry MS, Dunoyer C, Dean P, Bhatia S, Bavariya A, Ragheb J, et al. Predictors of seizure freedom after incomplete resection in children. Neurology. 2010;75(16):1448–53.

22. Benifla M, Rutka JT, Otsubo H, Lamberti-Pasculli M, Elliott I, Sell E, et al. Long-term seizure and social outcomes following temporal lobe surgery for intractable epilepsy during childhood. Epilepsy Res. 2008;82(2–3):133–8.
23. Benifla M, Otsubo H, Ochi A, Weiss SK, Donner EJ, Shroff M, et al. Temporal lobe surgery for intractable epilepsy in children: an analysis of outcomes in 126 children. Neurosurgery. 2006;59(6):1203–13; discussion 1213–4.
24. Spencer S, Huh L. Outcomes of epilepsy surgery in adults and children. Lancet Neurol. 2008;7(6):525–37.
25. Van Oijen M, De Waal H, Van Rijen PC, Jennekens-Schinkel A, van Huffelen AC, Van Nieuwenhuizen O, et al. Resective epilepsy surgery in childhood: the Dutch experience 1992–2002. Eur J Paediatr Neurol. 2006;10(3):114–23.
26. Ibrahim GM, Fallah A, Albert GW, Withers T, Otsubo H, Ochi A, et al. Occipital lobe epilepsy in children: characterization, evaluation and surgical outcomes. Epilepsy Res. 2012;99(3):335–45.
27. D'Argenzio L, Colonnelli MC, Harrison S, Jacques TS, Harkness W, Scott RC, et al. Seizure outcome after extratemporal epilepsy surgery in childhood. Dev Med Child Neurol. 2012;54(11):995–1000.
28. Miserocchi A, Cascardo B, Piroddi C, Fuschillo D, Cardinale F, Nobili L, et al. Surgery for temporal lobe epilepsy in children: relevance of presurgical evaluation and analysis of outcome. J Neurosurg Pediatr. 2013;11(3):256–67.
29. Trinka E, Dubeau F, Andermann F, Hui A, Bastos A, Li LM, et al. Successful epilepsy surgery in catastrophic postencephalitic epilepsy. Neurology. 2000;54(11):2170–3.
30. Trinka E, Dubeau F, Andermann F, Bastos A, Hui A, Li LM, et al. Clinical findings, imaging characteristics and outcome in catastrophic post-encephalitic epilepsy. Epileptic Disord. 2000;2(3):153–62.
31. Chen YJ, Fang PC, Chow JC. Clinical characteristics and prognostic factors of postencephalitic epilepsy in children. J Child Neurol. 2006;21(12):1047–51.
32. Duchowny M. Hemispherectomy for epilepsy: when is one half better than two? Neurology. 2004;62(10):1664–5.
33. Moosa AN, Gupta A, Jehi L, Marashly A, Cosmo G, Lachhwani D, et al. Longitudinal seizure outcome and prognostic predictors after hemispherectomy in 170 children. Neurology. 2013;80(3):253–60.
34. Limbrick DD, Narayan P, Powers AK, Ojemann JG, Park TS, Bertrand M, et al. Hemispherotomy: efficacy and analysis of seizure recurrence. J Neurosurg Pediatr. 2009;4(4):323–32.
35. Ramantani G, Kadish NE, Brandt A, Strobl K, Stathi A, Wiegand G, et al. Seizure control and developmental trajectories after hemispherotomy for refractory epilepsy in childhood and adolescence. Epilepsia. 2013;54(6):1046–55.
36. Devlin AM, Cross JH, Harkness W, Chong WK, Harding B, Vargha-Khadem F, et al. Clinical outcomes of hemispherectomy for epilepsy in childhood and adolescence. Brain. 2003;126(Pt 3):556–66.
37. Kossoff EH, Vining EP, Pillas DJ, Pyzik PL, Avellino AM, Carson BS, et al. Hemispherectomy for intractable unihemispheric epilepsy etiology vs outcome. Neurology. 2003;61(7):887–90.
38. Lee YJ, Kim EH, Yum MS, Lee JK, Hong S, Ko TS. Long-term outcomes of hemispheric disconnection in pediatric patients with intractable epilepsy. J Clin Neurol. 2014;10(2):101–7.
39. Duchowny M, Jayakar P, Resnick T, Harvey AS, Alvarez L, Dean P, et al. Epilepsy surgery in the first three years of life. Epilepsia. 1998;39(7):737–43.
40. Hemb M, Velasco TR, Parnes MS, Wu JY, Lerner JT, Matsumoto JH, et al. Improved outcomes in pediatric epilepsy surgery: the UCLA experience, 1986–2008. Neurology. 2010;74(22):1768–75.
41. Liava A, Mai R, Tassi L, Cossu M, Sartori I, Nobili L, et al. Paediatric epilepsy surgery in the posterior cortex: a study of 62 cases. Epileptic Disord. 2014;16(2):141–73.
42. Eriksson S, Malmgren K, Rydenhag B, Jonsson L, Uvebrant P, Nordborg C. Surgical treatment of epilepsy–clinical, radiological and histopathological findings in 139 children and adults. Acta Neurol Scand. 1999;99(1):8–15.

43. Sarkis RA, Jehi L, Najm IM, Kotagal P, Bingaman WE. Seizure outcomes following multilobar epilepsy surgery. Epilepsia. 2012;53(1):44–50.
44. Kral T, Kuczaty S, Blumcke I, Urbach H, Clusmann H, Wiestler OD, et al. Postsurgical outcome of children and adolescents with medically refractory frontal lobe epilepsies. Childs Nerv Syst. 2001;17(10):595–601.
45. Englot DJ, Wang DD, Rolston JD, Shih TT, Chang EF. Rates and predictors of long-term seizure freedom after frontal lobe epilepsy surgery: a systematic review and meta-analysis. J Neurosurg. 2012;116(5):1042–8.
46. Kasasbeh AS, Yarbrough CK, Limbrick DD, Steger-May K, Leach JL, Mangano FT, et al. Characterization of the supplementary motor area syndrome and seizure outcome after medial frontal lobe resections in pediatric epilepsy surgery. Neurosurgery. 2012;70(5):1152–68; discussion 1168.
47. Alkawadri R, So NK, Van Ness PC, Alexopoulos AV. Cingulate epilepsy: report of 3 electroclinical subtypes with surgical outcomes. JAMA Neurol. 2013;70(8):995–1002.
48. Park YS, Lee YH, Shim KW, Lee YJ, Kim HD, Lee JS, et al. Insular epilepsy surgery under neuronavigation guidance using depth electrode. Childs Nerv Syst. 2009;25(5):591–7.
49. Levitt MR, Ojemann JG, Kuratani J. Insular epilepsy masquerading as multifocal cortical epilepsy as proven by depth electrode. J Neurosurg Pediatr. 2010;5(4):365–7.
50. Chiosa V, Granziera C, Spinelli L, Pollo C, Roulet-Perez E, Groppa S, et al. Successful surgical resection in non-lesional operculo-insular epilepsy without intracranial monitoring. Epileptic Disord. 2013;15(2):148–57.
51. von Lehe M, Wellmer J, Urbach H, Schramm J, Elger CE, Clusmann H. Insular lesionectomy for refractory epilepsy: management and outcome. Brain. 2009;132(Pt 4):1048–56.
52. Binder DK, Von Lehe M, Kral T, Bien CG, Urbach H, Schramm J, et al. Surgical treatment of occipital lobe epilepsy. J Neurosurg. 2008;109(1):57–69.
53. Gibbs F, Gibbs E. Atlas of electroencephalography. 2nd ed. Cambridge, MA: Addison-Wesley Press; 1953.
54. Engel J, Pedley TA. Epilepsy: a comprehensive textbook, vol. 3. 2nd ed. Philadelphia: Lippincott Williams & Wilkins; 2008.
55. Jobst BC, Williamson PD, Thadani VM, Gilbert KL, Holmes GL, Morse RP, et al. Intractable occipital lobe epilepsy: clinical characteristics and surgical treatment. Epilepsia. 2010;51(11): 2334–7.
56. Tandon N, Alexopoulos AV, Warbel A, Najm IM, Bingaman WE. Occipital epilepsy: spatial categorization and surgical management. J Neurosurg. 2009;110(2):306–18.
57. Davis KL, Murro AM, Park YD, Lee GP, Cohen MJ, Smith JR. Posterior quadrant epilepsy surgery: predictors of outcome. Seizure. 2012;21(9):722–8.
58. Gleissner U, Kuczaty S, Clusmann H, Elger CE, Helmstaedter C. Neuropsychological results in pediatric patients with epilepsy surgery in the parietal cortex. Epilepsia. 2008;49(4):700–4.
59. Lee YJ, Kang HC, Bae SJ, Kim HD, Kim JT, Lee BI, et al. Comparison of temporal lobectomies of children and adults with intractable temporal lobe epilepsy. Childs Nerv Syst. 2010;26(2):177–83.
60. Skirrow C, Cross JH, Cormack F, Harkness W, Vargha-Khadem F, Baldeweg T. Long-term intellectual outcome after temporal lobe surgery in childhood. Neurology. 2011;76(15):1330–7.
61. Vadera S, Kshettry VR, Klaas P, Bingaman W. Seizure-free and neuropsychological outcomes after temporal lobectomy with amygdalohippocampectomy in pediatric patients with hippocampal sclerosis. J Neurosurg Pediatr. 2012;10(2):103–7.
62. Lopez-Gonzalez MA, Gonzalez-Martinez JA, Jehi L, Kotagal P, Warbel A, Bingaman W. Epilepsy surgery of the temporal lobe in pediatric population: a retrospective analysis. Neurosurgery. 2012;70(3):684–92.
63. Maton B, Jayakar P, Resnick T, Morrison G, Ragheb J, Duchowny M. Surgery for medically intractable temporal lobe epilepsy during early life. Epilepsia. 2008;49(1):80–7.
64. Smyth MD, Limbrick Jr DD, Ojemann JG, Zempel J, Robinson S, O'Brien DF, et al. Outcome following surgery for temporal lobe epilepsy with hippocampal involvement in preadolescent children: emphasis on mesial temporal sclerosis. J Neurosurg. 2007;106(3 Suppl):205–10.

65. Mittal S, Montes JL, Farmer JP, Rosenblatt B, Dubeau F, Andermann F, et al. Long-term outcome after surgical treatment of temporal lobe epilepsy in children. J Neurosurg. 2005;103(5 Suppl):401–12.
66. Brockhaus A, Elger CE. Complex partial seizures of temporal lobe origin in children of different age groups. Epilepsia. 1995;36(12):1173–81.
67. Cukiert A, Cukiert CM, Burattini JA, Lima AM, Forster CR, Baise C, et al. A prospective long-term study on the outcome after vagus nerve stimulation at maximally tolerated current intensity in a cohort of children with refractory secondary generalized epilepsy. Neuromodulation. 2013;16(6):551–6; discussion 556.
68. Lancman G, Virk M, Shao H, Mazumdar M, Greenfield JP, Weinstein S, et al. Vagus nerve stimulation vs. corpus callosotomy in the treatment of Lennox-Gastaut syndrome: a meta-analysis. Seizure. 2013;22(1):3–8.
69. Stigsdotter-Broman L, Olsson I, Flink R, Rydenhag B, Malmgren K. Long-term follow-up after callosotomy–a prospective, population based, observational study. Epilepsia. 2014;55(2):316–21.
70. Tanriverdi T, Olivier A, Poulin N, Andermann F, Dubeau F. Long-term seizure outcome after corpus callosotomy: a retrospective analysis of 95 patients. J Neurosurg. 2009;110(2):332–42.
71. Sunaga S, Shimizu H, Sugano H. Long-term follow-up of seizure outcomes after corpus callosotomy. Seizure. 2009;18(2):124–8.
72. Kwan P, Schachter SC, Brodie MJ. Drug-resistant epilepsy. N Engl J Med. 2011;365(10):919–26.
73. Kim SK, Wang KC, Hwang YS, Kim KJ, Chae JH, Kim IO, et al. Epilepsy surgery in children: outcomes and complications. J Neurosurg Pediatr. 2008;1(4):277–83.
74. Boshuisen K, Arzimanoglou A, Cross JH, Uiterwaal CSPM, Polster T, van Nieuwenhuizen O, Braun KPJ, 'TimeToStop' study group. Timing of AED withdrawal does not influence long-term seizure outcome after paediatric epilepsy surgery. The 'TimeToStop' study. Lancet Neurol. 2012;11(9):784–91.

Chapter 5
Long-Term Cognitive Outcomes After Epilepsy Surgery in Adults

Sallie Baxendale

Abstract The literature on the long-term (>5 years) changes in cognitive function in people who undergo epilepsy surgery is small and currently limited to series who have undergone temporal lobe resections. This reflects both pragmatic and cultural factors. Longitudinal studies suggest that the majority of epilepsy surgery candidates have stable memory functions at assessments conducted more than 5 years after surgery, with scores comparable to those they obtained 12–24 months after the operation. There is a subset of patients in whom ongoing seizures are associated with progressive memory impairment. These individual patterns of change are obscured in group analyses. Left temporal lobe resections are consistently identified as a risk factor for progressive deterioration in verbal memory decline, particularly in those with good preoperative function. However, "floor effects" on the standardized tests used to assess cognitive function, evident prior to surgery or soon afterwards, may mask long-term deterioration in a considerably larger proportion of these patients than the literature currently suggests. Some improvements in verbal memory function have been reported at long-term follow-up in patients who have undergone right temporal lobe resections. More research is urgently needed to identify those most at risk of long-term deterioration in memory function following a temporal lobe resection and to examine the long-term trajectories of cognitive function following extratemporal surgeries.

Keywords Memory • Temporal lobe epilepsy • Reliable change indices • Prediction • Long-term outcome • Cognitive function • Neuropsychological tests

---

Conflicts of Interest The author has no conflicts of interest to declare.

S. Baxendale, PhD, C.Psychol, AFBPsS
Department of Clinical and Experimental Epilepsy, National Hospital for Neurology and Neurosurgery, London, UK
e-mail: s.baxendale@ucl.ac.uk

K. Malmgren et al. (eds.), *Long-Term Outcomes of Epilepsy Surgery in Adults and Children*, DOI 10.1007/978-3-319-17783-0_5

Introduction

Although cognitive change is second only to seizure control with respect to the outcome literature in epilepsy surgery, long-term follow-up studies of cognitive outcome are scarce. A PubMed search using the terms "Epilepsy Surgery" and "Outcome" and "Cognitive" or "Memory" conducted in December 2014 returned a list of over 350 studies of potential interest. Of these, less than 3 % utilized a follow-up period of 5 years or more. Over 75 % of the studies of neuropsychological change following epilepsy surgery report results from assessments that have been conducted within 12 months of the surgery, with many reporting test results from assessments conducted within 6 months of the operation.

The prevalence of short-term follow-up studies reflects a number of pragmatic and cultural factors. Epilepsy surgery is a specialist procedure and surgical candidates may travel many miles for treatment at a national specialist center. While patients may be followed up by the surgical team for a year after surgery, they may revert to their local services for ongoing care after that, particularly if they are seizure free, and subsequently be lost to research follow-up. In some parts of the world, postoperative neuropsychological assessments may be seen as primarily a research tool, rather than a clinical requirement. The procedure is not always covered in countries that rely on medical insurance for health provision. This may explain, at least in part, the relative lack of long-term studies from North America, given the significant contribution that surgical series from the region have made to the neuropsychological outcome literature as a whole. It is also the case that neuropsychological follow-up studies are often the subject of PhD thesis; research projects that are typically completed over a 3-year time frame.

This chapter reviews the literature on long-term neuropsychological outcomes following epilepsy surgery. Long-term was defined as a 5-year follow-up or longer.

Search and Eligibility Criteria

To be included in this review, studies had to fulfil the criteria presented in Table 5.1.

Although some neuropsychological outcomes have been reported within more comprehensive reports of long-term surgical outcome, details tend to be limited and the specific follow-up periods for the postoperative neuropsychological assessments are not always clear or are based on earlier postoperative assessments [1–4]. These reports were not therefore included in the final review.

Table 5.1 Inclusion criteria for the review

1. Published in a peer review journal
Anecdotal or descriptive reports of neuropsychological function, published in book chapters were excluded
2. Include adult participants
Studies with mixed pediatric and adult samples whose outcomes could not be distinguished from each other were excluded, due to the difficulties in comparing adult neuropsychological outcomes to those in children where a developmental perspective is critical in the interpretation of changes in neuropsychological test scores
3. Have a follow-up period of at least 5 years
A number of studies have reported the results of patients who have been followed up over a mixed time frame (e.g., from 1 year to 20 years). These studies were included wherever meaningful data about the long-term follow-up could be extracted from the report. However, they were excluded where it was not possible to determine from the report when the neuropsychological follow-up had been conducted
4. Report standardized neuropsychological test results
Studies that reported qualitative neuropsychological outcomes such as parental ratings of intelligence were excluded
5. Reports on all types of elective epilepsy surgery were eligible for inclusion

Results

Seven studies met our eligibility criteria [5–11]. The results are summarized in the chapter Appendix. Excluding multiple reports from the same center, the long-term neuropsychological data on adults from just five different epilepsy surgery series have been reported to date, with data reported on a total of only 400 patients worldwide. Four of these series are from Europe (Germany [10], the Netherlands [5], Sweden [6, 7, 9], and the UK [8]) and one is from the USA [11]. All of the participants in these long-term outcome studies had undergone temporal lobe surgery. Althausen et al. [12] have recently reported long-term outcomes, including cognitive changes, in patients who underwent hemispherectomy, but the cognitive outcomes were based on data from a postal questionnaire rather than neuropsychological tests and so the study did not fulfil the inclusion criteria for this review.

Study Designs

It is inevitable that some patients will be lost to follow-up in longitudinal studies. However a number of these series are limited by systematic bias in the sample studied. Long-term neuropsychological follow-up was only a routine part of the postoperative follow-up in one surgical series (the Swedish studies). In the German study, patients were offered financial compensation to return for a follow-up neuropsychological assessment and comprised 70 % of the surgical series [10], while in the UK study, only 25 % of eligible postoperative candidates underwent a repeat neuropsychological assessment 5 years or more after their operation [8]. These participants were patients who remained under the care of the specialist hospital in London, a national center for epilepsy surgery, and therefore were more likely to have ongoing seizures than those who had been discharged back to their local neurology services. Only two of the studies used medically treated epilepsy controls [10, 11] and only the Swedish series employed a healthy control group [6, 7, 9].

Two long-term series, those from the Netherlands [5] and Sweden [6, 7, 9] report longitudinal data with neuropsychological assessments conducted at specified time intervals following surgery. In these series, the long-term outcome was assessed at 6 years and 10 years respectively. In the other series, the long-term assessments were conducted at different time points for the candidates with the greatest range being between 5 and 17 years following the surgery [8]. Combining data from a wide range of follow-up points since surgery into a single measure of "long-term follow-up" may obscure patterns in the trajectory of change over time.

All of the studies reported data from patients who had undergone both right and left temporal lobe resections. In the Swedish studies, the patients were dichotomized by language dominance rather than a right vs. left distinction, that is, dominant vs. non -dominant resection. In all but one of the studies, the surgical candidates had undergone a standard temporal lobe resection. The outcome data in the Dutch series is based upon a series of patients who underwent a selective amygdalohippocampectomy [5].

The majority of studies reported changes at a group level, that is, type of surgery by time of assessment. The German, UK, and Swedish studies also reported data using reliable change indices for individual patients.

Long-Term Neuropsychological Outcomes

The majority of patients in these series had stable memory function at the long-term follow-up assessment, although as Baxendale et al. [8] report, many were functioning below the 15th percentile on the test norms preoperatively with little capacity for further decline, particularly when defined by rigorous reliable change criteria.

There are conflicting findings regarding the relationship between progressive memory decline and continuing seizures in the long-term outcome literature. Generally, studies that have employed group level analyses have failed to find a significant relationship [5, 6] while those that have looked at individual trajectories suggest that ongoing seizures after surgery are associated with a progressive deterioration in memory skills [8, 10]. These findings suggest that there is a subset of surgical patients in whom ongoing seizures are associated with progressive memory impairments. These patterns are obscured in group analyses. Surgery on the left or language dominant side is consistently identified across the long-term outcome studies as a risk factor for progressive deterioration in verbal memory decline, particularly in those with ongoing seizures following surgery and good preoperative function. When compared to a medically treated control group, surgery appears to accelerate memory decline and exceeds it when performed on the left, or if seizures continue postoperatively [10].

Some improvements in verbal memory function have been reported at long-term follow-up in patients who have undergone right or non-dominant temporal lobe resections [7, 10] although Alpherts et al. [5] suggest that these improvements may not always be sustained in the long-term. Practice effects are rarely considered or adequately controlled for in longitudinal studies. Even when reliable change indices are employed to determine change over time, they are rarely based on the same time intervals as those used in the longitudinal study.

The long-term data suggests that the memory functions of most patients who undergo temporal lobe surgery for epilepsy, stabilize within the first few years after the operation and that they subsequently follow normal age-related decline gradients [13]. The extent of the stepwise postoperative decline, and its subsequent acceleration, will determine when the patient will eventually develop clinically significant memory deficits. (See Fig. 5.1.) The majority of patients who have been studied to date had surgery in their late twenties or early thirties. Even at their long-term follow-up they have a mean age (across the studies) in their forties. Normal age-related cognitive declines are noticed in healthy individuals toward the end of the fifth decade and accelerate thereon [14]. The effects of this normal age-related

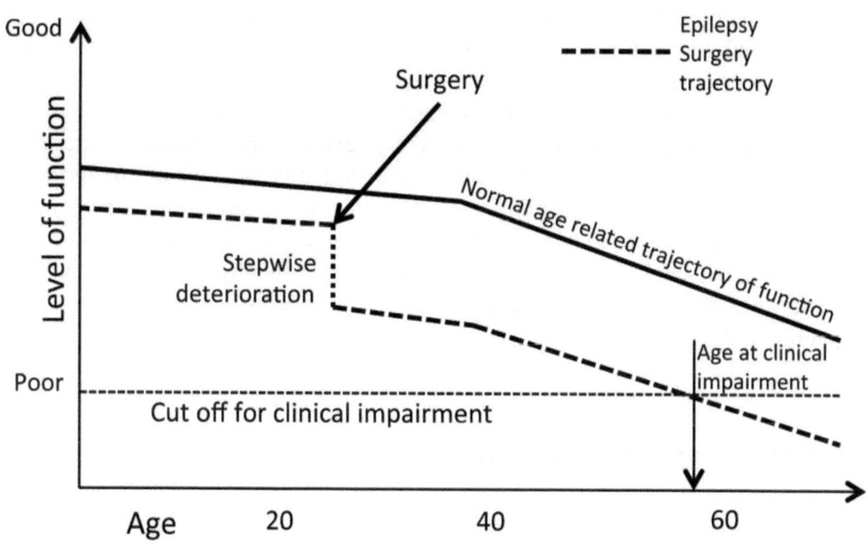

Fig. 5.1 Schematic of postoperative changes in memory function following surgery. Patients with temporal lobe epilepsy follow the same trajectories of age related decline in memory function but start from a lower level of function. Surgery precipitates a stepwise decline in function. Age related deterioration may continue at a similar rate to that in the healthy aging brain but the cut-off for clinical impairment is reached at an earlier age (See Elger et al. [13])

deterioration in function in the latter life of postoperative patients remain a critical unknown. Indeed, little is known about the trajectories of cognitive function in people with longstanding epilepsy in their seventh decade and beyond.

Limitations of the Literature

Many surgical candidates already function below the second percentile on standardized memory tests prior to surgery [8]. Postoperative deteriorations in memory function in either the short- or longer term will not be detected in group studies or in studies that utilize reliable change indices to measure individual change, as these patients are already functioning at, or very close to, the floor of standardized tests. It is therefore likely that outcome studies have underestimated the true extent of postoperative memory deterioration. There is a need to develop new measures that are sensitive to change in this group; these may well rely on more behaviorally based indices of function.

We know that postoperative memory capacity is a function of the integrity of the structures removed during surgery against the reserve of those left in situ [15]. A number of studies have utilized biomarkers to quantify this reserve and capacity in multivariate models to predict postoperative memory function [16–23]. These have yet to be employed in long-term outcome studies, which will also need to incorporate postoperative factors that indicate the likely focus of the postoperative seizures. The focus of postoperative seizures is likely to be a critical factor in determining postoperative memory patterns. Postoperative seizures with contralateral involvement may be associated with a progressive decline in memory function, whereas those with a residual focus in the operated hemisphere may experience less deterioration.

Despite over half a century of successful epilepsy surgery, knowledge of the long-term neuropsychological consequences of extra temporal resections remains limited to clinical experience. The long-term data that is available has focused primarily on memory and intellectual functions following temporal lobe surgery, very little is known about the long-term impact of the surgery on language and executive functions. The special considerations that have been highlighted in the outcome literature for those with a low IQ [24–26] or older patients [27, 28] have yet to be explored in the long-term cognitive literature.

Guidelines for Future Research

Generating large samples in longitudinal follow-up studies is challenging. Presurgical neuropsychological protocols may change over time, together with the clinical characteristics of patients who are offered surgery. Cumulative numbers of patients become lost to follow-up over time. These are not usually random losses. Patients who do well postoperatively, that is, those who become seizure free, and who eventually cease medication following surgery are less likely to keep in contact

Table 5.2 Ideal requirements for long-term cognitive outcome studies

1. Follow- up
(a) Fixed intervals after surgery
(b) Within specific time bands (eg 5–10 years; 10–15 years; 15–20 years)
(c) Mixed follow-up intervals after a specific time point (eg. >5 years)
(d) Mixed follow-up including patients assessed <1 year after surgery
2. Participants
(a) Whole population follow-up
(b) Random sample
(c) Biased sample
(d) Self-selected group (clinical referrals)
3. Neuropsychological measures
(a) Standardized tests, alternative versions at each assessment, measures that are sensitive to change and avoid floor effects
(b) Standardized clinical tests/z scores
(c) Qualitative measures (interview, questionnaire, unstandardized behavioral measures)
4. Analyses
(a) Must take into account capacity to decline, must include analyses of change at an individual level, must include widest possible range of predictors (neurophysiology, neuroimaging, pre and postoperative clinical history, psychiatric comorbidities)
(b) Group level analyses
5. Discussion
(a) Results should be set in the context of the wider outcome literature (<5 year follow-up)

(a) Gold standard
(b) Some useful information
(c) Use with caution, may limit the conclusions that can be drawn from the data
(d) May introduce significant confounds

with specialist epilepsy services and may be more likely to be lost to follow-up than patients who continue to experience seizures.

In order to ensure that surgical candidates are able to make as informed a choice as possible with respect to epilepsy surgery, we need to provide a longitudinal perspective on cognitive change. At present the evidence base for this advice is thin and limited to temporal lobe resections. In order to make a clinically meaningful contribution to the long-term literature, future studies should meet a number of minimum requirements. These are outlined in Table 5.2.

Conclusions

The literature on the long-term cognitive functions of patients who undergo epilepsy surgery is small and limited to series who have undergone temporal lobe resections. This reflects pragmatic and cultural factors. Longitudinal studies suggest that the majority of patients have stable memory function at the long-term follow-up assessment, with scores comparable to those they obtained 12–14 months after surgery. There is a subset of surgical patients in whom ongoing seizures are associated with progressive memory impairments. These patterns are obscured in group analyses. Surgery on the left or language dominant side is consistently identified as a risk factor for progressive deterioration in verbal memory decline, particularly in those with good preoperative function. However “floor effects” on the standardized tests, evident prior to surgery or soon afterwards, may mask long-term deterioration in a considerably larger proportion of these patients. Some improvements in verbal memory function have been reported at long-term follow-up in patients who have undergone right or non-dominant temporal lobe resections. More research is urgently needed to identify those most at risk of long-term deterioration in memory function following a temporal lobe resection and to delineate the long-term trajectories of cognitive function following other surgical procedures.

Appendix. Summary of Study Characteristics and Results from Long-Term Cognitive Outcome Series

Authors	Participants	Follow-up	Neuropsychological Tests	Analyses	Results
Andersson - Roswall et al. (2012) [7] Sweden	$N=51$ 23 DTL 28 NDTL	2 years 10 years	The Claeson–Dahl Learning and Retention Test (CD) – List learning task Cronholm–Molander Memory Test (CM) (word pair associations)	Reliable change indices to determine significant change	Most patients had stable verbal memory postoperatively. Some patients showed partial recovery, especially in the NDTL group. Fewer patients had reliable declines at 10 years than at 2 years. The only risk factor for decline both short- and long-term was DTL resection
Baxendale et al. (2012) [8] UK	$N=70$ 33 LTL 37 RTL	3 months 1 year >5 years (mean 9.1 years; range 5–17 years)	Wechsler Adult Intelligence Scales Adult Memory & Information Processing Battery Verbal Learning Visual Learning	Group changes over time Reliable change indices to determine significant change	The majority of patients had stable memory function across the assessments. However, many were functioning below the 15th percentile on the test norms preoperatively with little capacity for further decline. Progressive decline in cognitive function was associated with poor postoperative seizure control
Andersson - Roswall et al. (2010) [6] Sweden	$N=51$ 23 DTL 28 NDTL	2 years 10 years	The Claeson–Dahl Learning and Retention Test (CD) List learning task Visual memory task Rey Osterreith Complex Figure Task Cronholm–Molander Memory Test (CM) (word pair associations)	Group analyses	The DTL group had declined in verbal memory at the 10-year follow-up compared to the NDTL group and to the controls. However, this decline was detected already 2 years postoperatively, with no further decline from 2 to 10 years

(continued)

Appendix (continued)

Authors	Participants	Follow-up	Neuropsychological Tests	Analyses	Results
Alpherts et al. (2006) [5] Netherlands	34 LTL 54 RTL (SAH)	6 months 2 years 6 years	Wechsler Adult Intelligence Scales Rey Auditory Verbal Learning Test (Dutch Version)	Group analyses	LTL patients demonstrated a progressive decline in consolidation and acquisition of verbal material for up to 2 years after surgery. This decline is greater in patients with mesial temporal sclerosis. The RTL patients demonstrated an initial gain in both memory acquisition and consolidation, which vanished in the long-term Predictors of postoperative verbal memory performance at 6 years after surgery were side of surgery, preoperative memory score and older age. Memory outcome was not related to postoperative seizure control
Engman et al. (2006) [9] Sweden	$N=25$ 10 DTL 15 NDTL 25 healthy controls	2 years 10 years	Wechsler Adult Intelligence Scales Cronholm–Molander Memory Test (CM) – word pair associations Rey Osterreith Complex Figure Test	Group analyses	At the group level, there was a significant increment across time in IQ, partly due to practice effects. This was not seen in the memory scores. The analysis at the individual level of change from baseline to 2 years suggested a decline in memory scores which returned towards baseline level at the 10-year follow-up. These findings suggest that some deterioration in memory function recorded at the 2-year follow-up may not be stable in the long-term

Rausch et al. (2003) [11] USA	$N=21$ LTL 23 RTL $N=8$ Non surgical, epilepsy controls	1 year >9 year (mean 12.1, range 9.1–19 years)	Wechsler Adult Intelligence Scales Wechsler Memory Scales Paired associate learning Prose recall Visual reproduction	Group analyses	Patients with LTL surgery showed selective early decreases in verbal memory. At the long-term follow-up, further decreases in verbal memory and visual memory scores were seen for all patient groups. Non-memory scores remained stable over time. LTL surgery and initial high scores were predictors of verbal memory decreases seen at the early follow-up. Late memory declines were predicted by higher 1-year scores. LTL surgery was an additional predictor of late verbal memory decline
Helmstaedter et al. (2003) [10] Germany	$N=147$ surgical patients 72 LTL 75 RTL 102 non surgical, epilepsy controls	1 year 2–10 years (median=49 months)	Verbal learning memory test (German version) Figural memory test Letter cancellation task Phonetic word fluency task Vocabulary test	Group analyses Reliable change indices	Fifty percent of the medically treated and 60 % of the surgical patients showed significant memory decline at long-term follow-up with no significant change in non-memory functions. Surgery accelerated the decline seen in the medically treated group and exceeded it when surgery was performed on the left, or if seizures continued postoperatively. Seizure-free surgical patients showed recovery of non-memory functions at 1 year after surgery and of memory functions at long-term follow-up. Multiple regression indicated retest interval, seizure control, and mental reserve capacity as predictors of performance changes

References

1. Bujarski KA, Hirashima F, Roberts DW, Jobst BC, Gilbert KL, Roth RM, et al. Long-term seizure, cognitive, and psychiatric outcome following trans-middle temporal gyrus amygdalohippocampectomy and standard temporal lobectomy. J Neurosurg. 2013;119:16–23.
2. Keogan M, McMackin D, Peng S, Phillips J, Burke T, Murphy S, et al. Temporal neocorticectomy in management of intractable epilepsy: long-term outcome and predictive factors. Epilepsia. 1992;33:852–61.
3. Kirkpatrick PJ, Honavar M, Janota I, Polkey CE. Control of temporal lobe epilepsy following en bloc resection of low-grade tumors. J Neurosurg. 1993;78:19–25.
4. Paglioli E, Palmini A, Portuguez M, Paglioli E, Azambuja N, da Costa JC, et al. Seizure and memory outcome following temporal lobe surgery: selective compared with nonselective approaches for hippocampal sclerosis. J Neurosurg. 2006;104:70–8.
5. Alpherts WC, Vermeulen J, van Rijen PC, da Silva FH, van Veelen CW. Verbal memory decline after temporal epilepsy surgery?: A 6-year multiple assessments follow-up study. Neurology. 2006;67:626–31.
6. Andersson-Roswall L, Engman E, Samuelsson H, Malmgren K. Cognitive outcome 10 years after temporal lobe epilepsy surgery: a prospective controlled study. Neurology. 2010;74:1977–85.
7. Andersson-Roswall L, Malmgren K, Engman E, Samuelsson H. Verbal memory decline is less frequent at 10 years than at 2 years after temporal lobe surgery for epilepsy. Epilepsy Behav. 2012;24:462–7.
8. Baxendale S, Thompson PJ, Duncan JS. Neuropsychological function in patients who have had epilepsy surgery: a long-term follow-up. Epilepsy Behav. 2012;23:24–9.
9. Engman E, Andersson-Roswall L, Samuelsson H, Malmgren K. Serial cognitive change patterns across time after temporal lobe resection for epilepsy. Epilepsy Behav. 2006;8:765–72.
10. Helmstaedter C, Kurthen M, Lux S, Reuber M, Elger CE. Chronic epilepsy and cognition: a longitudinal study in temporal lobe epilepsy. Ann Neurol. 2003;54:425–32.
11. Rausch R, Kraemer S, Pietras CJ, Le M, Vickrey BG, Passaro EA. Early and late cognitive changes following temporal lobe surgery for epilepsy. Neurology. 2003;60:951–9.
12. Althausen A, Gleissner U, Hoppe C, Sassen R, Buddewig S, von Lehe M, et al. Long-term outcome of hemispheric surgery at different ages in 61 epilepsy patients. J Neurol Neurosurg Psychiatry. 2013;84:529–36.
13. Elger CE, Helmstaedter C, Kurthen M. Chronic epilepsy and cognition. Lancet Neurol. 2004;3:663–72.
14. Baxendale S. IQ and ability across the adult life span. Appl Neuropsychol. 2011;18:164–7.
15. Chelune GJ. Hippocampal adequacy versus functional reserve: predicting memory functions following temporal lobectomy. Arch Clin Neuropsychol. 1995;10:413–32.
16. Baxendale S, Thompson P, Harkness W, Duncan J. Predicting memory decline following epilepsy surgery: a multivariate approach. Epilepsia. 2006;47:1887–94.
17. Binder JR, Swanson SJ, Sabsevitz DS, Hammeke TA, Raghavan M, Mueller WM. A comparison of two fMRI methods for predicting verbal memory decline after left temporal lobectomy: language lateralization versus hippocampal activation asymmetry. Epilepsia. 2010;51:618–26.
18. Bonelli SB, Powell RH, Yogarajah M, Samson RS, Symms MR, Thompson PJ, et al. Imaging memory in temporal lobe epilepsy: predicting the effects of temporal lobe resection. Brain. 2010;133:1186–99.
19. Busch RM, Dulay MF, Kim KH, Chapin JS, Jehi L, Kalman CC, et al. Pre-surgical mood predicts memory decline after anterior temporal lobe resection for epilepsy. Arch Clin Neuropsychol. 2011;26:739–45.
20. Potter JL, Schefft BK, Beebe DW, Howe SR, Yeh HS, Privitera MD. Presurgical neuropsychological testing predicts cognitive and seizure outcomes after anterior temporal lobectomy. Epilepsy Behav. 2009;16:246–53.

21. Sherman EM, Wiebe S, Fay-McClymont TB, Tellez-Zenteno J, Metcalfe A, Hernandez-Ronquillo L, et al. Neuropsychological outcomes after epilepsy surgery: systematic review and pooled estimates. Epilepsia. 2011;52:857–69.
22. St-Laurent M, McCormick C, Cohn M, Misic B, Giannoylis I, McAndrews MP. Using multivariate data reduction to predict postsurgery memory decline in patients with mesial temporal lobe epilepsy. Epilepsy Behav. 2014;31:220–7.
23. Vulliemoz S, Prilipko O, Herrmann FR, Pollo C, Landis T, Pegna AJ, et al. Can postictal memory predict postoperative memory in patients with temporal lobe epilepsy? Epilepsia. 2012;53:e170–3.
24. Garcia P. Is seizure surgery an option for patients with very low IQ? Epilepsy Curr. 2008;8:150–1.
25. Davies R, Baxendale S, Thompson P, Duncan JS. Epilepsy surgery for people with a low IQ. Seizure. 2009;18:150–2.
26. Malmgren K, Olsson I, Engman E, Flink R, Rydenhag B. Seizure outcome after resective epilepsy surgery in patients with low IQ. Brain. 2008;131:535–42.
27. Bialek F, Rydenhag B, Flink R, Malmgren K. Outcomes after resective epilepsy surgery in patients over 50 years of age in Sweden 1990–2009–a prospective longitudinal study. Seizure. 2014;23:641–5.
28. Chapin JS, Busch RM, Silveira DC, Wehner T, Naugle RI, Ferguson L, et al. Memory performance in older adults before and after temporal lobectomy for pharmacoresistant epilepsy. Clin Neuropsychol. 2013;27:1316–27.

Chapter 6
Long-Term Cognitive Outcomes After Epilepsy Surgery in Children

Torsten Baldeweg and Caroline Skirrow

Abstract Here we examine the evidence for long-term changes in cognitive functions after epilepsy surgery in studies published mostly since 2010. Specifically, we looked for evidence of developmental "catch-up" as indicated by an increase in IQ scores in comparison with preoperative values. About half of the studies report significant increase in IQ scores in the surgical group over time or in comparison with a nonsurgical control group. Better cognitive outcomes are linked to greater overall level of seizure freedom and partially to medication reduction. When taking into account the large variability in sample sizes and seizure freedom between studies, a modest correlation of improved cognitive outcomes with longer follow-up duration can be observed. Further research is urgently needed which relates preoperative cognitive changes with postoperative development and identifies clinical and educational factors which facilitate cognitive outcomes after epilepsy surgery in children.

Keywords Cognition • Intelligence • Memory • Children • Epilepsy • Epilepsy surgery • Temporal lobe surgery • Hemispherectomy

T. Baldeweg, MD (✉) • C. Skirrow, PhD
Cognitive Neuroscience and Neuropsychiatry Section, Developmental Neurosciences Division, Institute of Child Health, University College London, London, UK

Great Ormond Street Hospital NHS Trust, London, UK
e-mail: t.baldeweg@ucl.ac.uk

K. Malmgren et al. (eds.), *Long-Term Outcomes of Epilepsy Surgery in Adults and Children*, DOI 10.1007/978-3-319-17783-0_6

Introduction

Surgical intervention may be offered as a treatment for children with epilepsy in whom seizures cannot effectively be controlled by medication. Neuropsychological function in these children is an area of significant concern, since cognitive impairment is frequently associated with childhood-onset epilepsy [1–3] and mounting evidence implicates continuing seizures in progressive deterioration of cognitive, academic, and adaptive skills [4–6]. However, the possible positive impact of relief from seizures must be weighed up against potential risks to cognitive function posed by resective brain surgery.

In children, in whom developmental changes are rapid and ongoing, long-term follow-up studies are required to assess the balance of risks and benefits of epilepsy surgery. Postsurgical cognitive development is subject to a multitude of intervening factors, such as potential seizure recurrence, fluctuating antiepileptic drug (AED) use, and importantly: different educational challenges, transition to adulthood, and independent living. These factors interact with continuing brain development and plasticity.

However, assessing cognitive change in children with epilepsy comes with specific challenges. Measures of intellectual function (IQ) are typically normed in relation to a healthy peer group, and to maintain IQ levels, a child must continuously acquire new skills and information over time. However, children with epilepsy may not acquire skills as rapidly or to the same level as healthy peers, as shown for IQ [7] and memory [8]. Moreover, while in adults, a decline in IQ mostly indicates a loss of skills, this is not the case for children (see Ref. [9] for a detailed discussion), where this may reflect either loss of skills, plateauing of skills (thereby failing to keep up with peers), or even developmental progress (increased skills but not in line with their peer group). In contrast, unchanged IQ scores post-surgery may indicate continuation of a child's previous trajectory or even an end to seizure-related cognitive decline and resumption of normal development.

In this context, Smith and colleagues [10] describe three categories of potential change in cognitive function after epilepsy surgery, which can be summarized as the following: (1) *no developmental change*: surgery has no impact and the child progresses at the same developmental rate as before; (2) *developmental slowing:* preoperative cognitive functions decline with seizures and surgery halts cognitive loss but the child nevertheless develops more slowly than healthy peers; and (3) *surgery-related cognitive impairment:* cognitive decline due to the removal of functionally intact brain tissue. Two further possibilities can be added in the context of long-term follow-up after surgery: (4) *"catch-up" development:* surgery-related seizure reduction enables accelerated brain maturation leading to cognitive improvement; and (5) *growing into a deficit:* cognitive deficits emerge over time, in the context of diminishing potential for brain plasticity, and late emerging skills and functions as children progress into adulthood [11].

In this chapter, we summarize recent evidence of cognitive outcome after epilepsy surgery. We aim to clarify patterns of postsurgical outcome at extended follow-up, and determine the consistency of evidence associating seizure freedom and AED withdrawal with improved cognition. We focus on change in intellectual/developmental function and memory function, which are most frequently reported. We start with the historical context of this research, followed by the main conclusions and issues highlighted in recent review articles of short-term postsurgical outcome, and then we conduct a review of the literature with an emphasis on identifying original research on long-term outcomes after surgical intervention (≥4 years post-surgery). Data from this research is then analyzed to evaluate if longer postsurgical follow-up times are associated with greater *"catch-up" development*. Our hypothesis is based on the consideration that a major alteration of developmental trajectory would require a considerable period of time and educational input, and has been supported by evidence from our own long-term follow-up study [12].

Historical Context and Overview of Research to Date

In 1890, Victor Horsley gave a detailed account of his experience of performing pioneering neurosurgery on patients with focal epilepsy. He observed (Ref. [13], p. 1291) an "immediate and progressive improvement in the mental condition." He further suggested that "a final answer can be given on the permanency of the freedom from epilepsy until each case has been observed for about five years, but if the attacks are only mitigated in severity, and not absolutely cured, a notable relief is at once the clearest evidence and the most desirable result."

Davidson and Falconer [14] were the first to document long-term outcomes in a cohort of children who had temporal lobe surgery in London hospitals, with follow-up periods of up to 25 years. Positive adaptations into adult life were reported in many patients, but no supporting neuropsychological evidence was presented. Similarly, Lindsay and colleagues [15] provided careful long-term observations from the Park Hospital for Children in Oxford. They noted (p. 584) that "of those who were tested (using neuropsychological assessments), none has demonstrated a significant fall in intelligence; indeed, in a small number we found a steady rise in IQ scores over five or six years. Our experience thereby accords with that of Sir Victor Horsley in 1890."

Subsequent studies, usually with much shorter follow-up periods, have been less conclusive in support of early observations of postsurgical cognitive improvement. The short- to intermediate-term cognitive outcomes (1–2 years) after epilepsy surgery are well documented and have been reviewed extensively [10, 16–18]. More general clinical outcomes in the context of surgery in adults and children, including cognition and behavior have also been previously discussed [19–22]. Here we summarize the three main points highlighted in previous reviews:

1. Is epilepsy a progressive cognitive disease? Lah [17] concluded that "intractable seizure disorders that start early in life and require aggressive pharmacological treatment have a cumulative, negative impact on cognitive development of individuals with epilepsy. This may not be the case for less aggressive seizure disorders." This view was confirmed by van Schooneveld and Braun [18] reviewing the evidence that presurgical cognitive function is determined by age at onset, underlying epileptogenic etiology, duration of epilepsy, presence of epileptic spasms, the number of AED trials, gender, and the development of an epileptic encephalopathy. The authors stressed that since postoperative outcome is closely correlated with preoperative levels, these variables may all determine postoperative functioning.
2. What is the short-term outcome after surgery? Most reviews conclude that there is very little change in intellectual functions at the group level. At an individual level, different patterns of cognitive change after surgery have been observed, which include the patterns of cognitive change outlined above (*no developmental change, developmental slowing, surgery related cognitive impairment,* and *"catch-up" development*). Seizure freedom and completeness of resection appear to benefit cognitive development most consistently [17, 18]. Very few studies have reported on outcomes after more than 4 years and the existing evidence is contradictory.
3. What are the primary methodological limitations? Most previous studies are subject to the common shortcomings of observational studies [23], such as retrospective designs (case note reviews), use of referral populations, small samples size, differing follow-up durations within samples, and wide inclusion criteria (i.e., samples with mixed etiologies). In addition, Smith et al. [10] requested that future studies report on risk-associated and protective factors, include a nonsurgical epilepsy control group, and report on longer follow-up periods.

Literature Review

This chapter focuses on studies that report cognitive outcome after childhood epilepsy surgery with a longer follow-up period nearing or beyond 4 years. We conducted a PubMed search with the terms of "epilepsy surgery in children" and "cognitive outcome" (including memory and intelligence, language or attention) supplemented by references from previous reviews. Studies of outcome in cognitive faculties other than memory and intelligence were few and even fewer long-term outcome studies were available. These other outcomes will therefore not be discussed here. Only studies of surgery in childhood (i.e., <18 years) with at least ten participants and which incorporated both pre- and postsurgical cognitive data (allowing the evaluation of postsurgical cognitive change) are reviewed, see Appendix.

Intellectual/Developmental Outcome

For intellectual/developmental outcome, we report on composite measures of cognitive function (full-scale intelligence quotient [FSIQ], or where this was unavailable verbal IQ [VIQ], or performance IQ [PIQ], as in previous work [18], or developmental quotient [DQ]). In Appendix, we present: (1) long-term studies with a mean follow-up nearing or beyond 4 years and (2) studies with shorter follow-up durations published since 2010, most of which have not been included in previous reviews (see above).

We identified a total of 31 studies fulfilling the above criteria. These studies contained a total of 1,119 patients (mean 37 per study). Twelve studies reported on long-term outcomes after epilepsy surgery. These studies contained a total of 312 patients (mean 27 patients per study). Mean follow-up ranged from 3.9 years to 10 years (average 6.1). Half of the studies investigated specific surgical targets such as anterior temporal lobe resections ($n=3$) or hemispherectomy ($n=3$). The remainder contained a mixture of surgical targets (including focal, multilobar, and hemispheric resections, $n=6$). Age at surgery was either early (<7 years, $n=6$), later (>7 years, $n=1$) or included a wide range of surgical ages ($n=5$). Not surprisingly, most of the focal surgery studies were in the older age group and conversely, more mixed surgery, and hemispherectomy cohorts had early surgery, reflecting the pathology mix of patients who present with severe epilepsy at different ages.

In addition, we identified 19 studies published since 2010 fulfilling the above criteria; except that they reported intellectual or developmental outcomes after a shorter interval post-epilepsy surgery (<3.9 years). These short-term outcome studies contained a total of 798 participants (mean 42 participants per study). Follow-up ranged from 1 year to 3.5 years (mean 1.8 years). These studies again contained cohorts with mixed ($n=9$) and specific surgical targets ($n=6$), and there was a greater focus on exploring outcomes after specific pathological diagnoses (total $n=4$, e.g., hypothalamic hamartoma $n=1$, dysembryoplastic neuroepithelial tumors (DNT) $n=1$, glioneuronal tumors $n=1$, tuberous sclerosis $n=1$). Mean age at surgery was later (>7 years) in all studies with the exception of Ref. [24], which focused on surgery in infancy and Ref. [25] which focused on outcomes after hemispherectomy only.

Intellectual/Developmental Outcome: Analysis of Published Studies

Pre- to Postoperative IQ/DQ Changes: Individual Data

First, we analyzed the association of follow-up period with respect to the proportion of patients with reported changes in their cognitive status. Definitions of individual change differed between studies (see Appendix, and Ref. [18] for common definitions). Data was therefore analyzed within all studies, and repeated in a subset of studies with a high IQ change cut-off: reporting individual changes of IQ with minimum increase or decrease of ten IQ points.

Individual change data was reported in 21 studies, across which 30 % of patients improved, 12 % deteriorated, and 58 % showed no significant change in IQ/DQ scores. More homogenous data was provided in 15 studies with a high IQ change threshold (≥10 IQ/DQ points). These provided more modest indices of IQ change (21 % improved, 14 % deteriorated). Postsurgical AED cessation was linked to rates of increase in IQ/DQ in all studies at a trend level ($r=.48$, $p=.09$), remaining so for the more homogeneous studies ($r=.53$, $p=.09$). A notable association was that across 14 studies in the homogeneous subsample, the reported percentage of seizure freedom correlated with increasing proportion of patients who improved cognitively ($r=.64$, $p=.01$).

Because the number of participants in each study varied widely (from 10 to 206), we also calculated indices of change weighted by sample size (by multiplying change rates [or group-level change] by participant numbers). Analysis using these weighted change indices confirmed correlations of increased IQ with AED withdrawal and seizure freedom. When examining the influence of follow-up duration after controlling for differences in seizure freedom between studies, we observed a positive correlation with percentage of participants who improved at follow-up ($r=.55$, $p=.009$). Equally, the relative proportion of patients who improved compared to those who declined positively correlated with longer follow-up duration ($r=.60$, $p=.007$).

Overall it appeared that greater improvements were seen in cohorts with focal resections or mixed surgical targets (including focal resections, hemispherectomy, and palliative surgeries) than in cohorts with hemispherectomy only. A greater proportion of patients from studies of focal resections and mixed surgical targets experienced increased IQ/DQ, and fewer losses were seen postsurgically compared with hemispherectomy-only studies (focal resection, $n=7$: increase 31 %, decline 9 %; mixed surgery, $n=8$: increase 37 %, decline 11 %; hemispherectomy, $n=6$: increase 15 %, decline 15 %). However, these differences were nonsignificant.

Pre- to Postoperative IQ/DQ Change: Group-Level Comparisons

Subsequently, we report on studies, which statistically tested at group level for changes in IQ/DQ across the follow-up period in the surgical sample or between surgical and nonsurgical patients. Among the 17 studies where a statistical comparison of IQ/DQ longitudinally within the surgical group was performed, six studies reported a significant change (all increases in IQ/DQ scores) in the surgical group, while 11 failed to do so. We tested if there were any systematic differences in basic study characteristics (number of patients, age at surgery, percentage seizure freedom, percentage of AED) between those studies, but failed to detect any. Across all studies reporting change in IQ over follow-up ($n=25$), there was a mean increase of 2.1 IQ/DQ points per participant. Studies with long-term follow-up were not more likely to find positive IQ change, which was noted only in two out of five studies. However, in line with the observed relationship with individual change in IQ noted above, duration of follow-up was also correlated with the weighted mean change in IQ scores ($r = .41$, $p = .028$).

Pre- to Postoperative IQ/DQ Change in Relation to Seizure Freedom

Among the eight studies which tested the effect of seizure freedom on cognition, four reported significant IQ improvements in seizure free surgical patients, while four failed to do so. Furthermore, 9 out of 20 studies reported either an IQ improvement in the surgical group or reported better outcomes in the seizure-free group compared to those with continuing seizures in the surgical sample. Again, there was no striking difference in terms of study characteristics compared to those studies that did not find such effects. The importance of postoperative seizure freedom for cognitive and adaptive/behavioral outcome was nevertheless demonstrated by a number of recent studies with larger samples sizes [24, 26, 27].

Pre- to Postoperative IQ/DQ Change: Effect of AED Withdrawal

Among the seven studies which formally tested the effect of postoperative AED withdrawal on cognition, only one reported such an effect. Notably, this study [12] reported this effect also in those patients who were seizure free, which removes the potential confound of seizure frequency. Van Eeghen et al. [6] reported a negative correlation between cognitive change and number of AEDs in a small surgical cohort with tuberous sclerosis ($n = 8$).

Memory Outcome After Epilepsy Surgery

Memory outcome within a few years after epilepsy surgery has been consistently evaluated and reviewed [11, 17] and here we report on four studies with a longer follow-up of at least 4 years after surgery [28–31]. In mixed cohorts of temporal and extratemporal surgery, no evidence for memory decrements was reported [29] while improvements were found for vocabulary [29] and verbal learning [30].

Studies which specifically evaluated the impact of temporal lobe surgery noted verbal memory decline shortly after left-sided resections [32, 33, 9]. Nevertheless, this verbal memory loss appears to normalize from about 1 year after surgery [11], supported by follow-up studies at 2 years [34], 4 years [31], and 9 years [28]. The study of Skirrow and colleagues examined two forms of declarative memory (episodic and semantic) function at a minimum of 5 years after surgery. While there were no significant pre-to postoperative memory decrements, there were, in contrast, significant gains in verbal episodic memory after right temporal lobe surgery, and visual episodic memory improved after left temporal lobe surgery. This indicates a functional release in the unoperated temporal lobe from the impact of seizure activity. Furthermore, similar release effects were seen for IQ-derived semantic memory scores in the left temporal surgery group. A detailed MRI-based analysis of extent of neocortical and hippocampal resections revealed that better verbal episodic memory at follow-up was linked to greater postsurgical residual hippocampal volumes, most robustly in left surgical participants. Better semantic memory at follow-up was associated with smaller resections and greater temporal pole integrity after left temporal surgery, in keeping with the role of the anterior temporal lobes in adult semantic memory dysfunction. Results were independent of postsurgical IQ and language lateralization. These findings indicate postsurgical material-specific improvement in memory functions in the intact temporal lobe. However, outcome was linked to the anatomical integrity of the temporal lobe memory system, indicating that compensatory mechanisms are constrained by the amount of tissue which remains in the operated temporal lobe.

Discussion

All reviewed studies agree that the majority of patients do not show significant changes in IQ scores postoperatively, i.e., they remain on a stable developmental trajectory in parallel with normal development (trajectory A in Fig. 6.1, modified after Ref. [18]). Although their preoperative trajectory is generally not reported, one could surmise from published reports [35] and clinical observations that a significant proportion of children who are being considered for neurosurgical treatment do in fact show progressive loss of IQ scores, often in parallel with exacerbation of their seizure disorder (see Fig. 6.1, labeled "epileptic encephalopathy"). In this context, the finding of unchanged IQ can be considered a positive effect of the treatment, as it indicates a normalization of cognitive development. This pattern has been reported in a proportion of children who showed preoperative IQ declines [36]. Clearly, the relationship of pre- and postoperative cognitive trajectories deserves further study.

Only a minority of patients showed a significant drop in IQ or developmental scores, more often in those studies that reported on surgery in younger children. Some authors have commented on those children who experienced a drop in standardized developmental scores (e.g., Ref. [24]) as they nevertheless often do show developmental progress albeit at a slower pace than their healthy peers (see limitations below). On the positive side is that about twice as many patients improved postoperatively than showed cognitive deterioration. Many studies reported a beneficial IQ effect of either surgery or seizure freedom associated with surgery. Nevertheless, the potential benefit of significant seizure reduction has not been sufficiently considered. The impact of AED withdrawal can be demonstrated in some studies but is not universally seen. This is likely due to the coarseness of the AED analysis conducted, e.g., reduction in number of drugs used and the contribution of individual drugs have not been considered. There is nevertheless compelling evidence of AED impacting on cognition [18].

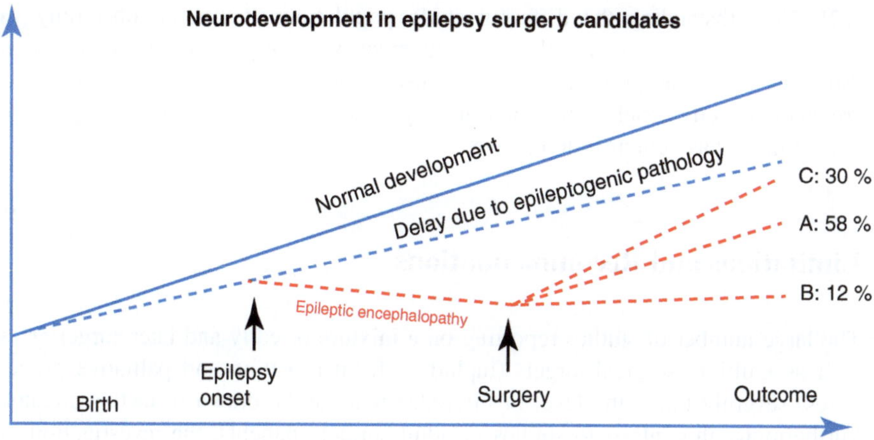

Fig. 6.1 Neurodevelopmental trajectories of epilepsy surgery candidates (Adapted from: van Schooneveld and Braun [18], by indicating proportions of children showing different postoperative cognitive trajectories): *A* stable development in parallel with healthy peers, no change in IQ scores, *B*: IQ decline: can indicate loss of skills or slower pace of development compared with healthy peers. *C*: "catch-up" development at a faster pace than healthy peers, resulting in IQ score increase. The indicated proportions are means derived from Appendix

A direct comparison of studies with long- versus short-term follow-up did not support our prediction of improved outcomes with longer follow-up. Although the expected trends were seen, those did not reach significance, perhaps due to the large variability in study characteristics. When taking into account the variability in participant numbers by computing weighted indices, modest support for this association was indeed observed, in particularly when statistically controlling for the large differences in reported seizure freedom between studies (from 35 to 100 %).

A key caveat is that the majority of studies did not specify a minimum follow-up time, which meant that most studies had a mixture of very short and very long post-surgical periods, with the inevitably possibility for bias (see limitations below). Two studies included a minimum follow-up period of over 5 years, but came to different conclusions regarding IQ change [12, 30]. The study of Skirrow and colleagues examined outcome in patients who had undergone temporal lobe surgery in childhood after a mean follow-up of 9 years (range 5–15 years). They report improved IQ in the surgical group, a change not observed in a non-surgery epilepsy control group. Greater IQ improvements were found among patients with lower IQs before surgery. Discontinuation of AEDs was a positive predictor of IQ change. An analysis of interim follow-up data points (available in a proportion of patients only) suggested that the IQ increase was only observed after 6 or more years post-surgery. In contrast, a 10-year follow-up of a heterogeneous cohort of 17 patients (including temporal and extratemporal resections, callosotomy, multiple subpial transections) by Viggedal and colleagues [30] did not report any significant group-level changes in IQ, although the absolute degree of change was similar to that of Skirrow et al.

[12]. Notwithstanding the differing study populations (temporal lobectomy vs mixed sample), the cohorts also differed much with respect to seizure freedom (86 % vs 35 %) and proportion of AED discontinuation (57 % vs 18 %). The discrepancy in study conclusions is not incompatible with the impact of those postoperative factors as demonstrated above.

Limitations and Recommendations

The large number of studies reporting on a mixture of early and later surgeries as well as multiple surgical targets (including focal resection and palliative procedures) severely limits the level of inference that can be drawn from this chapter. Furthermore, in contrast to studies of adult surgical patients, the investigation of children is complicated by the fact that epilepsy and surgery interact with rapid brain development. The inclusion of a nonsurgical control group, matched for basic illness characteristics at baseline assessment, would allow one to estimate the developmental trajectory without surgical intervention. In addition, such group is also helpful for estimation of retest effects and changes in test versions with progression into adulthood. Unfortunately, such comparison groups, however imperfect they might be, are rarely included in follow-up studies. In addition, a healthy control group (preferably siblings or otherwise closely matched, see Ref. [37]) would allow an estimation to which degree a restoration of the normal developmental trajectory can be achieved, which has not been reported for surgical samples.

The mode of participant recruitment is seldom clearly stated, and the inclusion of a very wide range of follow-up periods (months to over 10 years) suggests that retrospective chart review is the main source of data points. Neuropsychological assessments are often requested for clinical indication which can bias the sample toward the more severe end of the clinical and neuropsychiatric spectrum [6]. Few studies report on the representativeness of their sample for the wider clinical population seen at each institution. Finally, due to restrictions in sample size, the joint statistical estimation of different etiological and clinical factors such as duration of epilepsy, age at surgery, seizure control, and AED withdrawal is often not possible. Hence the inference made here about the impact of these factors is likely to be biased and limited. One more time we need to repeat the call made previously by Smith et al. [10] that better designed studies are urgently needed.

Nevertheless, the emerging evidence from the recent literature reviewed here and previously [10, 18] suggests that the majority of children show a stabilization of their cognitive trajectory after surgical treatment and that a significant proportion even do show signs of cognitive "catch-up." The degree of improvement appears to be correlated with postoperative seizure control and to some degree with antiepileptic medication reduction. There is suggestive evidence that compensatory processes for memory functions after temporal surgery are completed after 1–2 years, while change in intellectual functions require a more prolonged period of brain development unencumbered by seizure activity and polypharmacy. The impact of clinical factors which are likely to interact with developmental changes in brain plasticity, such as age at surgery and the extent of resection, requires further research.

Appendix. Summary of Study Characteristics and Results from Short- and Long-Term Cognitive Outcome Series in Children [9, 12, 24, 25, 30, 31, 33, 38–61]

Authors (year) [Ref.]	Number of participants (% of total sample)	Mean age, in years (range or sd): Epilepsy onset (range)	Mean age, in years (range or sd): Surgery (range)	Type of surgery	Measure	Individual change: Criteria	Individual change: Decline (%)	Individual change: Increase (%)	Groupwise IQ/DQ change (significance level, if reported)	Seizure free (%)	Postsurgical cognitive follow-up duration, in years (range)
Recent short-term follow-up studies (since 2011) with predominantly focal resections, including mixed surgical groups											
Ramantani et al. (2014) [38]	21	7.9 (0–15)	11.7 (0–15)	5 T, 12 TO, 9 F, 3P (all for glioneuronal tumors)	IQ	10 IQ points*	9.5	33.3	4.4 ($p = 0.052$)	86	1.8 (0–5)
Guan et al. (2014) [39]	16 (80 %)	5.7 (1–17)	8.9 (2–20)	20 H	IQ	–	–	–	6.8 ($p < .001$)	80	1.0 (–)
Meekes et al. (2013) [9]	21 (100 %)	7.3 (0–13)	13.9 (8–18)	21 T	VIQ	–	–	–	3.0 (n.s)	86	2.0 (–)
Lew et al. (2013) [40]	27 (54 %)	2.1 (0–13)	9.1 (0–21)	27 H	IQ	≥1 sd change	18.5	3.5	–2.5 (n.s.)	80	3.5 (0–7)
Oitment et al. (2013) [33]	75	6.0 (sd 4.2)	12.7 (–)	41 T, 13 ET, 21 ML	IQ	–	–	–	–1.2 (–)	56	1.5 (sd 1.0)
Viggedal et al. (2013) [41]	94 (100 %)	4.9 (–)	11 (0–18)	31 T, 20 F, 7 P, 3 O, 12 ML, 10 H, 7 C, 2 Dis, 2 MST	IQ/DQ	–	–	–	–3.0 (median) (–)	50	2.0 (–)
Villarejo-Ortega et al. (2013) [42]	17 (100 %)	5.4 (0–8)	7.6 (1–10)	17 H	IQ/DQ	10 IQ/DQ points	17.6	5.9	–2.6 (n.s)	67	3.1 (1–5)

(continued)

Appendix (continued)

Authors (year) [Ref.]	Number of participants (% of total sample)	Mean age, in years (range or sd)		Type of surgery	Measure	Individual change			Groupwise IQ/DQ change (significance level, if reported)	Seizure free (%)	Postsurgical cognitive follow-up duration, in years (range)
		Epilepsy onset (range)	Surgery (range)			Criteria	Decline (%)	Increase (%)			
Ramantani et al. (2013) [24]	28 (93 %)	0.4 (0–1)	1.7 (0–2)	4 T, 5 ET, 5 ML, 14 H	IQ	Categorical change	25	0	– (–)	70	1.3 (0–2)
Wethe et al. (2013) [43]	12	0.8 (0–5)	12.2 (3–39)	Hypothalamic hamartoma resection	IQ	Reliable change indices	0	42	8.3 (p = .001)	69	2.0 (0–3)
Fay-McClymont et al. (2012) [44]	13 (31 %)	1.4 (0–16)	10.8 (4–16)	3 T, 4 F, 1P (all for DNT)	IQ	Reliable change indices	15.4	15.4	– (–)	92	1.4 (0–2)
Liang et al. (2012) [45]	206 (100 %)	3.6 (–)	11.3 (6–14)	84 T, 75 F, 14 O, 9 P, 24 ML (additional C in 28 cases)	IQ	≥10 % Change of preoperative scores	5.3	40.3	6.9 (–)	72	1.0 (–)
D'Argenzio et al. (2011) [46]	31 (46 %)	–	–	47 F, 13 P, 6 O	VIQ/DQ	15 IQ points	16.1	9.6	–4.4 (n.s)	52	1.6 (0–7)
Chieffo et al. (2011) [47]	24 (100 %)	5.6 (0–14)	7.5 (1–17)	12 F 12 T	IQ/DQ	10 IQ points	20.8	–	– (–)	92	2.1 (1–7)
Datta et al. (2011) [48]	57	– (0–16)	11.7 (3–17)	30 T, 11 F, 7 P, 3 O, 9 ML, 1 C	IQ	–	–	–	0.0 (n.s)	67	– (all ≥1 year)
Garcia-Fernandez et al. (2011) [49]	21	7.14 (sd 4.93)	11.4 (2–19)	13 T, 2 F, 2 PR, 1 O, 1 P, 2 PC	IQ	10 IQ points*	19.1	28.5	3.4 (n.s)	86	1.0 (1–1)

Thomas et al. (2010) [25]	16	3.4 (0–11)	6.6 (0–13)	14 H, 2 Q	IQ	–	–	–	0.2 (n.s.)	94	3.0 (3–3)
Liang et al. (2010a) [50]	25	1.8 (0–13)	14.0 (6–23)	17 resective surgeries, 8 resections + C all for tuberous sclerosis	IQ	–	–	–	5.6 ($p<.01$)[a]	60	2.0 (2–2)
Liang et al. (2010b) [51]	60	3.3 (0–13)	16.7 (6–29)	30 T and 30 T + C	IQ	+4 and −2 IQ points	16.7	60	2.2 (n.s.)	67	2.0 (2–2)
Boshuisen et al. (2010) [52]	34 (79 %)	1.2 (0–11)	4.1 (0–14)	34 H	IQ/DQ	10 IQ points	8.8	26.5	–	77	1.8 (1–2)
Long-term follow-up studies (nearing or beyond 4 years post-surgery)											
Viggedal et al. (2012) [30]	16	(0–13)	12.0 (4–20)	11 T, 1 P, 2 H, 1 C, 1MST	IQ/DQ	10 IQ points	12.5	25	7.0* (–)	35	10 (10–10)
Battaglia et al. (2012) [53]	12	8.7 (5–12)	10.1 (6–16)	5 P, 3 PO, 4 O	IQ	10 IQ points*	0	0	2.0 (n.s*)	67	4.1 (2–9)
Skirrow et al. (2011) [12]	42	4.0 (0–14)	13.3 (4–18)	42 T	IQ	10 IQ points	2	41	7.9 ($p=.05$ at 6 years, $p<.001$ at 8+ years)	86	9.4 (5–15)
Dunkley et al. (2011) [54]	23 (48 %)	Med 0.38 (0–1)	1.7 (0–3)	27 H, 4 ML, 4 F, 3 T, 4 focal (location not further specified)	IQ/DQ	15 IQ/DQ points	21.7	8.7	– (–)	48	5.25 (2–13)
Roulet-Perez et al. (2010) [55]	10 (90 %)	0.9 (0–2)	2.8 (0–4)	3 T, 4 F, 3 Q, 1 H	IQ/DQ	10 IQ points*	10	50	13.6 (–)	100	4.9

(continued)

Appendix (continued)

Authors (year) [Ref.]	Number of participants (% of total sample)	Mean age, in years (range or sd)		Type of surgery	Measure	Individual change			Groupwise IQ/DQ change (significance level, if reported)	Seizure free (%)	Postsurgical cognitive follow-up duration, in years (range)
		Epilepsy onset (range)	Surgery (range)			Criteria	Decline (%)	Increase (%)			
Lettori et al. (2008) [56]	19 (100 %)	0.2 (0–2)	2.3 (0–5)	19 H	IQ/DQ	10 IQ/DQ points*	10.5	10.5	−2.1 (−)	73	6.5 (2–11)
Bourgeois et al. (2007) [57]	27	2.6 (0–12)	6.1 (0–16)	2 T, 4 O, 3P, 10ML, 8 H for Sturge-Weber syndrome	IQ/DQ	Categorical change	3.7	59	– (–)	70	7.3 (0–17)
Battaglia et al. (2006) [58]	45	0.5 (1–4)	2.3 (0–6)	19 H, 9 ML, 9 T, 4 F, 4 PO,	IQ/DQ	10 IQ/DQ points*	17.8	15.6	−1.3 (n.s)*	71	6.4 (2–14)
Pulsifer et al. (2004) [59]	53 (75 %)	3.6 (0–12)	7.2 (0–20)	53 H	IQ/DQ	15 IQ/DQ points	20.7	15.1	−2.14 (−)	65	5.4 (2.4–37)
Maehara et al. (2002) [60]	14 (100 %)	0.2 (<1 year)	2.4 (0–6)	14 H	DQ	10 DQ points*	7.1	28.6	6.4 (−)	43	3.9 (2–6)
Lewis et al. (1996) [31]	23 (100 %)	4.8 (sd 2.5)	14.5	23 T	IQ	–	–	–	3.5 ($p<0.05$)	74	4.8 (−)
Meyer et al. (1986) [61]	37 (74 %)	7.5 (1–14)	15.8 (7–18)	37 T	IQ	–	–	–	0.2 (n.s.)	75	4.5 (0–10)

Table 1: Short- and long-term outcome studies included in this review.

T – temporal, F- frontal, O – Occipital, P – parietal, TO –temporo-occipital, PO – Parieto-Occipital, FO – frontoparietal, TPO – temporoparietooccipital, ET – extratemporal, PR – perirolandic, PC – pre and post-cingulum, ML – multilobar, H – Hemispherectomy or Hemispherotomy, Q – functional quadrantectomy, C – Callosotomy, Dis – Disconnection, MST Multiple Subpial Transection, Categorical change *Derived from individual scores, n.s. – non-significant, a p-value derived from comparison with epilepsy control group, DNT – dysembryoplastic neuroepithelial tumours

References

1. Berg AT, Langfitt JT, Testa FM, Levy SR, DiMario F, Westerveld M, et al. Global cognitive function in children with epilepsy: a community-based study. Epilepsia. 2008;49:608–14.
2. Reilly C, Atkinson P, Das KB, Chin RF, Aylett SE, Burch V, et al. Neurobehavioral comorbidities in children with active epilepsy: a population-based study. Pediatrics. 2014;133:e1586–93.
3. Huttenlocher PR, Hapke RJ. A follow-up study of intractable seizures in childhood. Ann Neurol. 1990;28:699–705.
4. Hoie B, Mykletun A, Sommerfelt K, Bjornaes H, Skeidsvoll H, Waaler PE. Seizure-related factors and non-verbal intelligence in children with epilepsy. A population-based study from Western Norway. Seizure. 2005;14:223–31.
5. Dunn DW, Johnson CS, Perkins SM, Fastenau PS, Byars AW, deGrauw TJ, et al. Academic problems in children with seizures: relationships with neuropsychological functioning and family variables during the 3 years after onset. Epilepsy Behav. 2010;19:455–61.
6. van Eeghen AM, Chu-Shore CJ, Pulsifer MB, Camposano SE, Thiele EA. Cognitive and adaptive development of patients with tuberous sclerosis complex: a retrospective, longitudinal investigation. Epilepsy Behav. 2012;23:10–5.
7. van Iterson L, Zijlstra BJ, Augustijn PB, van der Leij A, de Jong PF. Duration of epilepsy and cognitive development in children: a longitudinal study. Neuropsychology. 2014;28:212–21.
8. Helmstaedter C, Elger CE. Chronic temporal lobe epilepsy: a neurodevelopmental or progressively dementing disease? Brain. 2009;132:2822–30.
9. Meekes J, Braams O, Braun KP, Jennekens-Schinkel A, van Nieuwenhuizen O. Verbal memory after epilepsy surgery in childhood. Epilepsy Res. 2013;107:146–55.
10. Smith ML, Lah S, Elliott I. Pediatric epilepsy surgery: neuropsychological outcomes and measurement issues. In: C. Helmstaedter et al., editors. Neuropsychology in the care of people with epilepsy. Paris: John Libbey Text; 2011. p. 239–50.
11. Gleissner U, Sassen R, Schramm J, Elger CE, Helmstaedter C. Greater functional recovery after temporal lobe epilepsy surgery in children. Brain. 2005;128:2822–9.
12. Skirrow C, Cross JH, Cormack F, Harkness W, Vargha-Khadem F, Baldeweg T. Long-term intellectual outcome after temporal lobe surgery in childhood. Neurology. 2011;76:1330–7.
13. Horsley V. Remarks on the surgery of the central nervous system. Br Med J. 1890;2:1286–92.
14. Davidson S, Falconer MA. Outcome of surgery in 40 children with temporal-lobe epilepsy. Lancet. 1975;1:1260–3.
15. Lindsay J, Glaser G, Richards P, Ounsted C. Developmental aspects of focal epilepsies of childhood treated by neurosurgery. Dev Med Child Neurol. 1984;26:574–87.
16. Helmstaedter C, Lendt M. Neuropsychological outcome of temporal and extratemporal lobe resections in children, chapter 24. In: Jambaque I et al., editors. Neuropsychology of childhood epilepsy. New York: Kluwer Academic/Plenum publishers; 2001. p. 215–27.
17. Lah S. Neuropsychological outcome following focal cortical removal for intractable epilepsy in children. Epilepsy Behav. 2004;5:804–17.
18. van Schooneveld MM, Braun KP. Cognitive outcome after epilepsy surgery in children. Brain Dev. 2013;35:721–9.
19. Ryvlin P, Cross JH, Rheims S. Epilepsy surgery in children and adults. Lancet Neurol. 2014;13:1114–26.
20. Perry MS, Duchowny M. Surgical versus medical treatment for refractory epilepsy: outcomes beyond seizure control. Epilepsia. 2013;54:2060–70.
21. Sherman EM, Wiebe S, Fay-McClymont TB, Tellez-Zenteno J, Metcalfe A, Hernandez-Ronquillo L, et al. Neuropsychological outcomes after epilepsy surgery: systematic review and pooled estimates. Epilepsia. 2011;52:857–69.
22. Spencer S, Huh L. Outcomes of epilepsy surgery in adults and children. Lancet Neurol. 2008;7:525–37.

23. Beghi E, Tonini C. Surgery for epilepsy: assessing evidence from observational studies. Epilepsy Res. 2006;70:97–102.
24. Ramantani G, Kadish NE, Brandt A, Strobl K, Stathi A, Wiegand G, et al. Seizure control and developmental trajectories after hemispherotomy for refractory epilepsy in childhood and adolescence. Epilepsia. 2013;54:1046–55.
25. Thomas SG, Daniel RT, Chacko AG, Thomas M, Russell PS. Cognitive changes following surgery in intractable hemispheric and sub-hemispheric pediatric epilepsy. Childs Nerv Syst. 2010;26:1067–73.
26. Moosa AN, Jehi L, Marashly A, Cosmo G, Lachhwani D, Wyllie E, et al. Long-term functional outcomes and their predictors after hemispherectomy in 115 children. Epilepsia. 2013;54:1771–9.
27. Althausen A, Gleissner U, Hoppe C, Sassen R, Buddewig S, von Lehe M, et al. Long-term outcome of hemispheric surgery at different ages in 61 epilepsy patients. J Neurol Neurosurg Psychiatry. 2013;84:529–36.
28. Skirrow C, Cross JH, Harrison S, Cormack F, Harkness W, Coleman R, et al. Temporal lobe surgery in childhood and neuroanatomical predictors of long-term declarative memory outcome. Brain. 2015;138(Pt 1):80–93. doi:10.1093/brain/awu313. Epub 2014 Nov 12.
29. Smith ML, Olds J, Snyder T, Elliott I, Lach L, Whiting S. A follow-up study of cognitive function in young adults who had resective epilepsy surgery in childhood. Epilepsy Behav. 2014;32:79–83. doi:10.1016/j.yebeh.2014.01.006. Epub 2014 Feb 7.
30. Viggedal G, Kristjansdottir R, Olsson I, Rydenhag B, Uvebrant P. Cognitive development from two to ten years after pediatric epilepsy surgery. Epilepsy Behav. 2012;25:2–8.
31. Lewis DV, Thompson Jr RJ, Santos CC, Oakes WJ, Radtke RA, Friedman AH, Namsoo L, Scott Swartzwelder H. Outcome of temporal lobectomy in adolescents. J Epilepsy. 1996;9(3):198–205.
32. Gleissner U, Sassen R, Lendt M, Clusmann H, Elger CE, Helmstaedter C. Pre- and postoperative verbal memory in pediatric patients with temporal lobe epilepsy. Epilepsy Res. 2002;51:287–96.
33. Oitment C, Vriezen E, Smith ML. Everyday memory in children after resective epilepsy surgery. Epilepsy Behav. 2013;28:141–6.
34. Smith ML, Elliott IM, Lach L. Memory outcome after pediatric epilepsy surgery: objective and subjective perspective. Child Neuropsychol. 2006;12:151–64.
35. Bjornaes H, Stabell K, Henriksen O, Loyning Y. The effects of refractory epilepsy on intellectual functioning in children and adults. A longitudinal study. Seizure. 2001;10:250–9.
36. Bjornaes H, Stabell KE, Henriksen O, Roste G, Diep LM. Surgical versus medical treatment for severe epilepsy: consequences for intellectual functioning in children and adults. A follow-up study. Seizure. 2002;11:473–82.
37. Hermann B, Jones J, Sheth R, Dow C, Koehn M, Seidenberg M. Children with new-onset epilepsy: neuropsychological status and brain structure. Brain. 2006;129:2609–19.
38. Ramantani G, Kadish NE, Anastasopoulos C, Brandt A, Wagner K, Strobl K, et al. Epilepsy surgery for glioneuronal tumors in childhood: avoid loss of time. Neurosurgery. 2014;74:648–57.
39. Guan Y, Zhou J, Luan G, Liu X. Surgical treatment of patients with Rasmussen encephalitis. Stereotact Funct Neurosurg. 2014;92:86–93.
40. Lew SM, Koop JI, Mueller WM, Matthews AE, Mallonee JC. Fifty consecutive hemispherectomies: outcomes, evolution of technique, complications, and lessons learned. Neurosurgery. 2014;74:182–94.
41. Viggedal G, Olsson I, Carlsson G, Rydenhag B, Uvebrant P. Intelligence two years after epilepsy surgery in children. Epilepsy Behav. 2013;29:565–70.
42. Villarejo-Ortega F, Garcia-Fernandez M, Fournier-Del CC, Fabregate-Fuente M, Alvarez-Linera J, De Prada-Vicente I, et al. Seizure and developmental outcomes after hemispherectomy in children and adolescents with intractable epilepsy. Childs Nerv Syst. 2013;29:475–88.

43. Wethe JV, Prigatano GP, Gray J, Chapple K, Rekate HL, Kerrigan JF. Cognitive functioning before and after surgical resection for hypothalamic hamartoma and epilepsy. Neurology. 2013;81:1044–50.
44. Fay-McClymont TB, Hrabok M, Sherman EM, Hader WJ, Connolly MB, Akdag S, et al. Systematic review and case series of neuropsychological functioning after epilepsy surgery in children with dysembryoplastic neuroepithelial tumors (DNET). Epilepsy Behav. 2012;23:481–6.
45. Liang S, Wang S, Zhang J, Ding C, Zhang Z, Fu X, et al. Long-term outcomes of epilepsy surgery in school-aged children with partial epilepsy. Pediatr Neurol. 2012;47:284–90.
46. D'Argenzio L, Colonnelli MC, Harrison S, Jacques TS, Harkness W, Vargha-Khadem F, et al. Cognitive outcome after extratemporal epilepsy surgery in childhood. Epilepsia. 2011;52:1966–72.
47. Chieffo D, Lettori D, Contaldo I, Perrino F, Graziano A, Palermo C, et al. Surgery of children with frontal lobe lesional epilepsy: neuropsychological study. Brain Dev. 2011;33:310–5.
48. Datta AN, Snyder TJ, Wheatley MB, Jurasek L, Ahmed NS, Gross DW, et al. Intelligence quotient is not affected by epilepsy surgery in childhood. Pediatr Neurol. 2011;44:117–21.
49. Garcia-Fernandez M, Fournier-Del CC, Ugalde-Canitrot A, Perez-Jimenez A, Alvarez-Linera J, De Prada-Vicente I, et al. Epilepsy surgery in children with developmental tumours. Seizure. 2011;20:616–27.
50. Liang S, Li A, Zhao M, Jiang H, Yu S, Meng X, et al. Epilepsy surgery in tuberous sclerosis complex: emphasis on surgical candidate and neuropsychology. Epilepsia. 2010;51:2316–21.
51. Liang S, Li A, Zhao M, Jiang H, Meng X, Sun Y. Anterior temporal lobectomy combined with anterior corpus callosotomy in patients with temporal lobe epilepsy and mental retardation. Seizure. 2010;19:330–4.
52. Boshuisen K, van Schooneveld MM, Leijten FS, de Kort GA, van Rijen PC, Gosselaar PH, et al. Contralateral MRI abnormalities affect seizure and cognitive outcome after hemispherectomy. Neurology. 2010;75:1623–30.
53. Battaglia D, Chieffo D, Tamburrini G, Lettori D, Losito E, Leo G, et al. Posterior resection for childhood lesional epilepsy: neuropsychological evolution. Epilepsy Behav. 2012;23:131–7.
54. Dunkley C, Kung J, Scott RC, Nicolaides P, Neville B, Aylett SE, et al. Epilepsy surgery in children under 3 years. Epilepsy Res. 2011;93:96–106.
55. Roulet-Perez E, Davidoff V, Mayor-Dubois C, Maeder-Ingvar M, Seeck M, Ruffieux C, et al. Impact of severe epilepsy on development: recovery potential after successful early epilepsy surgery. Epilepsia. 2010;51:1266–76.
56. Lettori D, Battaglia D, Sacco A, Veredice C, Chieffo D, Massimi L, et al. Early hemispherectomy in catastrophic epilepsy: a neuro-cognitive and epileptic long-term follow-up. Seizure. 2008;17:49–63.
57. Bourgeois M, Crimmins DW, de Oliveira RS, Arzimanoglou A, Garnett M, Roujeau T, et al. Surgical treatment of epilepsy in Sturge-Weber syndrome in children. J Neurosurg. 2007;106:20–8.
58. Battaglia D, Chieffo D, Lettori D, Perrino F, Di RC, Guzzetta F. Cognitive assessment in epilepsy surgery of children. Childs Nerv Syst. 2006;22:744–59.
59. Pulsifer MB, Brandt J, Salorio CF, Vining EP, Carson BS, Freeman JM. The cognitive outcome of hemispherectomy in 71 children. Epilepsia. 2004;45:243–54.
60. Maehara T, Shimizu H, Kawai K, Shigetomo R, Tamagawa K, Yamada T, et al. Postoperative development of children after hemispherotomy. Brain Dev. 2002;24:155–60.
61. Meyer FB, Marsh WR, Laws ER, et al. Temporal lobectomy in children with epilepsy. J Neurosurg. 1986;64:371–6.

Chapter 7
Long-Term Psychiatric Outcomes After Epilepsy Surgery in Adults

Andres M. Kanner

Abstract Psychiatric aspects of epilepsy surgery are very complex and have a pleomorphic expression, as an anterotemporal lobectomy (ATL) can be followed by remission, exacerbation in severity or recurrence of a presurgical psychiatric disorder, or the development of de novo psychopathology. Furthermore, presurgical psychiatric history appears to be associated with postsurgical persistence of epileptic seizures.

There is a dearth of studies on the long-term (>5 years) psychiatric trajectories of epilepsy surgery candidates. Most studies in this field report follow-up periods of 2 years or less. Postsurgical depression and/or anxiety disorders are the most frequent psychiatric disorders identified after resective surgeries, particularly following ATL, as 30 % are expected to experience depressive and/or anxiety episodes within the first 3–6 months. A presurgical psychiatric history has been found to be associated with an increased risk of postsurgical recurrences or exacerbations. In a majority of patients, symptoms are expected to remit by 1 year, though persistent psychopathology has been found in up to 15 % of patients. De novo postsurgical psychotic episodes and psychogenic non-epileptic seizures (PNES) on the other hand have been identified with a relatively low frequency.

Despite the relatively high frequency of postsurgical psychiatric complications (PPC), they remain under-recognized and undertreated. Furthermore, patients and families are often not informed of their potential occurrence. In this chapter, we review the prevalence of the various postsurgical psychiatric complications and their risk factors.

Keywords Major depressive episodes • Generalized anxiety disorder • Postictal psychosis • Treatment-resistant epilepsy • Mesial temporal sclerosis

---

A.M. Kanner, MD, FANA
Department of Neurology, Miller School of Medicine, University of Miami, Room #1324, NE 14th Street, Miami, FL 33136, USA
e-mail: a.kanner@med.miami.edu

K. Malmgren et al. (eds.), *Long-Term Outcomes of Epilepsy Surgery in Adults and Children*, DOI 10.1007/978-3-319-17783-0_7

Introduction

The lifetime and cross-section prevalence rates of psychiatric comorbidities in epilepsy are relatively high in patients with epilepsy (PWE), ranging between 30 and 35 % [1, 2] and it is even higher in patients who are being evaluated for epilepsy surgery, ranging from 43 to 80 % [3–6]. In fact, psychiatric comorbidities and epilepsy have a very complex relation, which is clearly illustrated in the pleomorphic psychiatric aspects of epilepsy surgery. For example, anterotemporal lobectomies (ATLs) can be associated with a remission of presurgical psychiatric disorders or postsurgical psychiatric complications (PPC), which include a recurrence and/or an exacerbation in severity of presurgical psychiatric disorders, or the development of de novo psychiatric episodes. Postsurgical psychiatric complications were initially reported by Hill et al. in 1957 [7], who described depressive episodes occurring independently of seizure outcome and which remitted within 18 months.

In the last 30 years, epilepsy surgery has been recognized as a leading therapeutic modality in the management of treatment-resistant focal epilepsy. Postsurgical psychiatric complications have been recognized in approximately 30 % of patients undergoing an ATL [8, 9]. Yet despite this relatively high prevalence, they remain unrecognized and untreated in many epilepsy surgery programs worldwide. In this chapter, we review the negative and positive impacts of epilepsy surgery on presurgical psychiatric disorders as well the available data on the development of de novo postsurgical psychopathology.

Postsurgical Psychiatric Complications: A Relatively Frequent Occurrence

Postsurgical mood and anxiety disorders are the most commonly recognized PPC, and with significantly lower frequency psychotic episodes, obsessive-compulsive disorders (OCDs), and psychogenic non-epileptic seizures (PNES). The following study illustrates the pleomorphic aspects of psychiatric aspects of epilepsy surgery:

The study included 100 consecutive patients (60 men and 40 women) age, who had undergone an anterotemporal lobectomy (ATL) for the management of treatment-resistant temporal lobe epilepsy (TLE) at the Rush Epilepsy Center in Chicago. Patients were followed postsurgically for a period of 8.3 ± 3.3 years [10, 11]. During their presurgical evaluation, a lifetime psychiatric history was identified in 56 patients; 21 had a depressive disorder, and 25 mixed depression and anxiety disorders, while 12 patients had other (non-psychotic) psychiatric disorders. Among the 100 patients, 41 experienced a PPC: 22 developed a de novo psychiatric episode, which consisted of a depressive/anxiety disorder in nine, a psychotic episode in four, PNES in seven and somatoform disorder in two. Twenty-six patients experienced an *exacerbation* in severity or recurrence of a presurgical depressive/anxiety disorders. Among the four patients who developed a de novo psychotic episode, these occurred within the first 6 months after an ATL, consisting of a manic episode in two and a paranoid episode in the other two patients. Two of these patients had lesional epilepsy, caused by a dysembryoplastic neuroepithelioma (DNET) in one and a ganglioglioma in the other. Symptoms remitted in two patients with pharmacotherapy without the need for hospitalization while the other two had to be hospitalized in a psychiatric unit. In one patient, symptoms remitted after the first admission, whereas the second patient had to be hospitalized twice. Two years after the ATL, psychiatric disorders were reported by 30, consisting of depressive with and/without anxiety episodes in 26 patients, while 11 had other type of psychiatric disorders (several patients had more than one psychiatric disorder). In 18 of these 30 patients, the PPC were severe and persistent despite multiple therapeutic interventions. At the time of the last contact (mean follow-up period of 8.3 ± 3.3 years), 16 patients continued to experience a persistent psychiatric disorder, 15 of whom had a depressive/anxiety disorder. Multivariate regression model identified a presurgical history of depression as predictors of persistent and severe postsurgical psychiatric complications. The ATL was associated with a reduction in the prevalence of psychiatric disorders by 40 % 2 years after surgery and by 71 % by the last contact.

Among the 100 patients, 7 developed de novo PNES. A presurgical lifetime psychiatric history was significantly associated with the development of postsurgical PNES. Interestingly enough, PNES were not reported in seizure-free patients; in fact, persistent seizures were significantly associated with the development of de novo PNES. Furthermore, failure to obtain gainful employment was not associated with the development of PNES. These findings differ from long-held assumptions that the development of a postsurgical PNES must be caused by the "stress" associated with a "seizure-free" life in patients with chronic epilepsy who are not "emotionally, physically, or economically ready to face their own or their families" increased expectations.

Likewise, the presurgical lifetime history of depression was associated with a worse postsurgical seizure outcome. Indeed, only 12 % of patients who became free of auras and disabling seizures after surgery were found to have a lifetime history of depression; in contrast, 79 % of patients with less than 90 % seizure reduction had a presurgical lifetime history of depression [11]. The findings of this study have been replicated in other studies, as shown below.

Postsurgical Depressive and Anxiety Disorders

As stated above, depressive and anxiety disorders are the most frequent PPCs. Most case series had a relatively short postsurgical follow-up period that ranged between 3 months and 1 year. In a recent review of prospective studies published in the literature, Rayner and Wilson concluded that postsurgical major depressive and anxiety episodes are likely to occur in approximately 30 % of patients undergoing an ATL. Most depressive episodes are diagnosed within the first 3–6 months after surgery and may persist for periods ranging between 6 and 12 months [9]. A presurgical history of mood and anxiety disorders has also been found to be a risk factor for the development of postsurgical anxiety episodes. While some authors have associated persistent postsurgical symptoms of depression with failure to achieve a seizure-free state [12], this has not been a uniform finding.

Postsurgical depressive and anxiety symptoms can be identified within the first 4–6 weeks after surgery. For example, in a study of 62 patients, 43 who had an ATL and 19 an extratemporal lobectomy (ETL), Wrench et al. identified symptoms of anxiety and/or depression in 66 % of ATL and 19 % of ETL patients, respectively [13]. At 3 months, 54 % of ATL and 33 % of ETL patients were still symptomatic with 30 % of ATL and 17 % of ETL patients still experiencing a depressive episode. By that time, 13 % of ATL patients had developed a de novo depressive episode and 15 % a de novo anxiety disorder, whereas 18 % had developed other types of de novo psychiatric disorders. In contrast, only 17 % of ETL patients had developed de novo anxiety, but not depression or other psychopathology. Likewise, Ring et al. [14] found that 45 % of 60 consecutive patients who underwent an ATL experienced emotional lability and anxiety in the first 6 weeks after surgery; in 22 % of these patients, it presented as a de novo phenomenon. These symptoms had remitted by 3 months or improved significantly. In a study of 44 patients who underwent an ATL, Glosser et al. [15] found that by the first month after surgery, 12 patients (31 %) had developed de novo depression and/or anxiety disorders or recurrence of a disorder that had been in remission during the 6 months preceding the surgical procedure. By 6 months, they were still symptomatic but significantly improved, and by 1 year all but two patients had become free of symptoms.

Can postsurgical depressive and anxiety disorders be anticipated?

As stated above, a presurgical history of mood and/or anxiety disorder has been identified in patients who go on to develop postsurgical episodes. For example, a preoperative history of depression and poor postoperative family dynamics (at 1, 6, and 12 months) were predictive of depression after surgery in the study by Wrench et al. cited above [13]. In a separate study of 107 patients, 90 of whom underwent an ATL and 17 an ETL, and who had a postsurgical follow-up period of 1 year, Quigg et al. [16] found that preoperative depressive traits predicted worse postoperative scores on scales measuring symptoms of depression. Likewise, in a study of 150 patients who underwent epilepsy surgery, Barbieri et al. found that the only predictive variable included a presurgical history of depressive episodes and older age at surgery [17].

Other potential predictive variables include epilepsy-related signs and symptoms such as *ictal* fear. For example, Kohler et al. found that, compared to patients without auras or with auras different than ictal fear, patients with preictal fear were more likely to exhibit postsurgical depressive and anxiety episodes [18]. Furthermore, while postoperative mood and anxiety disorders were more common in patients with persistent seizures, they were equally frequent in seizure-free patients who had experienced presurgical ictal fear. In addition, a majority of patients with ictal fear required the use of psychotropic medication after surgery.

Suicide is a PPC which has also been identified more frequently among patients who undergo an ATL than in the general population. For example, 27 of 360 patients who underwent an ATL died during a 5-year follow-up period [19]. Four of these deaths resulted from suicide, yielding a standardized mortality ratio (compared with suicides in the US population and adjusted for age and gender) of 13.3 (95 % CI = 3.6–34.0). Accordingly, a presurgical psychiatric evaluation in every surgical candidate is of the essence to identify those patients who may have a potential risk of postsurgical depressive and anxiety episodes. Prevention of postsurgical episodes of depression and anxiety can be achieved in such patients by introducing antidepressant medication with a selective-serotonin reuptake inhibitor or a selective serotonin-norepinephrine reuptake inhibitor at the first manifestation of the psychiatric symptomatology. Unfortunately, to date there are no studies on the pharmacologic treatment of postsurgical mood and anxiety disorder and this recommendation is based on expert consensus [20].

Obsessive-Compulsive Disorder (OCD)

Obsessive-compulsive disorder (OCD) is a rare postsurgical complication reported following ATL. Indeed, the development of de novo or aggravation of OCD was reported in a small case series of five patients with treatment-resistant TLE and "obsessive traits," who were followed after undergoing an ATL [21]. Within the first 2 months after surgery, two patients fulfilled OCD diagnostic criteria. While all of these patients became seizure free, they reported a significant worsening of their quality of life after surgery. In a separate case report, a 31-year-old man with dual pathology consisting of right mesial temporal sclerosis (MTS) and right occipital encephalomalacia experienced de novo obsessive-compulsive symptoms following resection of the right hippocampus and right occipital pole. He started to experience compulsions consisting of fear of contamination, constant hand washing, checking things, repeating rituals, and his symptomatology met criteria for OCD [22].

Postsurgical Psychotic Complications

Postsurgical psychotic complications have been identified in an average of 3 % with some case series of patients undergoing an ATL reporting frequencies of 1 % and others up to 10 % [11, 23–32]. Most consist of de novo postsurgical psychotic episodes presenting as schizophreniform-like disorders, manic episodes, and postictal psychotic episodes. Psychotic symptomatology tends to appear within the first year in all patients [23]. In some case series, postsurgical psychotic episodes occur after seizure remission [24], while in others they are associated with persistent seizures.

Postsurgical manic episodes are also psychiatric complications of ATL, as demonstrated in a study of 415 consecutive patients, 16 of whom (3.8 %) experienced a de novo manic episode [29] within the first year after an ATL. These episodes were short-lived in all but one patient.

In addition, the risk of postsurgical psychotic episodes has been associated with right temporal seizure foci. For example, Mace and Trimble [26] reported seven consecutive patients who developed de novo psychotic episodes following an ATL, six of whom had an epileptogenic area in the right temporal lobe: one developed a delusional depression, four developed a schizophrenic-like psychosis, and one patient was diagnosed with Capgras syndrome.

The presence of gangliogliomas or DNET has also been associated with the development of de novo postsurgical psychotic disorders. Andermann et al. reported six patients from four centers who experienced a de novo psychotic disorder and estimated a risk of 2.5 % for the development of de novo psychosis (1 in 39) in patients with this type of lesion who undergo an ATL [27].

A schizotypal personality disorder has also been identified as a potential risk for the development of de novo postsurgical psychotic episodes in a small case series of three patients with MTS who after undergoing an ATL developed an acute psychotic episode the first year after surgery, diagnosed as "a schizoaffective disorder," "a brief psychotic disorder," and "a delusional disorder," respectively [28]. Of note, all patients were free of seizures after surgery. Whether or not the development of de novo postsurgical psychotic episodes reflects a phenomenon of forced normalization has been the source of significant debate that has yet to be settled.

Psychogenic Non-epileptic Seizures

Ferguson and Rayport were the first authors to describe the occurrence of postsurgical de novo PNES [33]. In all case series, the prevalence rates of postsurgical PNES have been low, ranging between 1.8 and 12 %. For example, Ney et al. identified de novo postsurgical PNES in 5 out of 96 patients who underwent epilepsy surgery [34]. They suggested that a low full-scale IQ, preoperative psychiatric comorbidity, and major surgical complications could be potential risk factors. In a study of 220 patients, 22 (10 %) developed postsurgical de novo PNES [35]. In this study, preoperative psychopathology was not identified, in contrast to the other studies and our own data (see above) [11].

Somatoform Disorder

Somatoform disorder is a rare (but possibly under-recognized) PPC. To date there has been one case series of 10 patients who developed a somatoform disorder after an ATL [36]. Seven of the 10 patients developed an undifferentiated somatoform disorder, one had pain and body dysmorphia, another had pain disorder, and another had body dysmorphia alone. Of note, among the 10 patients, nine had undergone a right ATL.

The Therapeutic Effect of Epilepsy Surgery on Presurgical Psychiatric Disorders

Several studies have demonstrated that in a significant number of patients, presurgical psychiatric disorders may improve significantly or even remit following an ATL. For example, 6 of 44 patients who underwent an ATL had been found to suffer from depression and anxiety before surgery became asymptomatic postsurgically [15]. Twenty-one patients were unchanged in their psychiatric status: eight who were symptomatic and 13 who were asymptomatic before surgery. Among the patients who continued to be symptomatic after surgery, their symptom severity measured with the Brief Psychiatric Rating Scale had improved significantly. In a study by Altshuler et al. [37], 17 out of 49 patients (35 %) had a lifetime history of at least one major depressive episode. Eight of these patients never experienced another major depressive episode postsurgically. Devinsky et al. reported the results of a study of 360 patients from seven epilepsy centers in the USA; 89 % underwent an ATL [12]. Psychiatric syndromes were identified at baseline and 2 years after surgery with a structured interview, the Composite International Diagnostic Interview (CIDI). Presurgically, 75 patients (22 %) met criteria for a diagnosis of depression, 59 (18 %) of anxiety disorders, and 12 (4 %) of other psychiatric disorders, including bipolar illness and schizophrenia. At the 2-year postsurgical evaluation, only 26 patients (9 %) met diagnostic criteria for depression, 20 (10 %) for anxiety, and 3 patients (1 %) met criteria for other psychiatric diagnoses. Thus, epilepsy surgery had resulted in symptom remission in more than 50 % of patients. In this study, the presence of an anxiety or depressive disorder postsurgically was not associated with seizure outcome.

Remission of OCD identified presurgically has been reported to remit following an ATL. For example, a 35-year-old woman with a 28-year history of treatment-resistant TLE secondary to right mesial temporal sclerosis had also had been suffering from a 10-year history of treatment-resistant OCD, consisting of obsessions of an urge to hurt her children every time she saw a sharp object [38]. Three weeks after a right ATL, she reported a complete remission of her obsessive symptoms and has remained symptom- and seizure-free. A second case consisted of a 28-year-old patient with treatment-resistant TLE who developed OCD symptoms shortly after the onset of TLE associated with a lesion in the right posterior temporal region [39]. After undergoing a lesionectomy and right ATL, she became seizure free and exhibited almost complete remission of her OCD.

The impact of ATL on the postsurgical course of the psychotic disorder has varied from unchanged (in a majority of cases), though some authors have reported an improvement of the presurgical psychotic disorder and/or level of functioning. For example, in a case series of six patients with a presurgical psychotic disorder who became seizure free after an ATL, Marchetti et al. found a relative improvement in the psychotic disorder of five of these patients [40]. These same authors reported an additional case of a 45-year-old female patient with a 30-year history of epilepsy and recurrent postictal psychotic episodes since the age of 35, which evolved to a chronic refractory interictal psychosis [41]. After having a right ATL she became seizure free, with remission of the psychotic disorder.

Improvement in psychogenic non-epileptic seizures after epilepsy surgery has also been reported. For example, Reuber et al. identified 13 patients with epileptic seizures and PNES before undergoing an ATL. After surgery, PNES improved significantly in 11 patients [42].

Impact of Presurgical Psychiatric Illness on Postsurgical Seizure Outcome

Several studies have documented an association between a presurgical psychiatric history and postsurgical seizure outcome as illustrated in our own study cited above [10, 43–45]. Furthermore in one study of 121 patients who underwent an ATL, those with a lifetime psychiatric history exhibited a worse postsurgical seizure outcome than those without [43]. In another study of 186 patients with treatment-resistant TLE secondary to MTS were followed for a 6-year period after undergoing an ATL [46]. Seventy-seven (41.4 %) patients had a presurgical Axis I diagnosis, including depression, interictal dysphoric disorder, interictal psychosis, postictal psychosis, anxiety disorders, and 23 had a personality disorder. The investigators found that preoperative anxiety disorders and personality disorders were associated with a failure of a seizure-free state. In two other studies that included 280 and 115 patients with TLE secondary to MTS, a preoperative psychiatric diagnosis was associated with a significantly lower postsurgical seizure-free state [8, 45]. This was not confirmed in a study of 72 patients with MTS only [46]. This study differed from the others by the shorter postsurgical follow-up period, which may account for the differences.

Concluding Remarks and Future Directions

The data reviewed in this chapter is indicative of a high prevalence of psychiatric comorbidity in epilepsy surgery candidates. This psychiatric comorbidity, whether present at the time of the presurgical evaluation or preceding it, has significant implications in the patients' risks of PPC, psychosocial adjustment as well as seizure outcome. Unfortunately, despite the relatively high prevalence of presurgical psychiatric comorbidities and PPC, most major epilepsy centers have failed to integrate a psychiatric evaluation into their presurgical workup. Instead, most centers have relied on neuropsychological evaluations, which while complementing a psychiatric evaluation, are not a substitute for them. Accordingly, clinicians are ill-prepared in identifying patients at risk for PPC. Often, patients and families are not advised on the potential risk of these complications and hence, their consent for surgery is based on incomplete information (See Chaps. 16 and 17 in this volume). Needless to say, failure to prepare patients and families for such complications can result in potential medicolegal problems.

The other side of the coin, however, is the remission of presurgical psychiatric comorbidities following ATL. As shown in our study, 40 % of patients with presurgical psychiatric disorders had become symptom free 2 years after their ATL and 70 % at the last contact (8.3 ± 3.3 years) [11]. This information must be also discussed with patients and their families as it constitutes another therapeutic benefit of epilepsy surgery.

Unfortunately, relative to the number of surgeries performed in major epilepsy centers, there is still a significant paucity of data on psychiatric aspects of epilepsy. This is reflected in the quasi absence of studies in extratemporal epilepsy surgery (in particular frontal lobe resections), all of which are another consequence of the failure to perform pre- and postsurgical psychiatric evaluations in *every* patient. In fact, this lack of data also limited our review to PPC occurring within the first 6–12 months after surgery and sadly, we could not achieve the aims to review the long-term PPC. Alas, these data are not available! Given the fluctuating nature of psychiatric conditions, longitudinal data are critical to accurately track the long-term trajectories in this patient population.

The field of psychiatric aspects of epilepsy surgery is still in its infancy, with most questions yet to be answered in a comprehensive manner. These include the identification of prevalence rates and risks factors of PPC in the different age groups and in particular in children and adolescents, and in elderly patients. In addition, the impact of epilepsy surgery on premorbid psychiatric disorders and the association (if any) of any previous psychiatric history on the postsurgical seizure outcome needs to be examined in prospective studies. The association of extratemporal epilepsy surgery (in particular in frontal lobe structures) with PPC, including the identification of their risk factors, remains practically unknown. Finally, the data reviewed in this chapter illustrates the complex relations between psychiatric disorders and epilepsy. A better understanding of the risks factors for PPC or the remission of presurgical psychiatric disorders after an ATL can yield valuable data on our understanding of potential pathogenic mechanisms operant in both types of disorders.

In summary, epilepsy surgery is associated with PPC which should be openly discussed with patients and family members with as much detail as the other surgical risks. Patients should be advised of the risk of postsurgical depressive and anxiety episodes occurring within the first 3–6 months which have a tendency to remit by 12–24 months in particular, in patients with a previous history of a mood disorder. However, patients need to be warned about the risk of de novo depressive and anxiety disorders and psychotic disorders.

References

1. Hesdorffer DC, Ishihara L, Mynepalli L, Webb DJ, Weil J, Hauser WA. Epilepsy, suicidality, and psychiatric disorders: a bidirectional association. Ann Neurol. 2012;72:184–91.
2. Tellez-Zenteno JF, Patten SB, Jetté N, Williams J, Wiebe S. Psychiatric comorbidity in epilepsy: a population-based analysis. Epilepsia. 2007;48:2336–44.
3. Kanner AM. Depression in epilepsy: prevalence, clinical semiology, pathogenic mechanisms and treatment. Biol Psychiatry. 2003;54:388–98.
4. Toone BK, Garralda ME, Ron MA. The psychoses of epilepsy and the functional psychoses: a clinical and phenomenological comparison. Br J Psychiatry. 1982;141:256–61.
5. McDermott S, Mani S, Krishnaswami S. A population-based analysis of specific behavior problems associated with childhood seizures. J Epilepsy. 1995;8:110–8.
6. Koch-Stoecker S. Psychiatric effects of surgery for temporal lobe epilepsy. In: Trimble M, Schmitz B, editors. The neuropsychiatry of epilepsy. Cambridge: Cambridge University Press; 2002. p. 266–82.
7. Hill D, Pond DA, Mitchell W, Falconer MA. Personality changes following temporal lobectomy for epilepsy. J Ment Sci. 1957;103:18–27.
8. Cleary RA, Thompson PJ, Fox Z, Foong J. Predictors of psychiatric and seizure outcome following temporal lobe epilepsy surgery. Epilepsia. 2012;53(10):1705–12.
9. Rayner G, Wilson SJ. Psychiatric care in epilepsy surgery: who needs it? Epilepsy Curr. 2012;12:46–50.
10. Kanner AM, Byrne R, Chicharro AV, Wuu J, Frey M. A lifetime psychiatric history predicts a worse seizure outcome following temporal lobectomy. Neurology. 2009;72:793–9.
11. Balabanov AJ, Kanner AM. Psychiatric outcome of epilepsy surgery. In: Luders HO, editor. Textbook of epilepsy surgery. London: Informa Healthcare; 2008. p. 1254–62.
12. Devinsky O, Barr WB, Vickrey BG, et al. Changes in depression and anxiety after resective surgery for epilepsy. Neurology. 2005;65:1744–942.
13. Wrench J, Wilson SJ, Bladin PF. Mood disturbance before and after seizure surgery: a comparison of temporal and extratemporal resections. Epilepsia. 2004;45:534–43.
14. Ring HA, Moriarty J, Trimble MR. A prospective study of the early postsurgical psychiatric associations of epilepsy surgery. J Neurol Neurosurg Psychiatry. 1998;64:601–4.
15. Glosser G, Zwill AS, Glosser DS, et al. Psychiatric aspects of temporal lobe epilepsy before and after anterior temporal lobectomy. J Neurol Neurosurg Psychiatry. 2000;68:53–8.
16. Quigg M, Broshek DK, Heidal-Schultz S, et al. Depression in intractable partial epilepsy varies by laterality of focus and surgery. Epilepsia. 2003;44:419–24.
17. Barbieri V, Cardinale F, Luoni A, Russo GL, Francione S, Tassi L, Sartori I, Castana L, Scarone S, Gambini O. Risk factors for postoperative depression in 150 subjects treated for drug-resistant focal epilepsy. Epidemiol Psychiatr Sci. 2011;20(1):99–105.
18. Kohler CG, Carran MA, Bilker W, et al. Association of fear auras with mood and anxiety disorders after temporal lobectomy. Epilepsia. 2001;42:674–81.
19. Hamid H, Devinsky O, Vickrey BG, Berg AT, Bazil CW, Langfitt JT, Walczak TS, Sperling MR, Shinnar S, Spencer SS. Suicide outcomes after resective epilepsy surgery. Epilepsy Behav. 2011;20(3):462–4.
20. Kerr MP, Mensah S, Besag F, et al. International consensus clinical practice statements for the treatment of neuropsychiatric conditions associated with epilepsy. Epilepsia. 2011;52(11):2133–8.
21. Kulaksizoglu IB, Bebek N, Baykan B, Imer M, Gürses C, Sencer S, Oktem-Tanör O, Gökyigit A. Obsessive-compulsive disorder after epilepsy surgery. Epilepsy Behav. 2004;5(1):113–8.
22. Roth RM, Jobst BC, Thadani VM, Gilbert KL, Roberts DW. New-onset obsessive-compulsive disorder following neurosurgery for medication-refractory seizure disorder. Epilepsy Behav. 2009;14(4):677–80.

23. Shaw P, Mellers J, Henderson M, Polkey C, David AS, Toone BK. Schizophrenia-like psychosis arising de novo following a temporal lobectomy: timing and risk factors. J Neurol Neurosurg Psychiatry. 2004;75:1003–8.
24. Leinonen E, Tuunainen A, Lepola U. Postoperative psychoses in epileptic patients after temporal lobectomy. Acta Neurol Scand. 1994;90:394–9.
25. Jensen I, Larsen JK. Mental aspects of temporal lobe epilepsy. Follow-up of 74 patients after resection of a temporal lobe. J Neurol Neurosurg Psychiatry. 1979;42:256–65.
26. Mace CJ, Trimble MR. Psychosis following temporal lobe surgery: a report of six cases. J Neurol Neurosurg Psychiatry. 1991;54:639–44.
27. Andermann LF, Savard G, Meencke HJ, McLachlan R, Moshe S, Andermann F. Psychosis after resection of ganglioglioma or DNET: evidence for an association. Epilepsia. 1999;40: 83–7.
28. Calvet E, Caravotta PG, Scévola L, Teitelbaum J, Seoane E, Kochen S, D'Alessio L. Psychosis after epilepsy surgery: report of three cases. Epilepsy Behav. 2011;22(4):804–7.
29. Carran MA, Kohler CG, O'Connor MJ, Bilker WB, Sperling MR. Mania following temporal lobectomy. Neurology. 2003;61:770–4.
30. Stevens JR. Psychiatric consequences of temporal lobectomy for intractable seizures. a 20–30-year follow-up of 14 cases. Psychol Med. 1990;20:529–45.
31. Christodoulou C, Koutroumanidid M, Hennessy MJ, et al. Postictal psychosis after temporal lobectomy. Neurology. 2002;59:1432–5.
32. Manchanda R, Miller H, McLachlan RS. Postictal psychosis after right temporal lobectomy. J Neurol Neurosurg Psychiatry. 1993;56:277–9.
33. Ferguson SM, Rayport M. The adjustment to living without epilepsy. J Nerv Ment Dis. 1965;140:26–37.
34. Ney GC, Barr WB, Napolitano C, et al. New-onset psychogenic seizures after surgery for epilepsy. Arch Neurol. 1998;55:726–30.
35. Glosser G, Roberts D, Glosser DS. Nonepileptic seizures after resective epilepsy surgery. Epilepsia. 1999;40:1750–4.
36. Naga AA, Devinski O, Barr WB. Somatoform disorders after temporal lobectomy. Cogn Behav Neuro. 2004;17:57–61.
37. Altshuler L, Rausch R, Delrahim S, Kay J, Crandall P. Temporal lobe epilepsy, temporal lobectomy and major depression. J Neuropsychiatry Clin Neurosci. 1999;11:436–43.
38. Kanner Morris HH, Stagno S, Chelune G, Luders HL. Remission of an obsessive-compulsive disorder following a right temporal lobectomy. Neuropsychiatry Neuropsychol Behav Neurol. 1993;6(2):126–9.
39. Barbieri V, Lo Russo G, Francione S, Scarone S, Gambini O. Association of temporal lobe epilepsy and obsessive-compulsive disorder in a patient successfully treated with right temporal lobectomy. Epilepsy Behav. 2005;6(4):617–9.
40. Marchetti RL, Fiore LA, Valente KD, Gronich G, Nogueira AB, Tzu WH. Surgical treatment of temporal lobe epilepsy with interictal psychosis: results of six cases. Epilepsy Behav. 2003;4:146–52.
41. Marchetti RL, Tavares AG, Gronich G, Fiore LA, Ferraz RB. Complete remission of epileptic psychosis after temporal lobectomy: case report. Arq Neuropsiquiatr. 2001;59(3-B): 802–5.
42. Reuber M, Kurthen M, Fernandez G, et al. Epilepsy surgery in patients with additional psychogenic seizures. Arch Neurol. 2002;59:82–6.
43. Anhouri S, Brown RJ, Krishnamoorthy ES, Trimble MR. Psychiatric outcome following temporal lobectomy: a predictive study. Epilepsia. 2000;41:1608–15.
44. Guarnieri R, Walz R, Hallak JE, Coimbra E, de Almeida E, Cescato MP, Velasco TR, Alexandre Jr V, Terra VC, Carlotti Jr CG, Assirati Jr JA, Sakamoto AC. Do psychiatric comorbidities predict postoperative seizure outcome in temporal lobe epilepsy surgery? Epilepsy Behav. 2009;14(3):529–34.

45. de Araújo Filho GM, Gomes FL, Mazetto L, Marinho MM, Tavares IM, Caboclo LO, Yacubian EM, Centeno RS. Major depressive disorder as a predictor of a worse seizure outcome one year after surgery in patients with temporal lobe epilepsy and mesial temporal sclerosis. Seizure. 2012;8:619–23.
46. Adams SJ, Velakoulis D, Kaye AH, Corcoran NM, O'Brien TJ. Psychiatric history does not predict seizure outcome following temporal lobectomy for mesial temporal sclerosis. Epilepsia. 2012;53(10):1700–4.

Chapter 8
Long-Term Psychiatric and Behavior Outcomes in Children Following Epilepsy Surgery

Ailsa McLellan

Abstract Epilepsy surgery is undoubtedly effective in reducing seizure frequency, and in many cases stopping seizures, in carefully selected children with drug-resistant epilepsy. However, seizure control clearly is not the only outcome from epilepsy surgery, and there are other outcomes which are arguably more important in some children including improved development, behavior, and quality of life.

Mental health problems are common in children with epilepsy (CWE), and are very frequently seen in children undergoing epilepsy surgery. Following surgery, there can be improvements in the mental health of some children, but there are others for whom there is no improvement, or indeed deterioration in their preexisting psychiatric symptoms. Furthermore, there are children who develop new psychiatric problems postoperatively. In this chapter, mental health problems in children undergoing epilepsy surgery will be reviewed and psychiatric outcome considered, with particular emphasis on what is known about long-term outcomes.

Keywords Pediatric epilepsy • Psychopathology • Temporal lobe resection • Hemispherectomy • Extratemporal resection • Corpus callosotomy • Hypothalamic hamartoma • Psychiatric outcome • Behavior problems • Mental health services

---

A. McLellan, MBChB, FRCP, FRCPCH
Paediatric Neurosciences, Royal Hospital for Sick Children, Edinburgh, Scotland, UK
e-mail: ailsa.mclellan@luht.scot.nhs.uk

K. Malmgren et al. (eds.), *Long-Term Outcomes of Epilepsy Surgery in Adults and Children*, DOI 10.1007/978-3-319-17783-0_8

Mental Health Problems in Children with Epilepsy

Mental health problems are 4.7 times more common in children with epilepsy (CWE) compared to the general population [1]. Psychiatric disorders are reported in 28–58 % of CWE compared to 7–9 % in the general pediatric population and 11–12 % of children with chronic illnesses which do not involve the central nervous system [2, 3]. Psychiatric disorders are a significant problem for the child and family, often more so than the seizures themselves, and have a huge impact on quality of life. The range of psychiatric diagnoses seen in children with epilepsy includes conduct disorders, emotional disorders, attention deficit hyperactivity disorder (ADHD), pervasive developmental disorder (PDD), psychosis, and conversion disorders.

There are many risk factors associated with psychopathology in children with epilepsy including structural brain abnormality, seizure frequency, cognitive impairment, effects of antiepileptic drugs (AEDs), and social and family factors [4]. Children with structural brain abnormalities are at particular risk of psychopathology with reported rates of 58 % children having a psychiatric diagnosis [2] and therefore inevitably high rates of mental health problems are seen in children being considered for epilepsy surgery.

Identification of psychopathology in children with epilepsy is important in order to then consider appropriate treatments with anticipated benefit on quality of life and therefore access to effective psychiatric services is key. There may be some situations in which the symptoms may be improved by straightforward interventions such as a change in AED or treatment of electrical status epilepticus of sleep (ESES) and therefore it is important to consider all potentially reversible factors. However, the majority of mental health problems in children with epilepsy are multifactorial and multidisciplinary working with input from different professionals including pediatric neurology and mental health services is crucial.

Mental Health Problems in Children Undergoing Epilepsy Surgery

Children undergoing resective epilepsy surgery are presumed to have structural brain abnormalities and are therefore at very high risk of mental health problems. Psychiatric disorders have been reported in 36–80 % of children undergoing evaluation for epilepsy surgery [5, 6] with most series reporting rates of mental health problems at the upper end of this range [7, 8]. The range of psychiatric diagnoses in pediatric epilepsy surgery candidates include attention deficit hyperactivity disorder (ADHD), anxiety disorder, depression, pervasive developmental disorder (PDD), and disruptive behavior disorder (DBD). A significant proportion of children with mental health problems have more than one psychiatric diagnosis (28–57 %) [6–8].

Mental health problems in children contribute significantly to the overall disability experienced by CWE. Therefore, in evaluating outcomes from epilepsy surgery, it is important to consider the effects of epilepsy surgery on psychopathology. However, few prospective studies evaluating psychiatric outcome in the short and long terms after epilepsy surgery have been published historically and there is a lack of control data. A simple hypothesis would be that mental health problems will improve following epilepsy surgery if the seizures are controlled, and while some children have an improvement in behavior postoperatively [8–10], this is not universally the case. Given that psychopathology in CWE is due to a complex interplay of many factors, seizure freedom will not always be associated with improved mental health.

The nociferous cortex, or "neural noise" hypothesis suggests that seizure activity can disrupt more extensive neural networks that extend beyond the irritant zone of the seizure [11] and has been postulated as a mechanism for mental health problems in epilepsy. It has been suggested that in temporal lobe epilepsy, the epileptogenic cortex may adversely affect the extratemporal regions that mediate executive function abilities with resultant impact on behavior [12]. If this concept is correct then the abnormal brain tissue causing epilepsy can affect the function of normal brain and therefore removal of the abnormal brain should have a beneficial effect on behavior [13].

Given that there are few long-term prospective studies of psychiatric outcome following epilepsy surgery in children, information is limited with respect to specific surgeries. However, what is known about outcomes is summarized below with some further details on effects of age at surgery and long-term psychiatric outcomes. In addition, there are some cases illustrating some of the psychiatric outcomes following epilepsy surgery in children.

Psychiatric Outcomes Following Temporal Lobe Resections

Children undergoing temporal lobe resections have higher rates of preoperative psychiatric diagnoses than children with extratemporal lesions. In a study by Salpekar et al. [6] of children being evaluated for epilepsy surgery, 87 % of children with temporal foci had a clinically significant score on the Child Behavior Checklist (CBCL), compared with 63 % of children with extratemporal foci. There are few studies however looking at psychiatric outcome following temporal resection for epilepsy. In a study of 60 children undergoing temporal lobectomy reported by the Great Ormond Street Epilepsy Surgery Programme [8], 83 % of children had a psychiatric diagnosis at some stage – 72 % preoperatively and 72 % postoperatively. These children had a mean age of epilepsy onset of 3.4 years, underwent surgery at a mean age of 10.6 years, and had been followed up for a mean of 5.1 years (range 2–10 years). The range of psychiatric disorders is summarized in Table 8.1. Psychiatric comorbidity was common with 45 % of children having two or more psychiatric disorders preoperatively and 57 % postoperatively. Psychiatric disorders resolved postoperatively in 16 % but 12 % of children developed a psychiatric disorder for the first time postoperatively, having been free of mental health problems

Table 8.1 Great Ormond Street Epilepsy Surgery Programme [8]

	Preoperative (total 60)	Postoperative (total 57)	Affected at any time
PDD	23 (38 %)	21 (37 %)	23 (38 %)
ADHD	14 (23 %)	13 (23 %)	16 (27 %)
ODD/CD	13 (22 %)	12 (21 %)	16 (27 %)
DBD	24 (40 %)	25 (42 %)	30 (50 %)
Emotional disorder	5 (8 %)	12 (21 %)	15 (25 %)
Eating disorder	1 (2 %)	2 (4 %)	2 (4 %)
Conversion disorder	1 (2 %)	1 (2 %)	2 (4 %)
Psychosis	0	1 (2 %)	1 (2 %)

DSM-IV diagnosis preoperatively, postoperatively, and total at any point in children undergoing temporal lobe surgery for epilepsy

PDD Pervasive developmental disorder, *ADHD* attention deficit hyperactivity disorder, *ODD/CD* oppositional defiant disorder/conduct disorder, *DBD* disruptive behavior disorder

preoperatively. New psychiatric diagnoses emerged postoperatively in 37 % and psychiatric symptoms deteriorated postoperatively in 25 %. There was no relationship between the emergence of new psychiatric diagnoses and seizure control as had been reported in adult study of temporal lobectomy and mental health [14] or indeed a small series of 16 children undergoing temporal lobectomy [7]. Furthermore, a systematic review of psychiatric outcome following epilepsy surgery, which included predominantly studies in adults, found that one of the two main predictors of psychiatric outcome was seizure freedom [15]. However, another study in children with follow-up of 1 year also found no relation between seizure status postoperatively and psychiatric outcome [16], so the literature is inconsistent and there is a need for large, long-term prospective studies of psychiatric outcome in epilepsy surgery cases to further investigate this relationship.

In the Great Ormond Street study [8], there was an emergence of emotional disorders postoperatively with 20 % of children developing emotional disorders postoperatively, the majority of whom were children with normal cognition who were seizure free (see Case 1). It is not clear why some children develop new psychiatric disorders postoperatively, even if they are seizure free, but it could be related to a number of factors including the wider neural networks involved, the change in electrophysiology when seizure focus has been removed, or even psychosocial adjustments to life without epilepsy and possibly AEDs (Case 1).

Psychiatric Outcomes Following Extratemporal Lobe Resections

There is little data in the literature examining postoperative psychiatric outcome from extratemporal lesions in children. Rates of mental health problems appear lower than for children undergoing temporal lobectomy [6], but are still significant. In a study of psychiatric outcome at least a year following surgery (range 12 months to 12 years)

Table 8.2 Great Ormond Street Epilepsy Surgery Programme [17]

Diagnoses	Preoperative, *n* (%)	Postoperative, *n* (%)	Lost diagnosis postop	Developed diagnosis postop	No change
ADHD	4 (6)	7 (10)	0	3	4
ODD/CD	9 (13)	10 (14)	0	1	9
DBD (NOS)	4 (6)	4 (6)	1	1	3
Change of behavior due to a general medical condition	9 (13)	6 (9)	4	1	5
Emotional disorder	10 (14)	12 (17)	0	2	10
ASD	9 (13)	10 (14)	0	1	9
Other major disorder	2 (3)	3 (4)	0	1	2

DSM-IV diagnoses pre- and postoperatively in children undergoing extratemporal resections

in 71 children undergoing extratemporal resection (predominantly frontal resections), one or more psychiatric diagnoses was present in 31/71 (44 %) children preoperatively and 32/71 (45 %) postoperatively [17]. Mental health problems improved postoperatively in eight (11 %) children, of these, five (7 %) completely resolved; in 6/71 (9 %) children with no preoperative diagnosis, a DSM-IV diagnoses evolved postoperatively. The nature of the psychiatric diagnoses is summarized in Table 8.2. There was no association between any change in psychopathology (positive or negative) and seizure outcome, or indeed any other factors such as pathology, location of surgery, etc. As with surgery in the temporal lobe, the removal of the epileptic focus producing epileptic discharges could result in marked improvement in behavior, particularly in the frontal lobe cases. Equally removal of frontal lobe tissue could cause disinhibition and other problems leading to behavioral disturbance [18].

A smaller study of 34 patients undergoing extratemporal resection found high rates of behavior problems in the children that underwent neuropsychology testing (18/34) pre- and postoperatively (1 year postop) using the CBCL to assess behavioral problems [19]. Overall, these children were found to score highly in the domain of attentional problems reported by parents and greater than normal in domains of somatic complaints, social problems, and anxiety/depression. Postoperatively, there were no measureable improvements in these areas, despite overall seizure freedom of 68 % of patients though parents did report some improvements.

Psychiatric Outcomes Following Hemispherectomy

Children undergoing hemispherectomy seem to have better behavioral outcomes postoperatively than those undergoing temporal lobectomy. Historically, hemispherectomy was reported to lead to remarkable behavioral improvements with a report by Wilson [20] describing 50 patients of whom 80 % had behavioral problems of whom following surgery, 94 % had a normalization of behavior. In the more recent literature, Pulsifer et al. [21] reported a series of 71 patients with hemispherectomy, 53 of whom underwent follow-up at a mean of 5.4 years postoperatively. The CBCL was used to assess behavioral problems and the overall score was not consistent with clinical problems. However, on the subscales of clinical problems with attention and thought problems, the scores were consistent with a clinically significant problem, but these scales improved significantly after surgery. In another large series of pediatric hemispherectomy [5], with a median follow-up 3.4 years, behavior difficulties were present in 12 children (36 %). The most common problem was difficulty with concentration (75 %), followed by fluctuating mood with or without socially intrusive behavior (66 %). Ninety-two percent of children had improvement in behavior post hemispherectomy who had been found to have preoperative behavioral problems. Five children were reported to have behavioral problems postoperatively having not experienced them preoperatively. The emergence of behavioral problems was neither related to seizure outcome nor to the cognitive abilities of the child.

The mechanisms leading to behavioral problems in children undergoing hemispherectomy, as with other epilepsy surgery candidates, are likely to be multifactorial. The role of epileptic discharges may be important in hemispherectomy candidates, as frequent, widespread epileptic discharges are common. Hemispherectomy prevents the spread of epileptic discharges to the unaffected hemisphere and may be one reason why behavioral problems may improve postoperatively in some children (Case 2).

Psychiatric Outcomes Following Corpus Callosotomy

In palliative surgery for epilepsy, it is also important to consider wider outcomes than just seizure control. Corpus callosotomy is performed as a palliative procedure with the aim of stopping, or at least reducing "drop" seizures which are associated with injury. It would not be expected that this type of surgery would lead to seizure freedom as children who have "drop" seizures typically have other seizure types. No brain tissue is removed during surgery, so the concept of removing abnormal brain tissue and the epileptic focus thereby improving behavioral problems does not apply. However, corpus callosotomy can prevent the spread of epileptic discharges from one hemisphere to another, so the concept of limiting the extent of electrical disturbance and evaluating whether this leads to an improvement in functioning has been considered. Yonekawa et al. [22] investigated 15 children undergoing corpus callosotomy with EEG and used the CBCL to assess their behavior. They were followed after just under a year (mean 0.8 years). The attention problem scale and total CBCL score significantly improved in children who had an improvement postoperatively in their EEG. Other studies [23–26] have also demonstrated improvements in behaviors (particularly attention, hyperactivity, and aggressive behaviors) post callosotomy with mean periods of follow-up ranging from 19 to 40 months after surgery.

Hypothalamic Hamartoma Surgery and Psychiatric Outcome

Behavioral problems are seen frequently (50–62 %) in children under evaluation in epilepsy surgery programs who have hypothalamic hamartoma and epilepsy [27, 28]. Harvey [27] followed up a series of 29 children for a mean period of 30 months (range 12–70 months) and found that 18/29 (62 %) had behavioral problems preoperatively, which were associated with an improvement if they were seizure free postoperatively. There was an emergence of mood problems in a small number of children (3/29; 10 %) all of whom were seizure free, which has some similarities to the emergence of new mood problems postoperatively in children who have had temporal lobectomy. Two children (7 %) developed psychosis. Seizure freedom therefore seems to be associated with an improvement in behavior in the clinical syndrome of hypothalamic hamartoma, but there is the possibility of the emergence of new psychiatric disorders even if seizures are well controlled.

Age at Surgery and Behavioral Outcome

It is recognized that children, and indeed adults, are coming to epilepsy surgery many years after their presentation with epilepsy. The impact of ongoing epileptic seizures on the developing brain and the possibility of reorganization of function due to brain plasticity have led clinicians to consider surgery at an earlier stage than it has been historically, in order to improve developmental and psychosocial outcomes. It is reasonable to consider then whether earlier surgery does lead to better psychiatric outcome. One of the difficulties in evaluating this is the lack of long-term prospective studies with standardized assessments of psychopathology and other variables and the identification of an appropriate control group. The best current evidence of advantages of earlier surgery from the point of view of developmental and psychiatric outcomes is from positive outcomes in these areas following hemispherectomy in young children and the knowledge that longer duration of epilepsy correlates negatively with developmental and behavioral outcomes, whereas earlier age at surgery is associated with better outcomes [29].

Treatment of Mental Health Problems in Children Following Epilepsy Surgery

Children and families need careful counseling about the range of mental health outcomes from epilepsy surgery, and psychiatric assessment should be an integral part of a comprehensive epilepsy surgery program. It is particularly important to discuss the possibility of the late emergence of mental health problems, as children may not be under regular review by the epilepsy surgery center several years after surgery, and families need to know how to access appropriate mental health services. Close liaison between the psychiatrist in the comprehensive epilepsy surgery program and the local psychiatric services is crucial as the local team will take the lead role in providing ongoing assessment and management of any mental health problems and will be able to link in more effectively to local pediatric services and education. Mental health problems in children with epilepsy should be managed using the same treatments and management strategies as children who do not have epilepsy as there is no evidence that children with epilepsy respond differently to conventional psychiatric therapies. Behavioral problems have significant impact and therefore effective management of mental health problems can enhance quality of life and overall outcome from epilepsy surgery.

Summary

Mental health problems are common in children with epilepsy, and are very prevalent in children being evaluated for all types of epilepsy surgery. Psychiatric assessment therefore should be an integral part of an epilepsy surgery program. Psychiatric disorders significantly impact children and their families and contribute significantly to the overall disability experienced by children with epilepsy. While the primary outcome of epilepsy surgery is seizure control, cognitive, behavioral, and quality of life outcomes are also hugely important. Psychiatric outcomes, however, are not clearly predictable and children and their families need to be carefully counseled about this. Ongoing psychiatric assessment and access to evidence-based treatments and psychosocial support are important for children with epilepsy, particularly those in epilepsy surgery programs. There is a need for long-term, multicenter, prospective case-control studies in order to better understand the psychiatric outcomes in the longer term and provide accurate prognostic information with regard to psychiatric outcome.

Case 1

A previously well boy presented with focal epilepsy at the age of 7. MRI revealed a left temporal lesion, with characteristics of a developmental tumor. Epilepsy continued despite adequate trials of three AEDs and he was then evaluated in an epilepsy surgery program at the age of 8. Preoperative evaluation did not identify any psychiatric diagnosis. He underwent a lesionectomy of the left temporal lesion, a ganglioglioma. He became seizure free postoperatively and remains seizure free, off AEDs now 4 years postsurgery. There is no recurrence of his ganglioglioma. Nine months after surgery, he developed an anxiety disorder which improved initially following input from mental health services. This has deteriorated in the last year (nearly 3 years following surgery) and he has also developed depression.

Case 2

A 4-year-old girl with a congenital left hemiparesis (due to a hemispheric malformation of cortical development) presented with focal epilepsy. She had mild developmental delay. Epileptic seizures were initially controlled on her second AED. At the age of 6, she was struggling with schoolwork and reported to have poor attention. She also had impulsive behavior, was reviewed by mental health services, and fulfilled criteria for ADHD. Prolonged EEG revealed frequent right-sided epileptic discharges in the awake state, and in sleep she was in electrical status (ESES). Treatment with corticosteroids lead to a transient improvement in attention and abolishment of ESES. Attentional problems returned 3 months following steroids as did ESES on EEG and her clinical focal seizures. She was evaluated in an epilepsy surgery program and underwent a right hemispherotomy. Three months postoperatively, she was reassessed and her attentional problems had improved, there was no evidence of ESES on EEG, and she was seizure free. Two years postoperatively, she no longer fulfils the criteria for ADHD and remains seizure free off AEDs.

References

1. McDermott S, Mani S, Krishnaswami S. A population- based analysis of specific behavior problems associated with childhood seizures. J Epilepsy. 1995;8:110–8.
2. Rutter M, Graham P, Yule W. A neuropsychiatric study in childhood. In: Clinics in developmental medicine, vol. 35/36. London: Heinemann; 1970.
3. Davies S, Heyman I, Goodman R. A population survey of mental health problems in children with epilepsy. Dev Med Child Neurol. 2003;45:292–5.
4. Davies S, Heyman I. Psychiatric aspects. In: Wallace SJ, Farrell K, editors. Epilepsy in children. London: Arnold; 2004. p. 447–62.
5. Devlin AM, Cross JH, Harkness W, Chong WK, Harding B, Vargha-Khadem F, Neville BG. Clinical outcomes of hemispherectomy for epilepsy in childhood and adolescence. Brain. 2003;126(Pt 3):556–66.
6. Salpekar JA, Berl MM, Havens K, Cushner-Weinstein S, Conry JA, Pearl PL, Yaun AL, Gaillard WD. Psychiatric symptoms in children prior to epilepsy surgery differ according to suspected seizure focus. Epilepsia. 2013;54(6):1074–82.
7. Danielsson S, Rydenhag B, Uvebrant P, Nordborg C, Olsson I. Temporal lobe resections in children with epilepsy: neuropsychiatric status in relation to neuropathology and seizure outcome. Epilepsy Behav. 2002;3(1):76–81.
8. McLellan A, Davies S, Heyman I, Harding B, Harkness W, Taylor D, Neville BG, Cross JH. Psychopathology in children with epilepsy before and after temporal lobe resection. Dev Med Child Neurol. 2005;47(10):666–72.
9. Lendt M, Helmstaedt C, Kuczaty S, Schramm J, Elger C. Behavioural disorders in children with epilepsy: early improvement after surgery. J Neurol Neurosurg Psychiatry. 2000;69(6):739–44.
10. Danielsson S, Viggedal G, Steffenburg S, Rydenhag B, Gillberg C, Olsson I. Psychopathology, psychosocial functioning, and IQ before and after epilepsy surgery in children with drug-resistant epilepsy. Epilepsy Behav. 2009;14(2):330–7.
11. Penfield W, Jaspar HH. Epilepsy and the functional anatomy of the human brain. Boston: Little, Brown; 1954. p. 841–2.

12. Hermann B, Seidenberg M. Executive system dysfunction in temporal lobe epilepsy: effects of nociferous cortex versus hippocampal pathology. J Clin Exp Neuropsychol. 1995;17(6):809–19.
13. Shields WD. Effects of epilepsy surgery on psychiatric and behavioral comorbidities in children and adolescents. Epilepsy Behav. 2004;5 Suppl 3:S18–24.
14. Blumer D, Wakhlu S, Davies K, Hermann B. Psychiatric outcome of temporal lobectomy for epilepsy: incidence and treatment of psychiatric complications. Epilepsia. 1998;39(5):478–86.
15. Macrodimitris S, Sherman EM, Forde S, Tellez-Zenteno JF, Metcalfe A, Hernandez-Ronquillo L, Wiebe S, Jetté N. Psychiatric outcomes of epilepsy surgery: a systematic review. Epilepsia. 2011;52(5):880–90.
16. Smith ML, Elliott IM, Lach L. Cognitive, psychosocial, and family function one year after pediatric epilepsy surgery. Epilepsia. 2004;45(6):650–60.
17. Colonnelli MC, Cross JH, Davies S, D'Argenzio L, Scott RC, Pickles A, Hannan S, Harkness W, Heyman I. Psychopathology in children before and after surgery for extratemporal lobe epilepsy. Dev Med Child Neurol. 2012;54(6):521–6.
18. Besag FM. Psychopathological outcome of extratemporal lobe surgery: the need for international collaboration on data collection. Dev Med Child Neurol. 2012;54(6):486.
19. Sinclair DB, Aronyk K, Snyder T, McKean JD, Wheatley M, Gross D, Bastos A, Ahmed SN, Hao C, Colmers W. Extratemporal resection for childhood epilepsy. Pediatr Neurol. 2004;30(3):177–85.
20. Wilson PJ. Cerebral hemispherectomy for infantile hemiplegia. A report of 50 cases. Brain. 1970;93(1):147–80.
21. Pulsifer MB, Brandt J, Salorio CF, Vining EP, Carson BS, Freeman JM. The cognitive outcome of hemispherectomy in 71 children. Epilepsia. 2004;45(3):243–54.
22. Yonekawa T, Nakagawa E, Takeshita E, Inoue Y, Inagaki M, Kaga M, Sugai K, Sasaki M, Kaido T, Takahashi A, Otsuki T. Effect of corpus callosotomy on attention deficit and behavioral problems in pediatric patients with intractable epilepsy. Epilepsy Behav. 2011;22(4):697–704.
23. Cendes F, Ragazzo PC, da Costa V, Martins LF. Corpus callosotomy in treatment of medically resistant epilepsy: preliminary results in a pediatric population. Epilepsia. 1993;34(5):910–7.
24. Maehara T, Shimizu H. Surgical outcome of corpus callosotomy in patients with drop attacks. Epilepsia. 2001;42:67–71.
25. Yang TF, Wong TT, Kwan SY, Chang KP, Lee YC, Hsu TC. Quality of life and life satisfaction in families after a child has undergone corpus callosotomy. Epilepsia. 1996;37(1):76–80.
26. Gilliam F, Wyllie E, Kotagal P, Geckler C, Rusyniak G. Parental assessment of functional outcome following corpus callosotomy. Epilepsia. 1996;37:535–75.
27. Harvey AS, Freeman JL, Berkovic SF, Rosenfeld JV. Transcallosal resection of hypothalamic hamartomas in patients with intractable epilepsy. Epileptic Disord. 2003;5(4):257–65.
28. Fohlen M, Lellouch A, Delalande O. Hypothalamic hamartoma with refractory epilepsy: surgical procedures and results in 18 patients. Epileptic Disord. 2003;5(4):267–73.
29. Spencer S, Huh L. Outcomes of epilepsy surgery in adults and children. Lancet Neurol. 2008;7:525–37.

Chapter 9
Mortality After Epilepsy Surgery

Torbjörn Tomson

Abstract This chapter reviews publications on long-term mortality after epilepsy surgery. Overall, eight studies based on epilepsy surgery cohorts from six different centers in the USA, the UK, or Brazil were identified. In addition, two nationwide population-based studies, from Sweden and Norway, respectively, were reviewed. The number of surgery cases in the cohorts ranged from 202 to 596. The studies were very heterogeneous in terms of age groups, types of epilepsy and surgery, methods for reporting mortality outcomes as well as comparison groups.

The interpretation of studies is further hampered by their observational nature, whether comparisons are made with refractory epilepsy patients found unsuitable for surgery or between epilepsy surgery patients with favorable and unfavorable seizure outcomes.

In the surgery cohorts, the cause of death was epilepsy related in on average 50 % of the cases with sudden unexpected death (SUDEP) being the most common. Most studies report lower mortality among those rendered seizure free versus those with recurrent seizures after surgery, while the trend in the same direction was non-significant in the two population-based studies.

Keywords Epilepsy surgery • Outcome • Observational study • Mortality • Standardized mortality ratio • Survival • Cause of death

T. Tomson, MD, PhD
Department of Clinical Neuroscience, Karolinska Institutet, Stockholm SE 171 76, Sweden

Department of Neurology, Karolinska University Hospital, Stockholm SE 171 76, Sweden
e-mail: torbjorn.tomson@karolinska.se

K. Malmgren et al. (eds.), *Long-Term Outcomes of Epilepsy Surgery in Adults and Children*, DOI 10.1007/978-3-319-17783-0_9

Introduction

Life expectancy has been reported to be reduced [1] and overall mortality rate increased among people with epilepsy [2]. The latter is commonly described using the measure standardized mortality ratio (SMR), defined as the ratio of the observed numbers of deaths in the study population (with epilepsy) to the expected number of deaths estimated by standardization to the reference population. The SMR ranges from 2 to 3 in community-based studies of incident cases of epilepsy from high income countries [2] thus demonstrating a two- to threefold increased mortality rate among people with epilepsy in general. The highest SMRs are seen during the first years after seizure onset [2–5], and are to a large extent related to underlying causes and comorbidities of epilepsy [6]. However, a significant excess mortality is observed also decades after seizure onset [2–7]. Patients with chronic refractory epilepsy have particularly high mortality rates, and in such populations the causes of death are also more related to the epilepsy and the seizures than to the cause of epilepsy [8, 9]. The specific causes vary with the setting, but sudden unexpected death in epilepsy (SUDEP) and seizure-related accidents are more prevalent in particular among epilepsy surgery candidates [10–13]. As an example, the incidence of SUDEP has been reported to be as high as 9 per 1,000 patient years among epilepsy surgery candidates [14, for review see 15].

As this volume is about long-term outcomes, this chapter will not discuss the low perioperative mortality, but rather focus on mortality as reported in long-term follow-up after epilepsy surgery. An assessment of the long-term outcome of surgery in terms of mortality would ideally be based on a randomized controlled study comparing the outcome in those randomized to surgery versus those randomized to no surgery. The only available study of this kind randomized 80 patients to immediate surgery or after the regular one-year waiting list for surgery [16]. During the one-year follow-up one patient died (of SUDEP) in the non-surgery group versus none among those that had undergone surgery. The sample size and follow-up time is clearly insufficient for a meaningful comparison of mortality, which was not the primary end-point of the study. Other available information on mortality after surgery is based on prospective observational studies, or sometimes retrospective analyses of epilepsy surgery cohorts from individual centers or in a couple of cases data from nationwide epilepsy surgery registries. Outcome has unfortunately been reported in a non-standardized manner, as proportion deceased, as mortality rates, or SMRs. Some have not provided any comparisons, others have compared mortality in those who underwent surgery with epilepsy patients that for some reason were considered unsuitable for surgery or who declined the procedure. Due to this heterogeneity in study design each reviewed study is reported individually in the following.

Single Center Studies

An early report comprised a consecutive and complete cohort of adults and adolescents who had entered evaluation for surgery for intractable epilepsy at the University of California, Los Angeles (UCLA), from 1974 to early 1990. Overall outcome data were first reported in 1995 [17] and with some more elaboration on mortality in 1997 [18]. Of 248 patients admitted, 202 were considered surgery patients. Of these, one drowned before scheduled surgery, three died in complications of presurgical invasive diagnostic procedures, and one died from a complication of resective surgery outside the program; 175 had anterior temporal resections and 22 extratemporal resections. Of the remaining 46 non-surgery patients, an epileptogenic region could not be localized in 42, two had contraindications for surgery, and two eventually declined surgery. The mean follow-up time for surgery patients was 5.8 years (during which 11 patients had repeat operations) and for the non-surgery cases 5.7 years. There were overall 18 deaths during follow-up in addition to the 5 deaths during the presurgical or perioperative evaluation mentioned above. In total, 14 of the 202 surgery patients were dead at follow-up (7 %), 9 of which occurred during the extended follow-up of the 197 patients that had survived pre- or immediate postoperative period (5 %). In contrast 9 of the 46 non-surgery patients (20 %) were deceased at follow-up. Unfortunately, causes of death were not systematically analyzed in this study. Some information on seizure control was available for 16 of the 18 deaths during follow-up. Two or more seizures had been experienced by 13 of the 16 deceased patients (81 %) over the last year preceding follow-up compared with 47 % among the survivors.

Salanova et al. [19] included 215 consecutive patients (age 8–57 years at surgery) with refractory temporal lobe epilepsy that had been treated surgically by the same neurosurgeon at a single US center between 1984 and 1999. The follow-up time ranged from 1–15 years; mean 7 years. There was no immediate surgical mortality. Eleven of the 215 patients died during follow-up (5 %) 1–9 years after surgery. One patient died of breast cancer, two committed suicide, two died in accidents, three died during seizures, three "suddenly and for unexplained reasons." The latter six might be compatible with a diagnosis of SUDEP, but sufficient detail is lacking. Of the 11 deaths, 3 occurred among the 148 that were seizure free (2 %) compared with 8 of the 67 patients who continued to have seizures after surgery (12 %). The SMR for seizure free patients was calculated to 1.7 (0.35–5.0) compared with 7.4 (3.2–14.5) for those with continued seizures. These investigators did not provide any comparison with patients that had declined surgery or that were considered unsuitable.

A third US single center study from Jefferson Comprehensive Epilepsy Center in Philadelphia published follow-up data on 393 patients in 1999 [10] and an extended series from the same center in 2005 [11]. The latter publication comprised all 583 patients who had undergone epilepsy surgery for refractory seizures between February 1st, 1986 and June 30th, 2000. The neurosurgical procedures included resections, multiple subpial transections (altogether 521), and partial or complete corpus callosum sections ($n=62$). Follow-up after surgery ended on September 15, 2000. At the end of follow-up 19 of the 583 patients had died (3 %). One case died in the perioperative phase, SUDEP was the cause of death in 10, cancer outside the CNS in 3, suicide in 2, motor vehicle accident, pneumonia, and myocarditis, the cause of death in one case each. Twelve deaths were observed among the 265 patients with recurrent seizures after surgery (5 %), whereas, only one of the 256 seizure free patients died (0.4 %, in breast cancer). The SMR for patients with recurrent seizures was 5.75 (3.51–9.27) compared with 0.45 (0.02–2.94) among those rendered seizure free. SMR appeared to be higher among people with recurrent seizures after corpus callosotomy, 11.9 (4.84–27.36) compared with after resection or subpial transection, 4.56 (2.47–8.21), although the confidence intervals overlapped.

Bell and colleagues audited survival status in patients with intractable focal epilepsy evaluated for epilepsy surgery since 1989 at the National Hospital for Neurology and Neurosurgery in London, UK [20]. Two cohorts were included, (1) all 561 patients (aged 16–64 years) that undergone epilepsy surgery at the center, and (2) all 641 patients (aged 15–71 years) that were evaluated for epilepsy surgery but were deemed unsuitable after investigation, those who declined, those who died before surgery, and those still awaiting surgery. Included were only patients with a minimum follow-up of 0.8 years from the date of surgery or initial presurgical evaluation in the second group. The maximum follow-up time in the surgery group was 17.4 years and 15.4 years in the non-surgery group. Information on the types of surgical procedures is not provided. There were 40 known deaths in the nonsurgical group (during 3,365 years of follow-up) and 19 deaths in the surgery group (3,905 person years), the risk of dying being more than twice as high in the non-surgery cohort, Hazard Ratio 2.5 (1.5–4.4). Causes of death in the non-surgery group were considered to be epilepsy-related (SUDEP, drowning or status epilepticus) in 24 (20 of which in SUDEP), compared with in 7 for the surgery group. The surgery patients were divided according to seizure outcome after surgery into those who were completely seizure free or only had auras ("seizure free") versus those with seizures. Those with seizure at follow-up 1 year after surgery were 4.0 times (1.2–13.7, adjusted HR) more likely to die than those considered seizure free at 1 year follow-up.

Mortality outcomes have also been assessed in patients of all ages who underwent temporal resections for drug-resistant temporal lobe epilepsy at Maudsley Hospital, London, UK, between December 1st, 1975 and December 1st, 1995. The first report analyzed survival status of 299 of 305 consecutive patients followed up to December 1st 1997 [12]. At that time of follow-up 20 patients had died. Three deaths were considered a result of a direct operative complication. Thirteen of the deaths were considered to be epilepsy-related of which six were SUDEP, two in status epilepticus, two drowning, two in aspiration, and one accident. Only three of these 13 patients were seizure free after surgery until death. The overall SMR after surgery was 4.5 (3.2–6.6).

A second audit investigated late mortality in more or less the same cohort, epilepsy patients who had undergone temporal lobe surgery at Maudsley 1975–1995. In this audit deaths occurring after December 1st, 1997 until December 1st, 2009 were evaluated [21]. In the originally analyzed cohort of 305 patients, 21 were missing, but these were included in the extended follow-up. Excluded from the new analysis, however, were the 20 patients who died during the first audit period. The 306 patients included in this second analysis had an average follow-up of 11.7 years (range 2.3–12 years) adding up to a total of 3,569 patient-years. During this second audit period 19 patients died, of which 14 were males. The SMR was

2.01 (1.27–3.13) for male patients and 1.68 (0.70–4.03) among female patients. Six of the 19 deaths were considered epilepsy-related, all SUDEP. Only 2 of the 6 SUDEP patients were seizure free.

A single center study analyzed the incidence of SUDEP in a cohort of 550 patients with refractory epilepsy followed up by the Epilepsy Surgery Programme of the University Hospital of PUCRS, Porto Alegre, Brazil [22]. This cross-sectional study, carried out between January 1992 and July 2002, included 166 patients with refractory focal epilepsy that were epilepsy surgery candidates awaiting presurgical evaluation, and 384 patients that had already undergone epilepsy surgery (temporal lobe surgery in 221 and extratemporal in 163). The health status of the patients in the two groups was assessed by a telephone interview. There were no deaths secondary to the surgical procedure. Of the 384 surgery patients 14 (3.7 %) had died in probable SUDEP compared with 2 out of the 166 non-surgery patients (1.2 %).No other types of deaths were reported, but it is not clear if other deaths were excluded a priori. Of the 14 SUDEP cases in the surgery group, 12 were considered Engel Class I, i.e., seizure free (86 %). Among the 370 alive surgery patients 339 (92 %) were seizure free. However, the report does not state whether this refers to seizure outcome ever since surgery or a more limited time period. The observations from this study are indeed difficult to interpret as information on follow-up time and number of patient years in the two groups is missing. This is a major limitation since it is reasonable to assume that the observation time per patient in the surgery group is longer than for the patients awaiting presurgical assessment (non-surgery group).

Population-Based Studies

In contrast to these single center studies, Nilsson and collaborators [13] analyzed mortality in a population-based cohort of epilepsy surgery patients. The report is based on the nationwide Swedish National Epilepsy Surgery Register, which includes prospective data from all six operating centers in the country. All patients who were operated for epilepsy ($n = 596$, and 651 surgical procedures) or entered presurgical evaluation not leading to an operation ($n = 212$) between January 1990 and December 1998, were followed in the Cause-of-Death Register until December 1998. All ages were included. The most common surgical procedure was temporal lobe resections (57 %), followed by extratemporal resections (22 %) and callosotomies (12 %). Of the surgery patients 14 died during follow-up (2.3 %). One death was in a surgical complication, six of the deaths were in SUDEP, one in drowning, and the remaining in different malignancies. Among the non-surgery patients five died (2.4 %) of which four in SUDEP. In the surgery cohort, the SMR was 4.9 (2.7–8.3) compared with 7.9 (2.6–18.4) in the non-surgery group. The SUDEP incidence was 2.4 per 1,000 patient years in the surgery group and 6.3 per 1,000 patient years among non-surgery patients. Data on seizure outcome were limited to 2-year postoperative seizure control, which was available for 500 of the surgery patients.

This hampered attempts to evaluate mortality by seizure outcome, SMR was 3.8 (1.3–9.0) among those seizure free at 2-year follow-up compared to 4.3 (1.6–9.4) in the group with recurrent seizures. However, a more detailed analysis of the SUDEP cases including their medical records revealed that 5 of the 6 cases had recurrent seizures after surgery.

Another population-based nationwide study compared survival of patients that had been operated for focal epilepsy in Norway between 1948 and 1988, with a matched (for time, age, sex, seizure type) control group of patients with intractable focal epilepsy with medical management ($n=139$), and matched individuals from the general population ($n=196$) [22]. Out of the original 240 epilepsy surgery patients, 39 were excluded because the indication for surgery was a known brain tumor, and five that died from brain tumor within 5 years after surgery, leaving 196 surgery patients, aged 4–60 years at surgery, for evaluation. Only resective surgery for focal epilepsy was included. Resections were temporal in 106 (56 %), and frontal in 43 (23 %). The average follow-up time after surgery was 25 years and survival status determined by record linkage to the Death Certificate Register of Norway. The risk ratio for death in the surgery group was 0.63 (0.38–1.05) compared with the matched non-surgery epilepsy controls. For surgery patients that were seizure free 2 years after surgery, the risk ratio was 0.50 (0.17–1.18) compared with their matched controls ($n=50$ pairs). There were in total 34 deaths in the surgery group and 45 in the matched epilepsy group. The causes of death, in the two groups were considered similar based on ICD codes in the register. In the surgery group five died in accidents or suicide, four in SUDEP, and 4 in epilepsy (not further specified), these epilepsy-related death accounting for 39 % of the deaths.

Survival of the epilepsy surgery patients was lower than for the controls from the general population, risk ratio for death was 6.22 (3.08–12.58). The risk ration for those seizure free 2 years after surgery was 6.00 (1.34–26.81) compared with the matched general population, and 7.75 (2.74–21.96) for those with seizures at 2 years.

Conclusions

The interpretation of studies on mortality after surgery is hampered by their observational nature, whether comparisons are made with refractory epilepsy patients found unsuitable for surgery or between epilepsy surgery patients with favorable and unfavorable seizure outcome. Most of the single center studies attempted to assess mortality by seizure outcome (See Appendix). However, in many cases (including the Swedish and Norwegian population-based studies) seizure outcome status was assessed at a specific time point after surgery, typically 2 years, whereas follow-up of survival may extend over many decades.

Having more than one seizure over the last year was more common among the deceased compared with survivors [17], and deaths occurred more frequently in the group with seizures after surgery than among seizure free patients [11, 19, 20]. Although the population-based studies did not find a significant difference in overall mortality between those seizure free and those with seizures 2 years after surgery, the trend was in the direction of lower mortality among seizure free [13, 22].

During follow-up mortality was higher among patient found unsuitable for surgery compared with the surgery groups in the two single center studies where this was properly assessed [18, 20], whereas the two population-based studies showed nonsignificant trends for lower mortality in the surgery cohort compared with non-surgery controls of patients with refractory epilepsy [13, 22].

Causes of death in the surgery cohorts were reported in eight of the reviewed studies (See Appendix). Excluding one study that only reported SUDEP [23], the causes were epilepsy related (including SUDEP, seizures/status epilepticus, accidents, drowning, and suicide) in 50 % on average (range 37–91 %).

Overall, despite the methodological limitations with these observational studies, the data demonstrate that epilepsy surgery patients with refractory epilepsy to a large extent die from epilepsy- and seizure-related causes, and suggest that successful epilepsy surgery resulting in seizure freedom is likely to reduce the risk of premature mortality.

Appendix. Summary of Study Characteristics from Single Center Studies of Mortality After Epilepsy Surgery

Country and reference	Surgery cases, *n*	Age, years	Type of surgery/ epilepsy	Follow-up average, years	Comparison with non-surgery	Association with seizure outcome assessed	Causes of death analyzed
USA [18]	202	Adolescents and adults	All respective surgeries	5.8	Yes	Yes	Yes
USA [19]	215	8–57	TLE	7	No	Yes	Yes
USA [11]	521	11–66	All	4.9	No	Yes	Yes
UK [20]	561	16–64	Not known	6.9	Yes	Yes	Yes
UK[a][12]	305	All ages	TLE	9.1	No	Yes	Yes
UK[a][21]	306	All ages	TLE	11.7	No	Yes	Yes
Brazil [23]	384	All ages	All?	Not known	Yes	Yes	Only SUDEP, not clear

TLE Temporal lobe epilepsy
[a]Largerly the same cohort but different time spans of follow-up

References

1. Gaitatzis A, Johnson AL, Chadwick DW, Shorvon SD, Sander JW. Life expectancy in people with newly diagnosed epilepsy. Brain. 2004;127(Pt 11):2427–32.
2. Forsgren L, Hauser WA, Olafsson E, Sander JW, Sillanpaa M, Tomson T. Mortality of epilepsy in developed countries: a review. Epilepsia. 2005;46 Suppl 11:18–27.
3. Hauser WA, Annegers JF, Elveback LR. Mortality in patients with epilepsy. Epilepsia. 1980;21:399–412.
4. Lindsten H, Nystrom L, Forsgren L. Mortality risk in an adult cohort with a newly diagnosed unprovoked epileptic seizure: a population-based study. Epilepsia. 2000;41:1469–73.
5. Neligan A, Bell GS, Johnson AL, Goodridge DM, Shorvon SD, Sander JW. The long-term risk of premature mortality in people with epilepsy. Brain. 2011;134:388–95.
6. Lhatoo SD, Sander JWAS. Cause-specific mortality in epilepsy. Epilepsia. 2005;46 Suppl 11:36–9.
7. Sillanpaa M, Shinnar S. Long-term mortality in childhood-onset epilepsy. N Engl J Med. 2010;363:2522–9.
8. Mohanraj R, Norrie J, Stephen LJ, Kelly K, Hitiris N, Brodie MJ. Mortality in adults with newly diagnosed and chronic epilepsy: a retrospective comparative study. Lancet Neurol. 2006;5:481–7.
9. Rakitin A, Liik M, Oun A, Haldre S. Mortality risk in adults with newly diagnosed and chronic epilepsy: a population-based study. Eur J Neurol. 2011;18:465–70.
10. Sperling MR, Feldman H, Kinman J, Liporace JD, O'Connor MJ. Seizure control and mortality in epilepsy. Ann Neurol. 1999;46:45–50.
11. Sperling MR, Harris A, Nei M, Liporace JD, O'Connor MJ. Mortality after epilepsy surgery. Epilepsia. 2005;46 Suppl 11:49–53.
12. Hennessy MJ, Langan Y, Elwes RD, et al. A study of mortality after temporal lobe epilepsy surgery. Neurology. 1999;53:1276–83.
13. Nilsson L, Ahlbom A, Farahmand BY, Tomson T. Mortality in a population-based cohort of epilepsy surgery patients. Epilepsia. 2003;44:575–81.
14. Dasheiff RM. Sudden unexpected death in epilepsy: a series from an epilepsy surgery program and speculation on the relationship to sudden cardiac death. J Clin Neurophysiol. 1991;8:216–22.
15. Tomson T, Nashef L, Ryvlin P. Sudden unexpected death in epilepsy: current knowledge and future directions. Lancet Neurol. 2008;7:1021–31.
16. Wiebe S, Blume WT, Girvin JP, Eliasziw M. Effectiveness and efficiency of surgery for temporal lobe epilepsy study group. A randomized, controlled trial of surgery for temporal-lobe epilepsy. N Engl J Med. 2001;345(5):311–8.
17. Vickrey BG. Mortality in a consecutive cohort of 248 adolescents and adults who underwent diagnostic evaluation for epilepsy surgery. Epilepsia. 1997;38:S67–9.
18. Vickrey BG, Hays RD, Rausch R, et al. Outcomes in 248 patients who had diagnostic evaluations for epilepsy surgery. Lancet. 1995;346:1445–9.
19. Salanova V, Markand O, Worth R. Temporal lobe epilepsy surgery: outcome, complications, and late mortality rate in 215 patients. Epilepsia. 2002;43:170–4.
20. Bell GS, Sinha S, Tisi J, Stephani C, Scott CA, Harkness WF, McEvoy AW, Peacock JL, Walker MC, Smith SJ, Duncan JS, Sander JW. Premature mortality in refractory partial epilepsy: does surgical treatment make a difference? J Neurol Neurosurg Psychiatry. 2010;81(7):716–8.
21. Seymour N, Granbichler CA, Polkey CE, Nashef L. Mortality after temporal lobe epilepsy surgery. Epilepsia. 2012;53(2):267–71.
22. Stavem K, Guldvog B. Long-term survival after epilepsy surgery compared with matched epilepsy controls and the general population. Epilepsy Res. 2005;63(1):67–75.
23. Almeida AG, Nunes ML, Palmini AL, Costa JC. Incidence of SUDEP in a cohort of patients with refractory epilepsy: the role of surgery and lesion localization. Arq Neuropsiquiatr. 2010;68(6):898–902.

Chapter 10
Long-Term Educational and Vocational Outcomes of Adults After Epilepsy Surgery

Sarah J. Wilson and Honor Coleman

Abstract People with epilepsy typically have higher rates of unemployment and underemployment when compared to healthy peers or individuals with other chronic illnesses. It is unsurprising then, that patients often hope that epilepsy surgery will improve their postoperative vocational functioning. This chapter reviews published research examining the longer-term educational and vocational outcomes of adults undergoing epilepsy surgery. Since studies specifically investigating educational and vocational outcomes in adults are scarce, much of our knowledge comes from work looking at broader psychosocial outcomes. This makes it difficult to draw strong conclusions about factors, other than seizure outcome, that may impact vocational and employment outcomes after surgery, such as premorbid cognitive ability or behavioral coping strategies, among others. In general, seizure freedom is the strongest predictor of improvement in occupational status after surgery, followed by presurgical educational attainment and employment status, with those who are studying or working full-time before surgery continuing to show better functioning after surgery. Our review of the literature highlights the need for longer-term, longitudinal studies to accurately track individual trajectories of educational and vocational outcomes relative to medically treated patients and healthy controls to determine whether surgery results in significant improvements, or whether outcomes are primarily accounted for by presurgical functioning. The effectiveness of postoperative vocational rehabilitation strategies also requires systematic research. We argue that adopting a lifespan perspective is important for determining what constitutes a successful educational or vocational outcome for different individuals, and the range of factors that may lead to this outcome.

Keywords Employment • Education • Epilepsy surgery • Long-term outcome • Temporal lobe resection

---

S.J. Wilson, PhD (✉)
Melbourne School of Psychological Sciences, The University of Melbourne, Melbourne, VIC 3010, Australia

Comprehensive Epilepsy Program, Austin Health, Melbourne, VIC Australia
e-mail: sarahw@unimelb.edu.au

H. Coleman
Melbourne School of Psychological Sciences, The University of Melbourne, Melbourne, VIC 3010, Australia

K. Malmgren et al. (eds.), *Long-Term Outcomes of Epilepsy Surgery in Adults and Children*, DOI 10.1007/978-3-319-17783-0_10

Introduction

There are many studies examining the psychosocial and quality of life outcomes of adult patients undergoing epilepsy surgery within the early months to years after surgery [1]. Moreover, the range of postoperative psychosocial adjustment issues faced by patients and their families has been well documented, particularly within the first 24 months [2, 3]. These difficulties may prove disruptive to the process of acquiring and maintaining stable employment post-surgery, particularly if the individual has limited education or vocational skills before surgery. Consistent with this, studies have demonstrated that especially for patients who are unemployed before surgery, it can take more than 2 years following surgery to find employment [4]. Researchers have therefore acknowledged the importance of longer-term outcome studies (i.e., over 5 years post-surgery) to gain a more stable view of the vocational prognosis of epilepsy surgery [5–7]. In this chapter, we review published research examining the educational and vocational outcomes of adults 5 or more years after surgery.

At the outset, it should be noted that many studies follow patients from childhood or adolescence into adulthood, blurring the distinction between pediatric and adult vocational outcome studies. It is often important to traverse these age groups when considering a patient's progression in education and employment, as late adolescence and early adulthood represent the formative years of education, vocational training and employment, providing a foundation for later adulthood [8]. A further challenge to assessing longer-term vocational outcome studies is their frequent use of cross-sectional outcome designs, such that even if the average follow-up is 5 years, this can represent the combined educational and vocational outcomes of patients from 6 months to 10 years post-surgery [9]. In addition, those studies limiting their assessment of outcome to adult samples typically include patients ranging in age anywhere from 17 to 60 years at the time of surgery [10]. This is problematic because normal developmental processes and adjustment issues associated with life after surgery can differ widely across this age range, making it difficult to determine what constitutes a "successful" educational or vocational outcome for a given individual. For instance, the issues faced by a 17-year-old patient who is attempting to enter the workforce 5 years post-surgery, will differ markedly to those faced by a 60-year-old considering retirement, irrespective of their surgical outcomes. Lifespan-oriented, longitudinal studies therefore provide the ideal method of follow-up to track an individual's educational and vocational trajectory relative to preoperative levels of functioning and the developmental tasks associated with the individual's particular phase of the lifespan post-surgery [10].

Even when considering both cross-sectional and longitudinal studies, there is a scarcity of research directly examining the longer-term educational and vocational outcomes of adult epilepsy surgery patients. This is because the bulk of research to date has sought to examine broad, quantitative indices of psychosocial functioning, with questions pertaining to education and vocational opportunities briefly canvassed alongside of measures of personal or financial independence and driving [11,

12]. For example, studies often assign patients to broad categories of educational and vocational status, such as "student," "part-time employment," "full-time employment," or "sick-pay/ pension," to capture general changes pre- to post-surgery [12]. However, this provides minimal information about the nature of education or employment change for a given individual, or the factors most relevant to producing this change. Moreover, there is limited research comparing employment outcomes for different types of surgical resections or neuropathology, or associating employment outcomes with other post-surgery variables, such as psychiatric outcome [12, 13].

The Importance of Educational and Vocational Outcomes

Despite intellectual functioning predominantly within the average range, individuals with chronic epilepsy have a higher incidence of unemployment or underemployment [6, 14, 15]. Underemployment has been used to refer to an individual who is employed, but not in the desired capacity, in terms of remuneration, hours of employment, or level of skill and experience. Both unemployment and underemployment have been found to significantly impact on the quality of life of people with epilepsy [6]. Surveys from the United States and Great Britain suggest that between 25 and 46 % of people with epilepsy may be unemployed, compared with an estimate of 19 % for an age and sex-matched population without epilepsy [16]. Furthermore, a Canadian survey demonstrated that people with epilepsy show decreased rates of employment compared to both healthy peers and individuals with other chronic conditions. The number of annual disability days taken by people with epilepsy (41 ± 5) was much higher than those taken by people with other chronic illnesses (26 ± 1), the general population (17 ± 1), and healthy people (0.5 ± 0.25) [17].

Education and employment provide a range of benefits, from financial security, to social interaction, to improved feelings of independence and competence that can promote a positive self-image [15]. Employment has been positively correlated with quality of life [18, 19] and higher self-efficacy in people with epilepsy [20], while unemployment has been identified as a contributing factor to depression [21, 22]. It is not surprising then, that in adults deemed eligible for epilepsy surgery, employment is a commonly cited reason for electing to undergo surgery. Both patients and their families identify educational and vocational outcomes as important, with expectations of improvements post-surgery [7, 23–27]. Following the operation, studies have demonstrated that employment outcomes are directly relevant to patient satisfaction with surgery up to 10 years later [7].

When considering a patient's educational and vocational goals, the timing of surgery is often pertinent and should be evaluated relative to the patient's age and phase of psychosocial development [24, 28]. For instance, in some cases an adolescent or young adult may wish to delay undergoing surgery until the final year of school or university has been completed to minimize any disruption of surgery and postoperative recovery on educational outcomes. Alternatively, in other cases an earlier operation might be sought to minimize the effects of drug-resistant seizures and high dose pharmacotherapy on cognition, and therefore educational attainment. As for all treatment expectations, educational and vocational issues need to be carefully discussed between the treating team and the patient and family prior to surgery to ensure that expectations are realistic, that the timing of surgery is optimal, and that any relevant postoperative rehabilitation supports are in place [19, 24].

Educational and Vocational Outcomes: A Review of the Evidence

A recent systematic review of the long-term social outcomes following anterior temporal lobectomy (ATL) identified employment and driving as the two most commonly studied outcomes [12], yet there is still a relative paucity of data relating to these outcomes. This chapter reviews the available literature examining long-term educational and vocational outcomes following all types of epilepsy surgery (summarized in the Appendix). Databases including Medline, PubMed, PsychINFO, and ScienceDirect were searched for peer-reviewed studies published in English between 1980 and 2014 using various combinations of the following search terms: *long-term, psychosocial, education, vocational, employment, outcomes,* and *epilepsy surgery.* A total of 116 studies were identified. After duplicates were removed, studies were excluded if they had ≤20 participants, or participants aged ≤13 years at surgery. Inclusion criteria were an average follow-up time of 5 years or more, or an average close to 5 years and a range that extended beyond 5 years.

As shown in the Appendix, this resulted in a total of 16 studies included in the review, published between 1984 and 2013. Two of these studies relate to pediatric surgical candidates [9, 29], one to a mixed cohort of children and adults [30], and 13 to adult candidates [4, 7, 10, 32–41]. Ten (63 %) studies were conducted in the United States, two (13 %) in the United Kingdom, and one (6 %) each in Canada, France, Norway, and Sweden. Only three of the studies focused solely on employment status pre- to post-surgery [4, 33, 35]. The remaining 13 studies investigated employment outcomes alongside measures of quality of life [10, 36], driving and socioeconomic status [30–32, 37–39, 42], mood [7, 41] and social functioning [34, 40], or were part of a longer-term follow-up of pediatric patients, also investigating social and behavioral outcomes [9, 29]. Studies directly focusing on vocational outcomes allowed more in-depth descriptions of occupational histories or the utilization of more fine-grained categories of employment outcome, such as differentiating between patients who were voluntarily unemployed (homemakers) and those who were involuntarily unemployed after surgery [4, 33, 35].

Of the 16 studies, ten (63 %) studies assessed outcome after temporal lobectomy [4, 9, 10, 30, 32, 35, 37–40], while the remaining six (37 %) included both temporal and extratemporal resections [7, 33, 34, 36, 41] and/or hemispherectomies [29]. Only three (19 %) studies utilized a nonsurgical, medically managed control group, despite the importance of this group for assessing the impact of surgery over and above the impact of long-standing epilepsy and its pharmacological treatment [5, 6]. The use of healthy controls can help to contextualize patient vocational outcomes relative to healthy peers progressing through similar life stages. Despite this, only one study used a healthy control group [32]. They were able to demonstrate that up to 10 years post-surgery, even though patients who were seizure free were more likely to be employed than those with recurrent seizures, overall, patients were still working significantly less than healthy controls (61 % compared to 96 %) [32]. Across all studies, age of epilepsy onset ranged from 1 to 58 years, with an average age of 10.7 years,[1] while age at surgery ranged from 3 to 64 years, with an estimated average of 28.4 years. The average follow-up period across studies was 7 years (ranging from 1 to 28 years). In other words, while the literature on vocational outcomes of adult epilepsy surgery considers an "average" patient with chronic epilepsy (>15 years) undergoing surgery in young adulthood, there is substantial variation in both age at surgery and length of follow-up, limiting the strength of the conclusions that can currently be drawn for any particular age group.

Overall, the majority of studies (75 %) suggest improved vocational outcomes [7, 9, 10, 29–33, 35, 36, 38–40], however, one study reported a decline in the number of patients employed full-time following surgery [41], and three (19 %) suggested a mix of improvements and reductions in occupational status [4, 34, 37]. In particular, a study by Asztely and colleagues [41] demonstrated a reduction in full-time employment status from pre- to post-surgery; however, this was collapsed across seizure free and seizure recurrent patients. On closer inspection, those who attained seizure freedom following surgery maintained relative levels of employment from pre-surgery (82 %) to long-term follow-up (74 %), with a small increase in full-time employment (20 pre-surgery to 22 at long-term follow-up) [41]. In comparison, the number of employed patients with recurrent seizures was halved at long-term follow-up (30 %) compared to baseline levels (63 %). Studies reporting mixed findings also assessed vocational outcomes collapsed across all patients [37], used unique seizure outcome groupings [4], or extended follow-up periods without accounting for the impact of retirement [34].

Three studies investigated educational outcomes in pediatric samples [9, 29, 30], while three studies compared the percentage of adult patients studying pre- to post-surgery [35, 37, 41]. Two of the pediatric studies showed improvements in educational domains in ≥60 % of patients [9, 30], while all three adult studies demonstrated a decrease in the number of patients studying post-surgery [35, 37, 41]. The latter most likely reflects age-appropriate transitions from educational to vocational realms, again highlighting the importance of adopting a lifespan perspective. A cross-sectional study conducted by Mizrahi et al. [30] directly compared pediatric and adult outcomes, revealing that younger patients had greater improvements in educational and vocational status (62.5 %) compared to adult patients (37.5 %). This appears to be a consistent finding in the literature [8, 43]; however, prospective longitudinal studies are needed to map the translation of educational achievements to occupational gains from childhood to young adulthood.

---

[1] This, and other estimates, do not account for studies where age of onset/age at surgery were not reported.

In support of the efficacy of surgical treatment, the three studies comparing surgery to ongoing medical management demonstrate a trend towards higher employment following surgery [36, 38]. For two of these studies, however, there were significant baseline differences in seizure frequency, which was higher in the medically managed group [36, 38]. Nonetheless, following surgery, Jones et al. [38] reported a significantly higher number of patients (69 %) in full-time employment (69 % surgical, 39 % medical), while Vickrey and colleagues [36] reported a non-significant trend towards higher employment (59.6 % surgical, 51.1 % medical) after adjusting for those patients who had died. The third study by Guldvog and colleagues [34] found that a significant change in employment status was only observed in patients who were already in regular employment or education before surgery. In particular, around 60 % of surgically treated patients maintained full-time employment, compared to around 40 % of medically managed patients, leading the authors to conclude that surgical treatment, at the very least, ensures the maintenance of full-time employment [34]. These patients, however, underwent surgical treatment between 1949 and 1988 [34] and thus, may not reflect the benefits of recent advances in surgical techniques for cognition and vocational functioning [44, 45]. Despite the efficacy of surgery for improving vocational outcomes, long-term *full-time* employment rates vary between 54 and 74 % across studies [10, 38]. For those who experience seizure recurrence after surgery, lower rates of educational and vocational improvements are experienced [4, 7].

Predictors of Improved Vocational Outcomes After Surgery

Research to date has identified seizure control as the strongest predictor of employment status post-surgery [4, 7]. Both before and after surgery, educational and vocational functioning have been linked to seizure control in terms of the impact of habitual seizures on cognitive functioning [46], and their restrictions on employment and educational choices [14]. Patients who attain seizure freedom following surgery are significantly more likely to gain full-time employment or make progress in their employment when compared to those who continue to experience seizures following surgery [4, 7, 35]. For instance, one study indicated that the odds of working full-time 10 years following surgery are 9.5 times higher for seizure free patients compared to seizure recurrent patients. This improvement was not associated with side of resection, mood, nor impaired verbal memory, strongly implicating seizure outcome as the main driver of occupational change [32].

Differences in defining "seizure freedom" versus "seizure recurrence," however, make it difficult to compare findings across studies. For example, some studies define seizure freedom as a complete absence of seizures with or without auras [41], while others define seizure freedom as an absence of disabling seizures (allowing auras or nocturnal seizures) [37]. Alternatively, Sperling et al. [4] classified patients into three groups: (1) those completely seizure free following surgery, (2) those with a "mixed outcome" comprising some years of seizure freedom and some years with seizures, and (3) those with persistent seizures at around 5 years post-surgery. The seizure free group performed the best in terms of occupational outcomes, followed by the mixed group and finally, the persistent seizure group. No group differences were observed in pre-surgery education, occupational status, full-scale IQ, or global memory scores, leading the authors to propose an absence of confounding variables on the relationship between seizure control and occupational outcomes [4]. This suggests that studies utilising a stricter definition of seizure freedom may report greater improvements in vocational outcomes than those that adopt a less stringent definition, such as ≥75 % seizure improvement, or no disabling seizures.

In general, the relevance of other variables to vocational outcomes has been inconsistently reported. One study identified a number of factors significantly associated with postsurgical full-time work. These included presurgical education, work experience, employment factors, never having been in receipt of a disability pension, and postsurgical factors such as driving, further education, and improved seizure outcome. Of nine identified factors, those independently associated with full-time work following surgery included: (1) being a student or working full-time in the year before surgery (odds ratio of 16.2), (2) driving after surgery (odds ratio of 15.2), and (3) obtaining further education after surgery (odds ratio of 9.2) [37]. These point to the importance of having vocational skills in place before surgery, as well as providing vocational rehabilitation and support post-surgery [37].

Improving a patient's odds of gaining employment post-surgery via the use of postsurgical rehabilitation programs has only recently been investigated. In particular, Thorbecke and colleagues [13] conducted a two-year follow-up study assessing the effects of a rehabilitation program implemented over two stages. The first stage involved a broad, interdisciplinary program[2] provided in the first 3 weeks after surgery. The second stage was typically initiated around 6 months post-surgery and was oriented towards work integration and on-the-job-training for 2–3 weeks. The results were encouraging, with the rehabilitation group showing higher rates of postoperative employment compared to a control group, even after the significant effect of preoperative employment status had been taken into account [13].

In light of the significant advantages reported for patients with preoperative employment skills, Thorbecke and colleagues [13] suggested that patients who are unemployed before surgery may require a more intensive or extended intervention in order to acquire basic vocational skills and make gains post-surgery [13]. In particular, to maximize postsurgical vocational and educational outcomes, careful presurgical planning should be undertaken with the patient and the family. This may include engagement of the patient in prevocational counselling or skills training as well as postsurgical services such as those implemented by Thorbecke et al. [13]. Rehabilitation programs that provide comprehensive, multi-disciplinary services have been identified as creating the optimal environment for patients to realize their educational and vocational goals [47], and may directly contribute to perceptions of surgical success.

[2] Rehabilitation services included, among others, medical review, neuropsychological counselling, physiotherapy, speech therapy, social work counselling, and occupational therapy [13].

Conclusions

In summary, while surgery is generally thought to result in improvements in educational and vocational domains compared to medical therapy and, in particular, seizure freedom has been associated with the best outcomes, findings in the literature are mixed. Some studies support seizure outcome as the main driver of vocational change [4, 32], while others suggest that presurgical factors, such as educational and vocational attainments, play a similarly significant role [13, 37, 38]. Methodological limitations in the current literature, including limited use of comparison groups, and differences in age at the time of surgery and length of follow-up, likely contribute to variability in the current data.

There are still a number of relatively unexplored areas in the literature. For instance, while seizure freedom has been associated with improvements in occupational status, seizure freedom is also associated with improvements in self-esteem, reduced perceptions of stigma, and increased feelings of mastery [7]. Since gaining employment is dependent on a range of psychological and emotional skills, research is required to investigate the role that these psychological variables play over and above the cessation of seizures. Conversely, psychiatric comorbidities may have a negative impact on the ability of an individual to find and maintain employment, in line with broader findings from nonsurgical epilepsy studies [13]. This is particularly relevant for patients who experience seizure recurrence, as they tend to show poorer psychiatric outcomes, and thus, may benefit from increased psychological and vocational supports.

Finally, further research primarily focusing on educational and vocational outcomes is needed to enable clinicians to identify the factors most relevant to promoting positive changes in an individual's educational and vocational functioning post-surgery. A lifespan perspective provides a suitable framework for understanding the adjustment processes and life skills required by individuals to successfully achieve their educational and vocational goals after surgery. This, in turn, will assist in the development of more tailored rehabilitation programs that better equip patients for the changes that follow surgery relative to their phase of psychosocial development.

Appendix. Summary of Studies on Long-Term Educational and Vocational Outcomes of Adults After Epilepsy Surgery

Study	Sample	Design and follow-up period	Age at study	Age at onset	Age at surgery	Focus	Educational and vocational outcomes
Augustine et al. (1984) *USA*	32 temporal, frontal, or occipital-parietal resections	Cross-sectional, retrospective 3.9 years (1–10)	28.4 years (18–46)	11 years	NS	Employment status (pre- to post-surgery)	*FT Employment:* increased from 14 to 23 patients *Underemployed:* decreased from 8 to 0 patients *Unemployment:* stable, 10 pre-surgery to 9 post-surgery patients
Lindsay et al. (1984) *UK*	32 temporal lobectomy 10 hemispherectomy 8 extratemporal resections	Prospective 7 (<2 years) 12 (2–5 years) 22 (5–10 years) 9 (>10 years)	NS	Right-sided: 7.5 years Left-sided: 4.2 years	14 years (3–36)	Long-term psychosocial outcomes	*Educational:* for those studied in childhood, resolution of behavioral symptoms improved educational outcomes *Employment:* all 9 adult patients were employed post-surgery
Meyer et al. (1986) *USA*	50 temporal lobectomy	Cross-sectional, retrospective 4 years (0.6-10)	NS	7.5 years (1–14)	15.8 years (7–18)	Social and behavioral development	*Education/Employment:* 85 % in school or employed
Mizrahi et al. (1990) *USA*	22 temporal lobectomy (8 children, 14 adults)	Cross-sectional, retrospective 5 years (2–8)	NS	6 years (2–10)	21 years (7–36)	Educational, vocational and living status	*Employment:* 64 % of adults, and 25 % of children *Education:* 7 % of adults and 63 % of children in education at follow-up *Homemaker:* 7 % of adults and 13 % of children *Unemployed:* 21 % of adults

(continued)

Appendix (continued)

Study	Sample	Design and follow-up period	Age at study	Age at onset	Age at surgery	Focus	Educational and vocational outcomes
Guldvog et al. (1991) *Norway*	119 resective surgery 94 nonsurgical controls	Cross-sectional, retrospective Surgery: Md: 16 years (IQR: 12–27) Nonsurgery: Md: 17 years (IQR: 12–28)	NS	Surgery: Md: 10 years (IQR: 3–21) Nonsurgery: Md: 8 years (IQR: 3–13)	Md: 23 years (IQR: 14–33)	Functioning in daily social life	*Employment:* of those who were employed before treatment, 58.1 % of surgery patients remained in regular work, compared to 39.6 % of nonsurgical controls; 3.8 % of surgical patients moved to supported work, compared to 13.2 % of nonsurgical controls; 38.8 % of surgical patients became unemployed, compared to 47.2 % of nonsurgical controls. Working or educational situation was dependent on pretreatment status
Chovaz et al. (1994) *Canada*	42 ATL	Cross-sectional, retrospective 5 years (1–14)	NS	NS	31 years (17–60)	HRQOL, learned helplessness, psychosocial adjustment, driving and employment	*FT Employment:* increased from 36 to 54 %
Sperling et al. (1995) *USA*	86 ATL Group 1: 35 SF Group 2: 20 mixed (some SF years, some years with seizures) Group 3: 18 persistent seizures	Cross-sectional, retrospective Group 1: 4.8 years (*SD* = 1.6) Group 2: 5.3 years (*SD* = 1.7) Group 3: 5.0 years (*SD* = 1.1)	NS	NS	Group 1: 31.7 years (*SD* = 7.4) Group 2: 35.4 years (*SD* = 7.9) Group 3: 33.7 years (*SD* = 9.6)	Employment status	*Unemployment:* decreased from 25 to 11 % *Group differences:* Group 1 demonstrated the highest rate of improvement and the highest rate of FT employment. Group 3 patients rarely improved, and often deteriorated (17 %).

Vickrey et al. (1995) *USA*	176 temporal lobe resection 22 extratemporal resection 46 nonsurgical controls	Prospective Surgery: 5.8 years Nonsurgery: 5.7 years	NS	Surgery: 11.9 years Nonsurgery: 12.0 year	Age at evaluation: Surgery: 27.0 years Nonsurgery: 26.0 years	Employment abd HRQOL	*FT/PT Employment:* following surgery 60.1 % of surgery patients versus 48.6 % of controls was employed.
Sperling et al. (1996) *USA*	89 ATL	Prospective 5 years	NS	13.1 years (*SD*=9.2)	31.9 years (*SD*=9.1) (10–60)	Employment status (pre-to post-surgery)	*FT Employment:* increased from 34 to 63 % *PT Employment:* decreased from 18 to 11 % *Homemakers:* stable, from 8 to 9 % *Students:* decreased from 16 to 6 % *Unemployment:* decreased from 24 to 11 %
Reeves et al. (1997) *USA*	134 ATL	Cross-sectional, retrospective 4.2 y (2.5–6.5 y)	NS	12 years	31 year	Activities of daily living, driving, change in work outcome and income.	*FT/PT Employment:* changed for 19 % of patients. Seven patients (all SF) made occupational gains, whereas 10 patients lost FT or PT work after surgery. *Students:* of the 21 studying FT before surgery, 48 % were FT students after surgery, 43 % became employed FT, and 4.5 % were in a sheltered workshop.

(continued)

Appendix (continued)

Study	Sample	Design and follow-up period	Age at study	Age at onset	Age at surgery	Focus	Educational and vocational outcomes
Jones et al. (2002) *USA*	61 ATL 23 nonsurgical controls	Cross-sectional, retrospective Surgery: 5.8 years (2–9) Nonsurgery: 5.7 years (2–9)	NS	Surgery: 11.5 years (*SD*=10.3) Nonsurgery: 15.1 years (*SD*=12.4)	Surgery: 31.3 years (*SD*=8.9) Nonsurgery: 34.7 years (*SD*=10.3)	Employment, driving, independent living and financial independence	*FT Employment:* higher in surgery group (69 %) than control group (39 %). Improvements generally the same across surgery and control groups (17 % and 15 %, respectively). *Unemployment:* lower rates for surgery group (25 %) than for controls (52 %). This cohort was followed up at 12 and 17 years in Jones et al. (2013). *FT Employment:* At 12 year follow-up, 61 % of the surgery group and 33 % of the control group were employed FT At 17 year follow-up 43 % of the surgery group, and 22 % of the control group were employed FT.
Reid et al. (2004) *UK*	64 temporal lobectomy 3 extratemporal lesionectomies	Cross-sectional, retrospective 10.3 years (*SD*=1.97)	41.4 years (*SD*=9.4)	11.2 years (*SD*=8.7)	NS	HRQOL, depression, anxiety, impact of epilepsy, self-esteem, mastery, affect balance, stigma and health status.	*Employment:* following surgery, 49.3 % had obtained employment. SF patients were significantly more likely to be employed at follow-up

Erickson et al. (2005) *USA*	84 temporal lobectomy	Cross-sectional, retrospective 4.2 years (1–5)	NS	13.7 years (0–46)	31 years (5–64)	Employment and driving	*Employment:* employment rates significantly increased following surgery, however, not significantly associated with seizure outcome
Dupont et al. (2006) *France*	110 temporal lobectomy	Cross-sectional, retrospective 7 years (*SD*=4) (1–17)	42 years (*SD*=9)	11 years (*SD*=9)	35 years (*SD*=10)	Patient perceptions of the impact of surgery on driving, professional, familial, social and marital status	*Improvements:* self-reported occupational improvements in 47 %. Of those reporting improvements, 31 were SF since surgery and 43 were SF for at least one year since baseline assessment *Reductions:* self-reported reductions in occupational status in 14 %
Asztely et al. (2007) *Sweden*	54 temporal lobe resections 16 extratemporal resections	Cross-sectional, retrospective 12.4 years (8.6-16.2)	47 years (32–68)	16.7 years (1–58)	NS	Driving, QOL, presence of depressive symptoms, employment and living situation	*FT/PT Employment:* decreased from 74 to 55 % *Studying:* decreased from 5 to 0 % *Sick Pay/Pension:* increased from 22 to 43 % *Parental Leave:* increased from 0 to 2 %
Andersson-Roswall et al. (2013) *USA*	51 temporal lobe resections 23 healthy controls	Prospective 10 years	NS	NS	33.7 years (SD=10.1)	Vocational outcomes; Sick-pay/pension; Living Status; Driving; Mood	*Employment:* 61% of patients and 96% of healthy controls were working in some capacity at follow-up *FT Employment:* 41% of patients and 74% of healthy controls were employed FT at follow-up *PT Employment:* 20% of patients and 22% of healthy controls were employed PT at follow-up

Note. ATL anterior temporal lobectomy, *FT* full-time, *HRQOL* health-related quality of life, *IQR* inter-quartile range, *Md* median, *NS* not specified, *PT* part-time, *QOL* quality of life, *SD* standard deviation, *SF* seizure free, *TLE* temporal lobe epilepsy

References

1. Seiam A-HR, Dhaliwal H, Wiebe S. Determinants of quality of life after epilepsy surgery: systematic review and evidence summary. Epilepsy Behav. 2011;21(4):441–5.
2. Wilson SJ, Bladin PF, Saling MM, McIntosh AM, Lawrence JA. The longitudinal course of adjustment after seizure surgery. Seizure. 2001;10(3):165–72.
3. Wilson SJ, Bladin PF, Saling MM, Pattison PE. Characterizing psychosocial outcome trajectories following seizure surgery. Epilepsy Behav. 2005;6(4):570–80.
4. Sperling MR, Saykin AJ, Roberts FD, French JA, O'Connor MJ. Occupational outcome after temporal lobectomy for refractory epilepsy. Neurology. 1995;45(5):970–7.
5. Hemb M, Palmini A, Paglioli E, Paglioli EB, Costa da Costa J, Azambuja N, et al. An 18-year follow-up of seizure outcome after surgery for temporal lobe epilepsy and hippocampal sclerosis. J Neurol Neurosurg Psychiatry. 2013;84(7):800–5.
6. Perry MS, Duchowny M. Surgical versus medical treatment for refractory epilepsy: outcomes beyond seizure control. Epilepsia. 2013;54(12):2060–70.
7. Reid K, Herbert A, Baker GA. Epilepsy surgery: patient-perceived long-term costs and benefits. Epilepsy Behav. 2004;5(1):81–7.
8. Zarroli K, Tracy JI, Nei M, Sharan A, Sperling MR. Employment after anterior temporal lobectomy. Epilepsia. 2011;52(5):925–31.
9. Meyer FB, Marsh WR, Laws Jr ER, Sharbrough FW. Temporal lobectomy in children with epilepsy. J Neurosurg. 1986;64:371–6.
10. Chovaz CJ, McLachlan RS, Derry PA, Cummings AL. Psychosocial function following temporal lobectomy: influence of seizure control and learned helplessness. Seizure. 1994;3(3):171–6.
11. Téllez-Zenteno JF, Dhar R, Hernandez-Ronquillo L, Wiebe S. Long-term outcomes in epilepsy surgery: antiepileptic drugs, mortality, cognitive and psychosocial aspects. Brain. 2007;130(2):334–45.
12. Hamiwka L, Macrodimitris S, Téllez-Zenteno JF, Metcalfe A, Wiebe S, Kwon C-S, et al. Social outcomes after temporal or extratemporal epilepsy surgery: a systematic review. Epilepsia. 2011;52(5):870–9.
13. Thorbecke R, May TW, Koch-Stoecker S, Ebner A, Bien CG, Specht U. Effects of an inpatient rehabilitation program after temporal lobe epilepsy surgery and other factors on employment 2 years after epilepsy surgery. Epilepsia. 2014;55(5):725–33.
14. de Boer HM, Mula M, Sander JW. The global burden and stigma of epilepsy. Epilepsy Behav. 2008;12(4):540–6.
15. Falvo D. Chapter 6, Epilepsy and other conditions of the nervous system. In: Medical and psychosocial aspects of chronic illness and disability. 5th ed. Sudbury, Mass: Jones & Bartlett Publishers; 2013. p. 83–92.
16. Fisher RS, Vickrey BG, Gibson P, Hermann B. The impact of epilepsy from the patient's perspective I. Descriptions and subjective perceptions. Epilepsy Res. 2000;41(1):39–51.
17. Wiebe S, Eliasziw M, Bellhouse DR, Fallahay C. Burden of epilepsy: the Ontario health survey. Can J Neurol Sci. 1999;26(4):263–70.
18. Auriel E, Landov H, Blatt I, Theitler J, Gandelman-Marton R, Chistik V, et al. Quality of life in seizure-free patients with epilepsy on monotherapy. Epilepsy Behav. 2009;14(1):130–3.
19. Lv R, Wu L, Jin L, Lu Q, Wang M, Qu Y, et al. Depression, anxiety and quality of life in parents of children with epilepsy. Acta Neurol Scand. 2009;120(5):335–41.
20. DiIorio C, Osborne Shafer P, Letz R, Henry TR, Schomer DL, Yeager K. Behavioral, social, and affective factors associated with self-efficacy for self-management among people with epilepsy. Epilepsy Behav. 2006;9(1):158–63.
21. Lee S, No Y, Lee S. Factors contributing to depression in patients with epilepsy. Epilepsia. 2010;51(7):1305–8.

22. Reisinger EL, DiIorio C. Individual, seizure-related, and psychosocial predictors of depressive symptoms among people with epilepsy over six months. Epilepsy Behav. 2009;15(2):196–201.
23. Taylor DC, McMackin D, Staunton H, Delanty N, Phillips J. Patients' aims for epilepsy surgery: desires beyond seizure freedom. Epilepsia. 2001;42(5):629–33.
24. Wheelock I. Expectations and life changes associated with surgery for intractable epilepsy. J Epilepsy. 1998;11(1):48–57.
25. Wilson SJ, Saling MM, Lawrence J, Bladin PF. Outcome of temporal lobectomy: expectations and the prediction of perceived success. Epilepsy Res. 1999;36(1):1–14.
26. Wilson SJ, Saling MM, Kincade P, Bladin PF. Patient expectations of temporal lobe surgery. Epilepsia. 1998;39(2):167–74.
27. Baxendale SA, Thompson PJ. "If I didn't have epilepsy…": patient expectations of epilepsy surgery. J Epilepsy. 1996;9(4):274–81.
28. Wrench JM, Matsumoto R, Inoue Y, Wilson SJ. Current challenges in the practice of epilepsy surgery. Epilepsy Behav. 2011;22(1):23–31.
29. Lindsay J, Ounsted C, Richards P. Long-term outcome in children with temporal lobe seizures, V: indications and contra-indications for neurosurgery. Dev Med Child Neurol. 1984;26(1):25–32.
30. Mizrahi EM, Kellaway P, Grossman RG, Rutecki PA, Armstrong D, Rettig G, et al. Anterior temporal lobectomy and medically refractory temporal lobe epilepsy of childhood. Epilepsia. 1990;31(3):302–12.
31. Jones JE, Blocher JB, Jackson DC. Life outcomes of anterior temporal lobectomy: serial long-term follow-up evaluations. Neurosurgery. 2013;73(6):1018–25.
32. Andersson-Roswall L, Engman E, Samuelsson H, Malmgren K. Psychosocial status 10 years after temporal lobe resection for epilepsy, a longitudinal controlled study. Epilepsy Behav. 2013;28(1):127–31.
33. Augustine EA, Novelly RA, Mattson RH, Glaser GH, Williamson PD, Spencer DD, et al. Occupational adjustment following neurosurgical treatment of epilepsy. Ann Neurol. 1984;15(1):68–72.
34. Guldvog B, Løyning Y, Hauglie-Hanssen E, Flood S, Bjørnaes H. Surgical versus medical treatment for epilepsy. II. Outcome related to social areas. Epilepsia. 1991;32(4):477–86.
35. Sperling MR. Temporal lobectomy for refractory epilepsy. JAMA. 1996;276(6):470–5.
36. Vickrey BG, Hays RD, Rausch R, Engel J, Visscher BR, Ary CM, et al. Outcomes in 248 patients who had diagnostic evaluations for epilepsy surgery. Lancet. 1995;346(8988):1445–9.
37. Reeves AL, So EL, Evans RW, Cascino GD. Factors associated with work outcome after anterior temporal lobectomy for intractable epilepsy. Epilepsia. 1997;38(6):689–95.
38. Jones JE, Berven NL, Ramirez L, Woodard A, Hermann BP. Long-term psychosocial outcomes of anterior temporal lobectomy. Epilepsia. 2002;43(8):896–903.
39. Erickson JC, Ellenbogen RG, Khajevi K, Mulligan L, Ford GC, Jabbari B. Temporal lobectomy for refractory epilepsy in the US military. Mil Med. 2005;170(3):201–5.
40. Dupont S, Tanguy M-L, Clemenceau S, Adam C, Hazemann P, Baulac M. Long-term prognosis and psychosocial outcomes after surgery for MTLE. Epilepsia. 2006;47(12):2115–24.
41. Asztely F, Ekstedt G, Rydenhag B, Malmgren K. Long term follow-up of the first 70 operated adults in the Goteborg Epilepsy Surgery Series with respect to seizures, psychosocial outcome and use of antiepileptic drugs. J Neurol Neurosurg Psychiatry. 2007;78(6):605–9.
42. Keene DL, Loy-English I, Ventureyra ECG. Long-term socioeconomic outcome following surgical intervention in the treatment of refractory epilepsy in childhood and adolescence. Childs Nerv Syst. 1998;14(8):362–5.
43. Lendt M, Helmstaedter C, Elger CE. Pre- and postoperative socioeconomic development of 151 patients with focal epilepsies. Epilepsia. 1997;38(12):1330–7.

44. Wilson SJ, Engel J. Diverse perspectives on developments in epilepsy surgery. Seizure. 2010;19(10):659–68.
45. Engel J, McDermott MP, Wiebe S, Langfitt JT, Stern JM, Dewar S, et al. Early surgical therapy for drug-resistant temporal lobe epilepsy: a randomized trial. JAMA. 2012;307(9):922–30.
46. Baxendale S. The impact of epilepsy surgery on cognition and behavior. Epilepsy Behav. 2008;12(4):592–9.
47. Turner-Stokes L. Evidence for the effectiveness of multi-disciplinary rehabilitation following acquired brain injury: a synthesis of two systematic approaches. J Rehabil Med. 2008;40(9):691–701.

Chapter 11
Educational and Employment Outcomes Following Epilepsy Surgery in Childhood

Caroline Skirrow and Torsten Baldeweg

Abstract Childhood-onset epilepsy is associated with educational underattainment and underemployment. In some children, surgical intervention may be offered as treatment for medication-resistant seizures. Successful treatment may halt seizure-related cognitive and academic deterioration, providing opportunity for greater success in school and work. This chapter examines published research on four Indicators of educational and employment outcomes after epilepsy surgery in childhood (surgery age $\leq$ 18): (1) special educational provision (2) qualifications attained, (3) unemployment, and (4) financial independence. Few reports are available: research to date describes outcomes after temporal lobe surgery, hemispherectomy, and mixed surgical cohorts (resective and palliative surgeries). Better long-term outcomes across all four indicators are seen for patients who are seizure free postsurgically, and better outcome is associated with shorter lifetime duration of epilepsy. Long-term postsurgical employment outcomes in children are reported as superior to those of adults. Findings indicate that early surgery leading to seizure cessation may promote outcome. However, few studies compare outcomes of surgery with continued pharmacotherapy. Lack of longitudinal data makes it difficult to preclude that superior seizure and psychosocial outcomes simply reflect better presurgical function. More generally, duration of follow-up is often too brief to capture outcomes of epilepsy surgery in children, in whom these are continuing to emerge.

Keywords Education • Employment • Child • Epilepsy surgery • Temporal lobe surgery • Hemispherectomy

C. Skirrow, PhD (✉) • T. Baldeweg, MD
Cognitive Neuroscience and Neuropsychiatry Section, Developmental Neurosciences Division, Institute of Child Health, University College London, London, UK

Great Ormond Street Hospital NHS Trust, London, UK
e-mail: c.skirrow@ucl.ac.uk

K. Malmgren et al. (eds.), *Long-Term Outcomes of Epilepsy Surgery in Adults and Children*, DOI 10.1007/978-3-319-17783-0_11

Introduction

Seizures in childhood are linked to educational under-attainment and underemployment later in life [1–4]. Epilepsy impacts on school attendance, school performance, and academic attainment [5–7]. In turn, educational impairment, alongside the behavioral and cognitive problems and stigma associated with epilepsy, are likely to limit prospects for employment [8, 9].

Some children with medication-resistant epilepsy respond well to surgical intervention. Early intervention may protect children from the continual interruption of studies and the cognitive impact of seizures during critical periods of development, and allow them to complete schooling before their ability to study and work becomes compromised [8, 10–13].

Here we explore four key indicators of educational and employment outcomes which are frequently reported in the literature. These include: (1) special educational provision, (2) qualifications attained, (3) unemployment rates, and (4) financial independence/gainful employment. These outcome measures from studies focusing on surgery in childhood only (age $\leq$ 18) are presented in the Appendix.

Surgical and Clinical Variability

Children with epilepsy form a complex and diverse group [14] with varying seizure severity and heterogeneous clinical presentations, which can be caused by a range of underlying conditions. A variety of surgical procedures are available, which are tailored to the underlying pathology of each patient. These include temporal and extratemporal resections, hemispherectomy, multiple subpial transections, and corpus callosotomy [15]. Resective surgery can be offered as treatment for well-localized focal medication-resistant epilepsy, yielding seizure freedom in 50–60 % of children at $\geq$5 years postsurgery (temporal and extratemporal surgery, and hemispherectomy [16]). Multiple subpial transections and corpus callosotomy are primarily palliative measures, aiming to reduce rather than eliminate seizures [15].

Postsurgical cognitive and physical impairment, and seizure outcome vary in relation to different surgical interventions, and these factors are likely to influence long-term educational and employment prospects. The majority of studies on vocational and educational outcomes after epilepsy surgery in childhood focus on temporal lobe surgery [10, 17–22], fewer studies focus on outcomes after hemispherectomy exclusively [23–25], and some studies report on outcome in mixed cohorts of children who underwent different surgical interventions [26–29].

The Context of Childhood Epilepsy

Childhood epilepsy impacts on educational and occupational outcomes, even where seizures remit over time [1, 4, 30]. Seizures are not the only factor leading to psychosocial impairment: intellectual impairment, behavioral disorders, and social rejection also play major roles [8]. Intellectual disabilities are prevalent in childhood epilepsy [31–33] and are major determinants of outcome, since they place a cap on the course of an individual's educational and vocational trajectory [1, 3]. However, educational and occupational problems remain prevalent in individuals with childhood-onset epilepsy and normal intelligence [9], and academic impairments often exceed those expected by intellectual function [7]. Behavioral problems and disorders, which commonly co-occur with childhood epilepsy, are likely to be an important contributor to an academic and vocational underachievement [1, 7, 33].

Surgery for epilepsy may support behavioral recovery alongside seizure reduction (e.g., [19, 22, 34]), but it does not necessarily result in resolution of accompanying pre-morbid problems [34–36]. A comparison group is therefore vital to isolating potential benefits and costs associated with surgery in the context of seizures and the co-occurring problems associated with childhood epilepsy [37]. As outlined by Smith et al. [13], a medically treated comparison group is vital for identifying whether outcome is related to one or more of the following contributing factors: (a) epilepsy surgery, (b) ongoing development, (c) the natural course of the seizure disorder, or (d) effects of retesting. However, in practice, few studies include such a control group.

Educational Development and Special Educational Provision

Academic impairments often precede surgery: presurgical investigation of children with focal epilepsy show significant reading impairment in 38–47 %, with performance below levels predicted by intellectual function, and greater impairment in older children [38]. In line with these elevated rates of academic impairment, rates of special educational provision are high in children with intractable epilepsy (23–30 % [32, 39]), with population studies indicating a strong relationship of special educational provision with intellectual disability in childhood epilepsy [2, 40].

In children who undergo epilepsy surgery, rates of special education are higher in individuals with continuing seizures or more severe seizures postsurgery [17, 26, 28, 35]. A study by Gleissner and colleagues [39] reported little change in school placement after a 1-year follow-up in 63 children who underwent temporal lobe surgery. Decline in school placement was seen in five cases, with two individuals transferring to special education, one transferring to a lower type of secondary school, and two repeating a grade. These children were more likely to experience continuing seizures (4/5 cases).

Similarly, most research indicates that shortly after surgery, children are likely to continue progressing on the same educational trajectory. A 1-year follow-up study of children with temporal and extratemporal seizures found no differences in academic attainment between children who did and did not undergo surgery [13]. Another study of children and adults with focal epilepsy (excluding callosotomy, hemispherectomy, and IQ<77) found that 49 % of those in school at time of surgery became trainees or employees in positions which corresponded to their level of education, and another 42 % showed stable development in school at an average follow-up of 3 years [12].

Mizrahi et al. [21] report on eight children who underwent temporal lobe surgery, and returned to school postoperatively at the level of their preoperative placement. At follow-up, roughly 6 years later, of the four individuals who remained in education, two reported improved performances and two reported no change.

Hemispherectomy is a treatment which may best be considered separately from other resective surgeries, since it is associated with more marked cognitive and physical disability presurgically [24]. A study by Pulsifer and colleagues [41] in children and young adults (age at surgery ≤ 20) highlights that the underlying neural pathology may be an important contributor to educational outcome, documenting worse intellectual function, and more frequent provision of special education after hemispherectomy for dysplasia than for Rasmussen's encephalitis or vascular disorders. Moosa and colleagues [25] report on outcomes 6 years after hemispherectomy with favorable rates of seizure freedom (61 %). Their work highlights that special educational facilities may not be provided in a sufficient number of children who undergo hemispherectomy: only 27 % attend special schools, but basic reading abilities are not achieved in 54 %. Impaired reading was predicted by children with younger age of epilepsy onset, cortical abnormalities in the contralateral hemisphere on MRI, and seizure recurrence after surgery. However, findings by Althausen and colleagues [23] indicate that although intellectual function is impaired in many children who undergo hemispherectomy, many may also show improvements post surgery (38 % improvement vs only 9 % decline), with similar rates showing improvement in school performance (40 %).

Qualifications or Educational Level Attained

The studies reviewed indicate that persistent seizures lead to greater educational problems and increased the need for special educational provision. In line with these findings, studies also reveal that individuals with ongoing seizures tend to obtain fewer educational qualifications. This is shown across different surgical interventions [17, 26, 28].

However, there are two primary caveats that arise in the interpretation of results from these studies. First, intellectual disability has a strong relationship with medical intractability: prospects for postsurgical seizure freedom may be worse for patients with intellectual disability [39, 42] and presurgical intellectual dysfunction may be an important unexplored confounder in studies of educational outcome (e.g., [17, 26]). For example, as reported by Keene et al. [28], children with good postsurgical seizure outcome obtain higher educational qualifications, but also more commonly have normal intelligence (80 % with Engel I, vs 60 % with Engel II–IV). Second, the type of surgical intervention and the associated underlying pathology may strongly influence postsurgical outcome. Continuing seizures are more commonly experienced by children with palliative surgery (e.g., [26]). Moreover, better outcomes are reported in children with temporal and extratemporal resections than in children with hemispherectomy [29].

Two studies comparing educational qualifications in pharmacologically and surgically treated children report no significant differences between groups [22, 35]. Moreover, the study of temporal lobe epilepsy by Skirrow et al. [22] investigates only children with a temporal lobe lesion, and reports an absence of pre-morbid differences in intellectual function between groups. The Lach et al. [35] study indicates that benefits of temporal and extratemporal surgery may be seen only in individuals who become seizure free, with rates of higher education and recent engagement in education being lowest in individuals with surgery and continuing seizures. However, this study did not investigate pre- or postsurgical intellectual function.

Employment and Financial Independence

A general issue with most studies investigating outcome after surgical intervention for epilepsy in childhood is the lack of outcome data within employment-age adulthood. Most studies report on employment outcome when subjects are in their late teens and early twenties, excepting Jarrar et al. [18] who follow up patients with temporal lobe surgery for a minimum of 15 years. Overall, the long-term outcome of these patients is positive, with 78 % in gainful employment and only 9 % ($n=3$) unemployed. Continuing seizures are the primary reason for unemployment in only one individual, with severe arthritis and severe depression accounting for unemployment in the remaining two.

For studies with shorter follow-up durations, the overall rates of unemployment and independent living may not adequately reflect the long-term prospects for children with epilepsy surgery. For example, Engelhart et al. [26] identify rates of unemployment and financial independence as relatively low for individuals with epilepsy surgery and seizure remission (11 and 11 %, respectively) and those with continuing seizures (29 and 4 %, respectively). However, when they isolate those of employment-age and those for whom independent living would be age-appropriate, the rates of unemployment are comparatively elevated (seizure free: 21 % unemployed and 42.8 % independent living; continuing seizures: 53 % unemployed and 10 % independent living). Similar issues are revealed by Lewis et al. [19], where rates of unemployment after temporal lobe surgery are relatively low within the entire sample investigated (13 %), but of the nine individuals who graduated from high school and were not in higher education, only 55 % were in full-time employment.

Studies comparing employment or financial independence in relation to postsurgical seizure control find better employment outcome associated with seizure remission [17, 26, 28]. One study comparing temporal lobe surgery to pharmacological treatment found slightly higher rates of employment and independent living in surgically treated children, the majority of whom were seizure free [22]. This is supported by findings from another study [35], showing lowest unemployment rates in a cohort of seizure-free individuals who had undergone temporal or extratemporal surgery during childhood (19 %). Unemployment was elevated in a pharmacologically treated comparison group (26 %), but highest in those who were surgically treated with continuing seizures (36 %). Moreover, number of months employed was positively correlated with age at onset and inversely related to proportion of life with epilepsy.

In line with findings from educational outcome, prospects appear worse for individuals who undergo hemispherectomy than for those with extratemporal or temporal resections. The mixed surgical cohort study by Van Oijen et al. [29], reports that of patients followed up beyond age 16, 65 % are in paid employment, all of whom underwent temporal or extratemporal resection in childhood. Although patients who underwent hemispherectomy comprise nearly a third of this sample, none are employed at follow-up. In the study by Moosa and colleagues [25], no unemployment is seen after hemispherectomy. However, in those who were assessed at employment-age ($n=24$), only 20 % (all with right hemispherectomy) are gainfully employed. Unemployment rates are low due to provision of specialized education or day workshops which were attended by the remainder of the adult sample.

Surgery in childhood may be more beneficial than surgical intervention in adulthood. Two studies comparing employment rates after childhood and adulthood temporal lobe surgery find better employment rates after surgery in childhood [20, 21]. Jensen [20] reports that temporal lobe surgery prior to age 18 favorably influences postoperative working capacity. Similarly, Mizrahi et al. [21] report greater improvements in educational and vocational status after surgery in childhood (in 62.5 % vs 37.5 % in adult surgery). Larger studies with combined child and adult surgeries support these findings. Lendt et al. [12] report patients with a younger age of temporal and extratemporal surgery have a greater chance of finding or retaining a job at 1–5-year follow-up. More recently, Zarroli et al. [43] find that unemployment is associated with fewer years of seizure freedom postsurgery. The authors propose that the earlier age of surgery allows participants to complete schooling, providing the tools for gainful employment.

Discussion

Overall, research indicates that educational and employment outcomes are promoted after surgery which successfully eliminates seizures in childhood. Lower rates of special educational provision, higher academic attainment, less unemployment, and higher rates of financial independence are noted after surgery-related seizure cessation. Moreover, early onset of seizures and longer duration of epilepsy are consistently associated with worse outcomes. Comparisons with adult surgical cohorts also indicate that early surgery and reduction of seizures may be more beneficial. Findings are consistent with studies of childhood epilepsy reporting cognitive and academic impairment associated with early seizure onset [38, 44], and progressive deterioration of academic skills and cognitive function with ongoing seizures [45, 46].

However, there are a number of serious limitations of research to date that require further elucidation, which are outlined in turn below:

1. It is not clear whether benefits or risks of surgery exceed those of continuing pharmacotherapy, particularly in children in whom seizures persist postsurgically. Suggest that surgery without seizure remission may add an additional obstruction to educational and vocational development. In the study by Lach et al. [35], children with surgery and continuing seizures had educational qualifications, rates of employment, and income below those with nonsurgically treated epilepsy.
2. Almost all studies present outcomes without reference to presurgical educational or intellectual function. Children with impaired intellect may be less likely to be seizure free postsurgically [39, 42]. Moreover, better postsurgical psychosocial outcome has been associated with better presurgical function [12, 19, 27]. Group differences at outcome may therefore simply reflect differences which are present but unmeasured presurgically.
3. Evidence of outcomes after some surgical procedures (e.g., multilobar resections, callosotomy, and multiple subpial transections) is lacking, or cannot be isolated since they are reported only in the context of mixed surgical cohorts. Research is required to investigate outcomes after these interventions.
4. Studies are limited by the short duration of follow-up. Most studies report on outcomes in late adolescence and early adulthood, which is a time of transition in which many young adults are completing their education, and beginning their working career.
5. Further studies are required to establish whether employment is commensurate with education or training, pays adequately to sustain the costs of daily living, and provides adequate job satisfaction. With the exception of a few studies, most do not qualify employment beyond the level of whether a patient has a job or not.

Overall, research indicates that where seizures are successfully controlled by surgery, educational and employment outcomes are enhanced. Advantages of postsurgical seizure cessation may be greatest for individuals with earlier intervention and the shortest duration of epilepsy. However, in the context of surgical interventions which eliminate seizures in only a proportion of patients, much further research is required to provide clear indications on the long-term educational and employment prospects for children with epilepsy surgery in relation to continued pharmacological treatment.

Appendix. Summary of Studies on Educational and Employment Outcomes After Epilepsy Surgery in Childhood (Age ≤ 18)

Reference, year, country	Study design *response rate*	Participants and sample size	Age: At epilepsy onset	Age: At epilepsy surgery	Age at follow-up /duration of follow-up	Primary employment/ educational status at follow-up	Highest educational level completed or currently attending	% Special educational provision	% Unemployed	% Financially independent/ gainfully employed
Temporal lobe surgery										
[22], 2011, UK	Cross-sectional *Response rate: 70 %*	**42** surgically treated children 86 % seizure free	4.0	13.3	22.7	Skilled employment 10 % Unskilled employment 30 % In education 40 % Unemployed 20 %	No qualifications 35 % GCSE, NVQ, diploma 48 % A-levels, higher education 17 %	38 % (lifetime)	20 %	30 %
		11 pharmacologically treated children 36 % seizure free	3.7		20.8	Skilled employment 27 % Unskilled employment 27 % In education 18 % Unemployed 27 %	No qualifications 46 % GCSE, NVQ, diploma 46 % A-levels, higher education 9 %	45 % (lifetime)	27 %	9 %
[17], 2008, Canada	Cross-sectional *Response rate: 58 %*	**28** surgically treated children, Engel class I	3.3	11.7	Median follow-up 12 years (range 10–20)	Employed 54 % In education 25 % Homemakers 7 % Unemployed 14 %	Secondary/post-secondary 17 %	7 % (current)	14 %	
		14 surgically treated children, Engel class III-IV	3.8	12.8		Employed 36 % In education 21 % Unemployed 43 %	Post-secondary 7 %	14 % (current)	43 %	
[18], 2002, USA	Cross-sectional *Response rate 86 %*	**32** surgically treated children 53 % Engel class I	7.2	14.4	33.4	Employed gainfully 78 % Employed part-time 3 % Homemakers 9 % Unemployed 9 %			9 %	78 %
[19], 1996, USA	Cross-sectional *Response rate: 100 %*	**23** surgically treated children	4.8	14.5	19.3	Employed full-time 22 % Employed part-time 4 % In education 61 % Unemployed 13 %	9 % Grade school 82 % high school 9 % College		13 %	
[21], 1990 USA	Longitudinal *Response rate: N/A*	**8** surgically treated children	6.3	11.8	17.8	Employed 25 % In education 63 % Homemaker 13 %		38 % (current)	0 %	

		14 surgically treated adults	5.7	26.2	31.0	Employed 64 % In education 7 % Homemaker 7 % Unemployed 21 %			21 %	
[20], 1976, Denmark	Cross-sectional *Response rate: 100 %*	**18** surgically treated children		Age 4–17	Follow-up 7–16 years	Employed (or likely after finishing school) 61% Disablement pension 33 % In hospital/institution 6 %			39 %	
		56 surgically treated adults		Age 18–54		Employed (or likely after finishing school) 30 % Disablement pension 52 % In hospital/institution 11 %			63 %	
[10], 1975, UK	Cross-sectional *Response rate: 100 %*	**20** surgically treated children followed up 6+ years	Age ≤15	Age ≤15	Follow-up 6–24 years	Skilled employment or advanced training 15 % Unskilled employment 30 % Unemployed 40 % Data unavailable 15 %			40 %	
		20 surgically treated children followed up 1–5 years	Age ≤15	Age ≤15	Follow-up 1–5 years	Employed 35 % In education 50 % Unemployed 15 %			15 %	
Hemispherectomy										
[25],2013 USA	Cross-sectional *Response rate: 62 %*	**115** surgically treated children 61 % seizure free	1.7	6.7	12.7	Employed 5 % In education 71 % In training/unemployed 18 % Home care/minimally functional: 6 %		21 % (current)		5 %
[23], 2013, Germany	Cross-sectional *Response rate:75 %*	**61** surgically treated children 75 % seizure free	2.8	14.5	23.9	*In patients age 19+ (n=35)* Employed 21 % Sheltered employment 27 % Vocational training 27 % Unemployed 52 %	*In patients age 16+ (n = 40)* Graduation 45 % Special school degree 25 % No graduation 30 %	60 % *(Age 16+ only)*	52% *(Age 19+ only)*	41 % *(Age 19+ only)*
[24], 1987 UK	Longitudinal *Response rate: 100 %*	**17** Surgically treated children 70 % seizure free	5.3	11.9	24.5	Employed full-time 6 % Employed part-time 6 % In care, sheltered training, employment or rehabilitation 53 % In education 29 % Unemployed 6 %		17 % (current)	6 %	

(continued)

Appendix (continued)

Mixed surgical cohorts										
[26], 2013 the Netherlands	Cross-sectional *Response rate: 63 %*	**83** Surgically treated seizure free *(24 H, 44 TL, 15 E-T)*		7.7	14.8	Employed 39 % In education 10 % Pre-school age 40 % Unemployed 11 %	No qualifications: 8 % Primary: 27 % Secondary: 25 % Lower vocational: 22.9 % Higher vocational/university: 7 %	36.1 % (completed)	11 %	11 %
		28 Surgically treated, continuing seizures *(2 C, 10 H, 5 TL, 11 E-T)*		7.0	14.9	Employed 25 % In education 3.6 % Pre-school age 43 % Unemployed 29 %	No qualifications: 18 % Primary: 18 % Secondary: 46 % Lower vocational: 8.7 % Higher vocational/university: 0 %	50 % (completed)	29 %	4 %
[35],2010 Canada	Cross-sectional *response rate: 63 %*	**38** surgically treated seizure free *(24 TL, 14 E-T)*	6.1	13.2	22.2	Employed or in education 81 % Unemployed 19 %	High school: 63.2 % Vocational education: 21.1 % University: 15.8 %		19 %	
		33 surgically treated, continuing seizures *(18 TL, 15 E-T)*	5.5	13.9	22.6	Employed or in education 64 % Unemployed 36 %	High school: 78.8 % Vocational education: 15.2 % University: 6.1 %		36 %	
		31 pharmacologically treated continuing seizures	6.8	N/A	Matched in age to other groups	Employed or in education 74 % Unemployed 26 %	High school: 64.3% Vocational education: 17.9 % University: 17.9 %		26 %	
[29],2006 Netherlands	Cross-sectional *response rate: 93 %*	**64** surgically treated 59 % seizure and aura free *(19 H, 34 TL, 17 E-T)*	3.8	9.2	16.7	Employed 42 %	No qualifications/education 3 % Normal primary education 5 % Special education 44 % Occupational training 38 % University 11 %	44 % (completed)		33 %
[27]. 2004 USA	Cross-sectional *Response rate: 100 %*	**9**tuberous sclerosis and surgery, Engel 1 outcome *(7 L/M, 7 Tu)*	2.6	12.5	21.4	Employed 88 % In education 12 %	In education for at least 12 years 88 %		0 %	
		12tuberous sclerosis and surgery, Engel III-IV outcome *(2 C, 5 L/M, 5 Tu)*								

[28],1998, Canada	Cross-sectional *Response rate: 100 %*	**34** surgically treated Engel I	*(4 H, 43 TL, 17 E-T)*	5.6	11.7	19.6	Of patients who were able to work*: Employed full-time 17 % Employed part-time 16 % In education 56 % Unemployed 11 % *not clear whether this is determined by age, intellectual function, or both.	Grade school: 6 % Special education: 32 % High school: 38% Post-secondary: 23 %	32 % (compl eted)	Of those able to work 11% unemployed	40 %
		19 surgically treated Engel II-III		4.3	12.7	19.9		Grade school: 32% Special education: 37 % High school: 0% Post-secondary: 31 %	40 % (compl eted)		5 %
		11 surgically treated Engel IV		4.8	11.9	18.2		Grade school: 27 % Special education: 46 % High school: 27 % Post-secondary: 0 %	46 % (compl eted)		14 %

H Hemispherectomy, *C* callosotomy, *TL* temporal lobe surgery, *E-T* extratemporal resection, *L/M* lobar/multilobar, *Tu* tuberectomy, no data are available for diagonally shaded sections

References

1. Camfield CS, Camfield PR. The adult seizure and social outcomes of children with partial complex seizures. Brain. 2013;136:593–600.
2. Geerts A, Brouwer O, van Donselaar C, Stroink H, Peters B, Peeters E, Arts WF. Health perception and socioeconomic status following childhood-onset epilepsy: the Dutch study of epilepsy in childhood. Epilepsia. 2011;52(12):2192–202.
3. Kokkonen J, Kokkonen ER, Saukkonen AL, Pennanen P. Psychosocial outcome of young adults with epilepsy in childhood. J Neurol Neurosurg Psychiatry. 1997;62:265–8.
4. Sillanpaa M, Jalava M, Kaleva O, Shinnar S. Long-term prognosis of seizure with onset in childhood. N Engl J Med. 1998;338(24):1715–22.
5. Holdsworth L, Whitmore K. A study of children with epilepsy attending ordinary schools. I: their seizure patterns, progress and behaviour in school. Dev Med Child Neurol. 1974;16:746–58.
6. Aguiar BVK, Guerreiro MM, McBrian D, Montenegro MA. Seizure impact on the school attendance in children with epilepsy. Seizure. 2007;16:698–702.
7. Fastenau PS, Shen J, Dunn DW, Austin JK. Academic underachievement among children with epilepsy: proportion exceeding psychometric criteria for learning disability and associated risk factors. J Learn Disabil. 2008;41(3):195–207.
8. Lindsay J, Ounsted C, Richards P. Long-term outcome in children with temporal lobe seizures. I: social outcome and childhood factors. Dev Med Child Neurol. 1979;21:285–98.
9. Jalava M, Sillanpaa M, Camfield C, Camfield P. Social adjustment and competence 35 years after onset of childhood epilepsy: a prospective controlled study. Epilepsia. 1997;36(6):708–15.
10. Davidson S, Falconer MA. Outcome of surgery in 40 children with temporal-lobe epilepsy. Lancet. 1975;1(7919):1260–3.
11. Erba G, Winston KR, Adler JR, Welch K, Ziegler R, Hornig GW. Temporal lobectomy for complex partial seizures that began in childhood. Surg Neurol. 1992;38:424–32.
12. Lendt M, Helmsteadter C, Elger CE. Pre- and post-operative socioeconomic development of 151 patients with focal epilepsies. Epilepsia. 1997;38(2):1330–7.
13. Smith ML, Elliott IM, Lach L. Cognitive, psychosocial, and family function one year after pediatric epilepsy surgery. Epilepsia. 2004;45(6):650–60.
14. Camfield P, Camfield C. What happens to children with epilepsy when they become adults? Some facts and opinions. Padiatr Neurol. 2014;51(1):17–23.
15. Centeno RS, Yacubian EM, Sakamoto AC, Ferraz AFP, Carrete H, Cavalheiro S. Pre-surgical evaluation and surgical treatment in children with extratemporal epilepsy. Childs Nerv Syst. 2006;22:945–59.
16. Tellez-Zenteno JF, Dhar R, Wiebe S. Long-term seizure outcomes following epilepsy surgery: a systematic review and meta-analysis. Brain. 2005;128:1188–98.
17. Benifla M, Rutka JT, Otsubo H, Lamberti-Pasculli M, Elliott I, Sell E, RamachandranNair R, Ochi A, Weiss SK, Snead OC, Donner EJ. Long-term seizure and social outcomes following temporal lobe surgery for intractable epilepsy during childhood. Epilepsy Res. 2008;82:133–8.
18. Jarrar RG, Buchhalter JR, Meyer FB, Sharbrough FW, Laws E. Long-term follow-up of temporal lobectomy in children. Neurology. 2002;59:1635–7.
19. Lewis DV, Thompson RJ, Santos CC, Oakes WJ, Radtke RA, Friedman AH, Lee N, Swartzwelder HS. Outcome of temporal lobectomy in adolescents. J Epilepsy. 1996;9:198–205.
20. Jensen I. Temporal lobe epilepsy, social conditions and rehabilitation after surgery. Acta Neurol Scand. 1976;54:22–44.
21. Mizrahi EM, Kellaway P, Grossman RG, Rutecki PA, Armstrong D, Rettig G, Loewen S. Anterior temporal lobectomy and medically refractory temporal lobe epilepsy of childhood. Epilepsia. 1990;31(3):302–12.

22. Skirrow C, Cross JH, Cormack F, Harkness W, Vargha-Khadem F, Baldeweg T. Long-term intellectual outcome after temporal lobe surgery in childhood. Neurology. 2011;76:1330–7.
23. Althausen A, Gleissner U, Hoppe C, Sassen R, Buddewig S, von Lehe M, Schramm J, Elger CE, Helmstaedter C. Long-term outcome of hemispheric surgery at different ages in 61 epilepsy patients. J Neurol Neurosurg Psychiatry. 2013;84:529–36.
24. Lindsay J, Ounsted C, Richards P. Hemispherectomy for childhood epilepsy: a 36-year study. Dev Med Child Neurol. 1987;29(5):592–600.
25. Moosa ANC, Jehi L, Marashly A, Cosmo G, Lachhwani D, Wyllie E, Kotagal P, Bingaman W, Gupta A. Long-term functional outcomes and their predictors after hemispherectomy in 115 children. Epilepsia. 2013;54(10):1771–9.
26. Engelhart MCJM, van Schooneveld MMJ, Jennekens-Schinkel A, van Nieuwenhuizen O. 'With the benefit of hindsight': would you opt again for epilepsy surgery performed in childhood? Eur J Paediatr Neurol. 2013;17:462–70.
27. Jarrar RG, Buchhalter JR, Raffel C. Long-term outcome of epilepsy surgery in patients with tuberous sclerosis. Neurology. 2004;62:479–81.
28. Keene DL, Loy-English I, Ventureyra ECG. Long-term socioeconomic outcome following surgical intervention in the treatment of refractory epilepsy in childhood and adolescence. Childs Nerv Syst. 1998;14:362–5.
29. Van Oijen M, De Waal H, Van Rijen PC, Jennekens-Schinkel A, Van Huffelen AC, Van Niewenhuizen O. Resective epilepsy surgery in childhood: the Dutch experience 1992–2002. Eur J Paediatr Neurol. 2006;10:114–23.
30. Camfield CS, Camfield PR. Long-term social outcomes for children with epilepsy. Epilepsia. 2007;48 Suppl 9:3–5.
31. Berg AT, Langfitt JT, Testa FM, Levy SR, DiMario F, Westerveld M, Kulas J. Global cognitive functioning in children with epilepsy: a community-based study. Epilepsia. 2008;49(4):608–14.
32. Huttenlocher PR, Hapke RJ. A follow-up study of intractable seizures in childhood. Ann Neurol. 1990;28:699–705.
33. Reilly C, Atkinson P, Das KB, Chin RFMC, Aylett SE, Burch V, Gillberg C, Scott RC, Neville BGR. Neurobehavioural comorbidities in children with active epilepsy: a population based study. Pediatrics. 2014;133:e1586–93.
34. Macrodimitris S, Sherman EMS, Forde S, Tellez-Zenteno JF, Metcalfe A, Hernandez-Ronquillo L, Wiebe S, Jette N. Psychiatric outcomes of epilepsy surgery: a systematic review. Epilepsia. 2011;52(5):880–90.
35. Lach LM, Elliott I, Giecko T, Olds J, Snyder T, McCleary L, Whiting S, Lowe A, Nimigon J, Smith ML. Patient-reported outcome of pediatric epilepsy surgery: social inclusion or exclusion as young adults? Epilepsia. 2010;51(10):2089–97.
36. Smith LM, Kelly K, Kadis DF, Elliott IM, Olds J, Whiting S, Snyder T. Self-reported symptoms of psychological well-being in young adults who underwent respective epilepsy surgery in childhood. Epilepsia. 2011;52(5):891–9.
37. Tellez-Zenteno JF, Wiebe S. Long-term seizure and psychosocial outcomes of epilepsy surgery. Curr Treat Options Neurol. 2008;10(4):253–9.
38. Harrison S, Cross H, Harkness W, Vargha-Khadem F. Preoperative educational status of children with focal epilepsy. Epilepsy Behav. 2012;28(2):328.
39. Gleissner U, Clusmann H, Sassen R, Elger CE, Helmstaedter C. Postsurgical outcome in pediatric patients with epilepsy: a comparison of patients with intellectual disabilities, subaverage intelligence, and average-range intelligence. Epilepsia. 2006;42(2):406–14.
40. Wakamoto H, Nagao H, Hayashi M, Morimoto T. Long-term medical, educational, and social prognoses of childhood-onset epilepsy: a population-based study in a rural district of Japan. Brain Dev. 2000;22:246–55.
41. Pulsifer MB, Brandt J, Salorio CF, Vining EPG, Carson BS, Freeman JM. The cognitive outcome of hemispherectomy in 71 children. Epilepsia. 2004;45(3):243–54.
42. Yu HY, Shih YH, Su TP, Lin KN, Yiu CH, Lin YY, Kwan SY, Yen DJ. Preoperative IQ predicts seizure outcomes after anterior temporal lobectomy. Seizure. 2009;18(9):639–43.

43. Zarroli K, Tracy JI, Nei M, Sharan A, Sperling MR. Employment after anterior temporal lobectomy. Epilepsia. 2011;52(5):925–31.
44. Cormack F, Cross JH, Isaacs E, Harkness W, Wright I, Vargha-Khadem F, Baldeweg T. The development of intellectual abilities in pediatric temporal lobe epilepsy. Epilepsia. 2007;48:201–4.
45. Dunn DW, Johnson CS, Perkins SM, Fastenau PS, Byars AW, deGrauw TJ, Austin JK. Academic problems in children with seizures: relationships with neuropsychological functioning and family variables during the 3 years after onset. Epilepsy Behav. 2010;19(3): 455–61.
46. Van Iterson L, Zijlstra BJH, Augustijn PB, van der Leij A, de Jong PF. Duration of epilepsy and cognitive development in children: a longitudinal study. Neuropsychology. 2013;28(2): 212–21.

Chapter 12
Quality-of-Life Outcomes in Adults Following Epilepsy Surgery

Jana E. Jones and Melissa Hanson

Abstract People with epilepsy often report the negative impact of their condition on many aspects of quality of life (QOL). While surgical intervention is aimed at reducing or stopping seizures, there is an implicit assumption among both patients and physicians that successful surgery will result in beneficial changes in quality-of-life measures (see Chap. 16). This chapter reviews the quality-of-life (QOL) outcome literature in epilepsy surgery. The majority of studies in this field have utilized follow-up intervals of no more than 1–2 years. The literature is diverse and a wide range of surgical procedures, QOL measures, sample sizes, ages at onset, follow-up intervals, and controlled versus noncontrolled study designs have been reported. Improvements in QOL do not automatically accompany seizure freedom, in the short term at least. Psychiatric comorbidities, employment status, ability to drive, and antiepileptic drug (AED) cessation appear to be better predictors of health-related quality-of-life measures than seizure freedom alone. Improvements in QOL measures may be more common following right versus left temporal lobe resections. There is a complex relationship between measures of cognitive decline and seizure freedom following surgery with respect to their impact on QOL measures. At present, little is known about the impact of surgery at different stages in adulthood. It is likely that QOL changes are different for those who have surgery in the 20s compared to those in middle age or later. Future research in this area should incorporate standardized measures of seizure outcome and QOL measures with normative data. Studies must also employ valid measures that capture meaningful change in QOL from the patient's perspective at different time points after epilepsy surgery. It is likely that meaningful changes in QOL will take many years to develop after surgery, particularly for those patients who have lived most of their lives with epilepsy. Outcome studies with follow-up periods of 12–24 months are likely to underestimate the benefits of seizure freedom conferred by surgery. Only studies with longer-term follow-ups are able to accurately measure the impact in this domain.

Keywords Quality of life • Health-related quality of life • Epilepsy surgery • Surgical outcomes • Temporal lobectomy • Seizure freedom

---

J.E. Jones, PhD (✉) • M. Hanson, BS
Department of Neurology, University of Wisconsin School of Medicine and Public Health, 1685 Highland Ave Room 7229, Madison, WI 53705, USA
e-mail: jejones@neurology.wisc.edu

K. Malmgren et al. (eds.), *Long-Term Outcomes of Epilepsy Surgery in Adults and Children*, DOI 10.1007/978-3-319-17783-0_12

Abbreviations

ESI-55	Epilepsy Surgery Inventory-55
ILAE	International League Against Epilepsy
IQ	Intelligence quotient
QOL	Quality of life
QOLIE	Quality of Life in Epilepsy
SF-36	Short Form Health Survey-36
SHE	Subjective Handicap of Epilepsy
VNS	Vagus nerve stimulator
US	United States

Introduction

Epilepsy surgery is the treatment option of choice for a selected group of individuals with epilepsy, particularly those who have medically refractory seizures [1, 2]. Greatly reduced seizure frequency or seizure freedom is often the main outcome and focus of outcome studies in epilepsy. The literature has examined secondary outcomes like cognition, employment, driving, psychiatric aspects, and quality of life (QOL). Epilepsy disrupts many aspects of life and is commonly believed to reduce self-reported QOL [3, 4]. Notably, the literature reports some inconsistent findings regarding the impact of surgery on QOL. This chapter reviews the findings reported in the literature in order to understand the impact of surgery on QOL among adults with epilepsy, to identify gaps in the literature, and to make recommendations for future investigations.

The studies included in this chapter were selected based on the following criteria: (a) all studies included individuals at least 16 years of age, (b) use of validated measures of QOL, and (c) controlled and noncontrolled studies were included but were reviewed separately. We excluded the following studies: (a) mixed samples with children 15 years old and younger, (b) review articles, (c) inclusion of individuals with nonepileptic events, and (d) studies reporting overlapping participants. If the same research group had more than one publication, the most recent paper was reported.

Each study was characterized in terms of the following results: (a) longitudinal studies versus cross-sectional results; (b) types of surgery performed; (c) sample size; (d) description of control sample; (e) follow-up interval; (f) age at onset, age at surgery, and/or age at follow-up; (g) seizure outcome; (h) measures of QOL and results; and (i) predictors of QOL (see Appendices 12.1 and 12.2 where the characteristics and results of the reviewed studies are summarized).

Quality of Life After Surgery

Controlled Studies

Study Characteristics

A total of 32 studies were included in this chapter, and 17 studies were controlled (Appendix 12.1). Among the controlled studies, two studies were from randomized controlled trials [5, 6], 11 studies had either pre-surgery baseline and follow-up assessments or repeated follow-up evaluations, and six were cross-sectional studies. The majority of surgical procedures performed were temporal lobectomy, amygdalo-hippocampectomy, or anterior temporal lobectomy with four studies also reporting extratemporal resections as part of the sample [7–10], and two studies included one participant each with a hemispherectomy [10, 11]. Two studies did not report the type of surgical procedure performed [12, 13], and Stavem et al. [14] reported only that the surgical procedure used was for focal epilepsies. The mean sample size of the surgery group was 69.8 with sample sizes ranging from 10 to 202. Similarly, the mean sample size for the no-surgery control group was 57.5 with sample sizes ranging from 9 to 253. One study utilized a vagus nerve stimulator (VNS) comparison group [11]. Three studies also used a healthy control group in addition to a no-surgery group [9, 12, 15], and two studies specified utilizing waitlist control groups [15, 16]. In terms of the follow-up interval, studies reported a range from 3 months [5, 12] to an average of 15 years [14]. Most studies reported a follow-up interval of 1–2 years.

Surgical Outcomes

Age at Onset, Surgery, and Follow-Up

Age of onset of epilepsy was not reported in seven studies [5, 10–13, 15, 17] and ten studies reported age of seizure onset prior to age 18. Age at surgery or surgical evaluation was only provided in two studies [14, 16]. In terms of study age reported in the controlled studies, one study did not report an age [16], and the mean age in the surgery group across the remaining 15 studies was 32.2 years.

Seizure Free Versus Not Seizure Free

There was significant variability in the classification systems and definitions used to define “seizure freedom.” The Engel [18] and International League Against Epilepsy (ILAE) [19] surgical outcome seizure classification systems were only used in three studies [9, 10, 20]. The studies reported seizure freedom in the context of the previous year prior to the follow-up evaluation or since surgery. As a result of the varying definitions it is difficult to systematically compare seizure freedom across studies. However, based on each studies report of "seizure freedom" in the surgery group the rates range from 38 to 88 %, and the average rate of seizure freedom across all studies was 63.1 %. Notably, two studies did not report rates of seizure freedom [11, 12].

Quality of Life

There were 14 studies that used epilepsy-specific measures of quality of life (QOL) and three studies that used generic measures of QOL. Among these controlled studies, six used the Quality of Life in Epilepsy-89 (QOLIE-89) [21], and two used the QOLIE-31 [22], and one used the QOLIE-10 [23], six used the Epilepsy Surgery Inventory-55 (ESI-55) [24], three used the Short Form Health Survey (SF-36) [25], and one used the World Health Organization QOL-BREF-26 (WHOQOL-BREF-26) [26]. Kellet et al. [8] utilized a model of QOL proposed by Baker et al. [27] which uses multiple measures to assess QOL, including an overall QOL rating.

Overall among the controlled studies, QOL was found to be higher when comparing individuals who had surgery to those who did not have surgery. Interestingly, Vickrey et al. [7] examined a sample from the United States of 202 adults and adolescents who had surgery, and 46 individuals who did not have surgery and reported mixed results. Vickrey et al. [7] found significant differences in 5 of 11 subscales on the ESI-55 between the surgery and no-surgery groups, but there was no significant difference between the two groups in overall QOL or employment outcomes. Additionally, in a sample from Sweden, Taft et al. [10] followed 96 individuals who had surgery and 45 who did not have surgery at a 2-year follow-up using the SF-36 to measure QOL. Taft and colleagues reported mixed results with most QOL domains falling in the average range at follow-up with the exception that there was no improvement in the social functioning domain of QOL. Uniquely, Taft et al. [10] and Fiest et al. [6] examined QOL in the context of clinically meaningful change in order to more closely examine the extent of the improvement and not only the statistically significant differences between the surgery and no-surgery groups. Both studies reported higher rates of meaningful change in QOL in the surgery group compared to those in the medically managed group.

Frequently, QOL results were reported in the context of seizure freedom. Individuals who were considered seizure free had higher QOL compared to those who continued to have seizures. In addition, McLachlan et al. [28] followed a Canadian surgical group and a medically managed group over 24 months at baseline, 6, 12, and 24 months to monitor QOL using the ESI-55. Seizure freedom was defined as having no seizures over the study interval. Auras or simple partial seizures were excluded from the seizure-free group. Individuals who had a 90 % or greater reduction in seizures and individuals with less than 90 % reduction in seizures were also included in the analyses. At 24 months, it was reported that individuals who were seizure free and those who had a greater than 90 % seizure reduction had improved overall QOL. Additionally, it was reported that individuals who did not have at least a 90 % reduction in seizure frequency actually had a decline in QOL. In contrast,

Kellet et al. [8] followed 94 individuals who had surgery and 36 who did not have surgery in the United Kingdom, and used a theoretical model of quality of life [27]. It was reported that individuals in the surgery group who were still having seizures had improved QOL but to a lesser degree than those who were seizure free. Seizure freedom was defined as no seizures in the year prior to the follow-up evaluation, and auras or simple partial seizures were considered seizures and were excluded from the seizure-free group. On the contrary, Gilliam et al. [16] also used the ESI-55 in a sample of 125 individuals who had surgery and 71 wait-list controls from the United States. The authors reported they did not find a relationship between QOL and seizure freedom. Seizure freedom was defined as no seizures in the year prior to the follow-up evaluation, and auras or simple partial seizures were included in the seizure-free group. It is important to note that all three of the studies had different definitions for seizure freedom, which likely impacted the different findings reported.

Predictors of Quality of Life

Several of the controlled studies examined factors other than seizure freedom or reduced seizure frequency as predictors for improved quality of life. Gilliam et al. [16] reported that mood status, employment, driving, and antiepileptic drug (AED) cessation were better predictors of health-related quality of life than seizure freedom. IQ was also not associated with changes in QOL. In a sample from Turkey, Aydemir et al. [29] followed 21 individuals who had surgery compared to 20 individuals who were waiting to have surgery. The authors reported that in addition to seizure frequency that medical comorbidities and antiepileptic medications negatively impacted overall quality of life. In contrast to the findings of Taft et al. [10] reported above, social functioning improved in this sample. Helmstaedter et al. [30] followed 147 German individuals who had surgery and 102 medically managed individuals at baseline and 2–10 years after surgery. Helmstaedter and colleagues did not find a significant relationship between QOL and cognitive outcomes including memory, attention, and fluency. Additionally, there was no relationship between QOL and depression. In summary, when comparing individuals who had surgery with those who did not, QOL appears to be positively impacted by surgery and reduced seizure frequency and seizure freedom. However, there are indicators that other factors like employment, AEDs, and other medical conditions may have a greater influence on QOL than seizure freedom alone.

Noncontrolled Studies

Study Characteristics

As mentioned previously, a total of 32 studies were included in this chapter, and 15 studies were noncontrolled (Appendix 12.2). Among the noncontrolled studies, nine were longitudinal and six were cross-sectional studies. The majority of surgical procedures performed were temporal lobectomy, amygdalohippocampectomy, or anterior temporal lobectomy with six studies reporting extratemporal resections as part of the sample [31–36], and one study reported data on an adult sample with hemispherectomy as the only surgical procedure [37]. The mean sample size was 55.6 with sample sizes ranging from 21 to 132. In terms of the follow-up interval, studies reported a range from 3 months [38] to an average of 26 years [36]. Most studies reported follow-up intervals of 1–2 years.

Surgical Outcomes

Age at Onset, Surgery, and Follow-Up

Age of onset of epilepsy was not reported in four studies [34, 39–41]. The age of onset of epilepsy was in childhood for the majority of studies with a mean of 10.4 years for ten studies, and one study reported epilepsy onset in adulthood with an average onset age of 25 years [42]. Age at surgery was provided for nine of the studies with a mean age of 32 years reported at the time of surgery [31, 33, 35–39, 42, 43]. In terms of study age in the noncontrolled studies, the mean age across ten studies was 32.4 years, and a total of five studies did not report study age [36–39, 42].

Seizure Free Versus Not Seizure Free

As in the controlled studies, there was no uniform utilization of the classification systems or definition used to define "seizure freedom." Studies reported seizure freedom in the context of the previous year prior to the follow-up evaluation or seizures since surgery. The Engel [18] classification of surgical outcome seizure classification was most commonly used in seven studies [34, 36, 39–43] and one study [37] used the International League Against Epilepsy (ILAE) [19] surgical outcome seizure classification system, and one study [31, 44] utilized Vickrey et al. [7] seizure classification. As a result, it is difficult to systematically compare seizure freedom across the noncontrolled studies. However, based on each studies report of "seizure freedom" the rates range from 44 % to 100 %, and the average rate of seizure freedom across all studies was 62.9 %. Notably, one study did not report rates of seizure freedom [38].

Quality of Life

Among the noncontrolled studies, there were 12 studies that used epilepsy-specific measures of QOL, and three studies that used generic measures of QOL [31, 32, 38]. The following measures were used to measure QOL – in order of frequency: the QOLIE-31 [22] ($n=5$), Epilepsy Surgery Inventory-55 (ESI-55) ($n=3$) [24], Quality of Life in Epilepsy-89 (QOLIE-89) ($n=2$) [21], and just single studies employed the following measures, QOLIE-31 version [23], the Subjective Handicap of Epilepsy (SHE) [45], Short Form Health Survey (SF-36) [25], the Quality of Life Assessment Schedule (QOLAS) [32], and the World Health Organization QOL-BREF-26 (WHOQOL-BREF-26) [26]. Similar to one controlled study, Reid et al. [33] utilized a model of QOL proposed by Baker et al. [27], which utilizes multiple measures to factor into QOL, including an overall QOL rating.

In the noncontrolled studies, the majority of overall quality-of-life ratings improved following surgery. In a Canadian sample, Tanriverdi et al. [43] followed 63 individuals who had temporal lobe surgery at preoperative baseline, 6 months, 2 years, and 12 years after surgery using the QOLIE-10 to monitor the status of QOL overtime. Tanriverdi and colleagues reported that overall QOL was not better at 6 months compared to 12 years after surgery. There were only two QOL subscales that were improved at 12 years, which included reporting fewer medication side effects and fewer memory problems. Individuals who were seizure free had better QOL compared to those who continued to have seizures at all three time points. This study also noted ongoing social difficulties across all time points. In Germany, in a sample of 21 adults followed 1-year post-surgery, Buschmann et al. [34] reported that improvements in QOL, based on the SHE, were detected in individuals who were seizure free but also in those who continued to have seizures at a lower frequency after surgery. In a sample of 25 individuals with temporal lobe epilepsy from Portugal, Cunha, and Oliveira [41] followed these individuals at 1 month, 3 months, 6 months, and annually 1 year through 5 years post-surgery using the QOLIE-31 to monitor changes in quality of life. These authors reported both the seizure-free and the non–seizure-free groups demonstrated improved QOL after surgery, but those who were seizure free made greater gains in QOL. Among 36 individuals from India, Ahmad et al. [40] assessed QOL using the QOLIE-31 and reported significant improvement in overall QOL in both the seizure-free group and those who continued to have seizures. Additional QOL improvements were noted on subscales of seizure worry, emotional well-being, and social functioning. In contrast, Cankurtaran et al. [38] followed a sample of 22 individuals from Turkey preoperatively and postoperatively at 3 and 6 months, respectively, using the WHOQOL-BREF. The authors reported no difference in preoperative and postoperative QOL, but improvements were noted on social functioning scales.

Predictors of Quality of Life

A number of noncontrolled studies have examined factors other than seizure freedom or reduced seizure frequency as predictors for improved quality of life. In a Canadian sample of 47 individuals who had a temporal lobectomy, Rose et al. [44] used the ESI-55 preoperatively and at 24 months postoperatively, and the authors reported that preoperative QOL was a better predictor of postoperative QOL more so than seizure outcomes. Individuals with low or medium QOL at preoperative evaluation were likely to have the most improvement in reported QOL after surgery. Individuals with higher QOL scores preoperatively continued to endorse high QOL at both time points but did not have improved change scores postoperatively. In a sample from Germany, Elsharkawy et al. [35] reported that seizure freedom and no additional medical comorbidities were the most important predictors of improved quality of life even more so than AEDs and their side effects, which had a moderate impact on QOL. In this same sample, age at onset had only a small effect on QOL. Additionally, Tanriverdi et al. [43] also reported better quality of life in those individuals who had a discontinued or reduced AEDs at 2 and 12 years after surgery. Langfitt et al. [46] and Buschmann et al. [34] found no relationship between neuropsychological results and QOL. Langfitt et al. [46] also highlighted the additional finding that declines in cognition correlated with lower QOL only if seizures were not reduced. Cunha and Oliveira [41] reported that individuals without presurgical psychiatric problems had better QOL following surgery. Additionally, these authors reported better QOL in individuals with right temporal lobe resections as compared to left, and there was no relationship between QOL and age of onset or age at surgery.

In summary, noncontrolled studies report similar findings when compared to controlled studies; the majority of studies report that reduced seizure frequency and/or seizure freedom improve overall quality of life. Additional medical comorbidities also have a significant negative effect on QOL. AEDs appear to be consistent predictors of poorer QOL but cognitive changes do not appear to impact QOL after surgery.

Discussion

Despite the differences in surgical procedures, QOL measures utilized, sample sizes, age at onset, and follow-up intervals, or controlled versus noncontrolled study designs, QOL appears to improve after surgery particularly in the context of seizure freedom or significantly reduced seizure frequency. There were two studies that contradicted this finding of a relationship between seizure freedom and improved quality of life [16, 38]. Several studies [34, 41, 43] indicated that there was improvement in QOL postoperatively, and this finding did not require seizure freedom. Preoperative QOL was demonstrated as a predictor of improved postoperative QOL by Rose et al. [44] with the most improvement noted in those with low and medium QOL prior to surgery. AEDs and other medical comorbidities appear to negatively impact QOL postoperatively. Memory measures and other cognitive measures have not consistently been correlated with postoperative changes in QOL [30, 34]. Social aspects of quality of life were noted to improve in one study [40] but no improvement was noted in social aspects of QOL in a larger controlled study [10]. It is likely that meaningful changes in QOL will take many years to develop after surgery (see Chap. 10), particularly for those patients who have lived most of their lives with epilepsy. Outcome studies with follow-up periods of 12–24 months are likely to underestimate the benefits of the seizure freedom, conferred by surgery on measures of QOL. This is particularly the case with studies that assess outcome at 12 months. In most countries, patients will need to be seizure free for at least year before they can learn to drive or regain their driving license. The ability to drive is consistently listed by adult patients as one of their primary expectations of epilepsy surgery (see Chap. 14). The independence conferred by a driving license and the subsequent benefits to QOL will not be picked up in studies that only look at outcome at 1 year. Only studies with longer-term follow-ups are able to accurately measure the impact in this domain.

To continue to identify significant elements that impact QOL following epilepsy surgery, it will be important for researchers to incorporate several factors in future studies. First, as indicated in a systematic review of the QOL literature, Seiam et al. [3] stated that the most informative studies are those that are longitudinal with evaluations before and after surgery and illustrate comparisons to no-surgery controls. In addition and similar to Kim et al. [12] and Mikati et al. [9] studies, it will be equally important to consider the use of healthy controls as a comparison group in order to allow comparisons with healthy individuals in addition to the patient population. In an attempt to identify clinically significant changes in QOL, more than just statistically significant differences, Fiest et al. [6] and Taft et al. [10] examined minimum clinically important change, in order to capture this concept of a meaningful change in QOL from the patient's perspective. This is an important addition to the literature since it provides the individual's perspective of the importance of the changes in QOL. It is important to follow individuals over longer intervals to determine if there are different factors influencing QOL years after surgery. McLachlan et al. [28] monitored individuals with and without surgery at 6, 12, and 24 months after surgery and found more improvements in QOL at the 2-year follow-up, indicating that it may take more time to capture change or differences in QOL. At present, little is known about the impact of surgery at different stages in adulthood. It is likely that QOL changes are different for those who have surgery in the twenties compared to those in middle age or later. The current use of several classification systems, which may or may not include auras in the definition of seizure freedom, as well as the time frame that defines seizure freedom in the past year or total number of seizures since surgery, makes it difficult to understand the true impact of seizure freedom or reduced seizure frequency on QOL. There should be a debate regarding the selection of QOL measures to be utilized to capture postoperative outcomes. If healthy controls are to be utilized, this may broaden the debate regarding general or epilepsy-specific QOL measures. Epilepsy-specific measures may be more sensitive to detecting epilepsy-specific change, but a generic QOL measure like the WHOQOL [26] or SF-36 [25] allows for more cross-cultural comparisons, and it provides clinically meaningful change results of QOL compared to the general population and possibly other disease groups. This task could be accomplished in the context of a multicenter study designed to systematically compare frequently used QOL measures and make recommendations for particular outcome studies. Finally, it will be important to systematically examine predictor variables of QOL outcomes including psychiatric comorbidities, employment status, cognition, social support, and coping in order to better understand the factors that play a role in QOL after surgery, in the context of premorbid factors. These are inconsistently incorporated across studies at the present time.

Appendix 12.1. Summary of Study Characteristics and Results from Controlled Studies of Quality of Life after Epilepsy Surgery in adults

Author	Surgical procedure	Sample size	Age at onset	Age at surgery	Study age	Outcome measures	Seizure outcome	Summary of results	Follow-up interval
1. Kim et al. [12]	Not specified	19 surgery 21 no surgery 20 control	Not reported	Not reported	Surgery: 26.8 Control: 26.5	Korean version of QOLIE-89	Not reported	Individuals in surgery and no-surgery groups reported lower scores overall as compared to controls. The surgery group had improved postop QOL scores.	Pre-surgery and >3 mo. postop evaluation

2. Vickrey et al. [7]	Anterior temporal lobectomy ($n=175$) Extratemporal lobectomy ($n=22$)	202 surgery 46 no surgery	Surgery: 11.9 years No surgery: 12 years	Not reported	Surgery: 27 years No surgery: 26 years	ESI-55 (*at follow-up only*) Employment KAS AEDs Seizure outcome	Surgery: 60 % SF (no seizures, auras or 1 seizure) No surgery: 11 % SF	The surgery group scored significantly higher on 5 of 11 scales (seizure health perception, social function, pain, role limitations caused by physical problems and role limitations caused by emotional problems).	Pre-surgery, 5.8 years for surgery 5.7 years for no surgery

(continued)

Appendix (continued)

Author	Surgical procedure	Sample size	Age at onset	Age at surgery	Study age	Outcome measures	Seizure outcome	Summary of results	Follow-up interval
3. Kellet et al. [8]	48 % Anterior temporal lobectomy 25 % Amygdalohippocampectomy 18 % Temporal lesionectomy 9 % Extratemporal resection	94 surgery 36 no surgery	Surgery: 11.7 years No surgery: 12.4 years	Not reported	Surgery: 33.1 years No surgery: 33.6 years	Overall QOL Overall health Impact of epilepsy AEDs Seizure frequency Surgery satisfaction Stigma Mastery Anxiety Self-esteem Depression Affect balance Employment or education HRQOL model (Baker et al. [47])	Surgery: 47.9 % in the past year. (auras counted as seizures).	QOL outcomes were significantly better for SF group post-surgery than those with continuous seizures and the no-surgery group. QOL improved for participants with less frequent seizures, but to a lesser degree.	1986–1994 (years included in follow-up) No interval given.

4. McLachlan et al. [28]	Temporal lobectomy	51 surgery 21 no surgery	Surgery: 12.1 years No surgery: 17 years	Not reported	Surgery: 31.9 years No surgery: 34.2 years (baseline)	ESI-55	Surgery: 88 % >90 % reduction or SF Nonsurgery: 8 % >90 % reduction or SF (2-yr follow-up)	SF group and participants with at least 90 % seizure reduction improved in QOL post-surgery. This improvement was most evident at 2-yr follow-up. QOL deteriorated with < 90 % seizure reduction.	Pre-surgery, 6, 12, and 24 months

(continued)

Appendix (continued)

Author	Surgical procedure	Sample size	Age at onset	Age at surgery	Study age	Outcome measures	Seizure outcome	Summary of results	Follow-up interval
5. Gilliam et al. [16]	Anterior temporal lobectomy	125 surgery 71 waitlist control	Surgery: 12.3 years Waitlist: 14 years	Surgery: 31 years Wait-list: 33 years	Not reported	ESI-55 POMS Driving Employment/ school AEDs Seizure frequency Adverse events profile	Surgery: 65 % SF (no seizures or only auras)	Surgery group had better QOL scores in 8 or 11 scales. SF status and IQ not associated with better QOL. Mood status, employment, driving and AED cessation were associated with better QOL.	12 and 24 months
6. Markand et al. [20]	Anterior temporal lobectomy	53 surgery 37 no surgery	Surgery: 12.3 years No surgery: 13.4 years	Not reported	Surgery: 31 years No surgery: 36 9 year (baseline)	QOLIE-89	Surgery: 73.6 % SF No surgery: 0 % SF (Engel classification)	Overall QOL score and 10 of 17 scale scores improved in surgery group and was related to SF status	Pre-surgery, 1 and 2 years

7. Helmstaedter et al. [30]	Temporal lobectomy	147 surgery 120 no surgery	Surgery: 12 years No surgery: 17 years	Not reported	Surgery: 31 years No surgery: 35 years	QOLIE-10 VLMT DCS-R Employment or school BDI	Surgery: 63 % SF No surgery: 12 % SF	Seizure free improvement of non-memory functions in T1-T2 and improvement of memory in T2-T3 Seizure free less impaired QOLIE-10 scores and less depression	Pre-surgery, 1 year and 2–10 years
8. Aydemir et al. [29]	Temporal lobectomy	21 surgery 20 pre-surgery	Surgery: 8 years Pre-surgery: 6.3 years	Not reported	Surgery: 27 years Pre-surgery: 24.8 years	SF-36 BDI STAI Stigma Perceived impact of epilepsy Opinions on epilepsy and surgery	Surgery: 47.6 % SF	QOL of post-surgery was better than scores before surgery	6 months to 4 years Average 27 months

(continued)

Appendix (continued)

Author	Surgical procedure	Sample size	Age at onset	Age at surgery	Study age	Outcome measures	Seizure outcome	Summary of results	Follow-up interval
9. Bien et al. [15]	Temporal lobectomy	131 surgery 105 waitlist control 99 presurgical candidates 49 no surgery	Not reported	Not reported	Surgery: 31.1 years Waitlist: 35.3 years Presurgical: 31.9 years No surgery: 36.5 years	ESI-55 Seizure questionnaire AEDs	Surgery: 52 % SF Waitlist: 5 % SF Presurgical: 14 % SF No surgery: 24 % SF	QOL scores of SF higher than those who were not SF	Minimum 1 year
10. Mikati et al. [9]	75 % Temporal lobectomy 25 % Extratemporal resections	20 surgery 17 no surgery 20 controls	Surgery: 9.3 years No surgery: 14.82 years	Not reported	Surgery: 30.5 years No surgery: 31.5 years Control: 29.2 years	ESI-55	Surgery: 85 % SF No surgery: 35 % SF (Engel classification)	QOL was significantly better in surgery group than in nonsurgery group and reached similar levels to healthy controls at 3-year follow-up	3 years
11. Stavem et al. [14]	Resective surgery for focal epilepsy	70 surgery 70 matched controls	Surgery: 9.4 years No surgery: 9.6 years	Surgery: 24 years	Surgery: 37 years No surgery: 37 years	QOLIE-89	Surgery: 48 % SF No surgery: 19 % SF	Surgery patients had higher HRQOL scores than nonsurgery patients	Average 15 years

12. McGlone et al. [11]	Anterior temporal lobectomy ($n=8$) Amygdalohippocampectomy ($n=1$) Hemispherectomy ($n=1$)	16 VNS, 10 surgery 9 no surgery	Not reported	Not reported	VNS: 35 years Surgery: 36 years No surgery: 37 years	QOLIE-89 GDS WMS, MOQ	Not reported	QOL improved more in surgery group than in VNS or medically managed group	Pre-surgery and 1 year
13. Choi-Kwon et al. [17]	Anterior temporal lobectomy ($n=22$) Other ($n=10$)	32 surgery 32 no surgery	Not reported	Not reported	Surgery: 30.6 years No surgery: 31.4 years	Korean ESI-55 Seizure outcome AEDs Seizure stigma Korean version of HADS	Surgery: 84 % SF No surgery: 45 % SF (2-yr follow-up)	QOL improved in surgery group but not in nonsurgery group. At 6 months, SF was an important factor in QOL, while at 2 years, AEDs and depression were important	Pre-surgery, 6 months and 2 years

(continued)

Appendix (continued)

Author	Surgical procedure	Sample size	Age at onset	Age at surgery	Study age	Outcome measures	Seizure outcome	Summary of results	Follow-up interval
14. Engle et al. [5]	Temporal lobectomy	15 surgery 23 no surgery	Not reported	Not reported	Surgery: 37.5 years No surgery: 30.9 years (baseline)	QOLIE-89 QOLIE AD-48 Seizure outcome	Surgery: 73 % SF No surgery: 0 % SF	QOL scores were higher in the surgery group than the no-surgery group, but this difference was not significant	Pre-surgery, and every 3 months for 2 years
15. Kanchanatawan [13]	Not specified	60 surgery 60 no surgery	Not reported	Not reported	Surgery: 36.1 years No surgery: 29.3 years	Thai version of WHOQOL-BREF-26 Thai version of HDRS	Surgery: 66.7 % SF No surgery: 5 % SF	Surgery group had better QOL scores than nonsurgery group and had similar QOL scores compared to the general Thai population	Minimum 1 year

16. Fiest et al. [6]	Temporal lobectomy	40 surgery 40 no surgery	Surgery: 14.3 years No surgery: 16.2 years	Not reported	Surgery: 35.5 years No surgery: 34.4 years (baseline)	QOLIE-89 QOLIE-31 SF-36 HUI-III GHQ	Surgery: 38 % SF No surgery: 3 % SF	More surgery group had meaningful improvement in QOL than nonsurgery group. No surgery group had worsening of QOL at follow-ups	Pre-surgery, 6 and 12 months
17. Taft et al. [10]	Temporal lobectomy ($n=80$) Frontal lobectomy ($n=12$) Parietal lobectomy ($n=1$) Multilobe resection ($n=1$) Hemispherectomy ($n=1$) Multiple subpial transection ($n=1$)	96 surgery 45 no surgery	Not reported	Not reported	Surgery: Median 33 years No surgery: Median 33 years (baseline)	SF-36 Seizure freedom HADS Surgery satisfaction	Surgery: 55 % SF No surgery: 11 % SF (ILAE classification)	QOL scores of SF surgery group reached norm at follow-up except in social functioning No change in not SF groups	Pre-surgery and average 2 years follow-up

Abbreviations: *AEDs* antiepileptic drugs, *BDI* Beck Depression Inventory, *BPRS* Brief Psychiatric Rating Scale, *DCS-R* Diagnostikum für Zerebralschädigung revised (visual memory test), *ESI-55* Epilepsy Surgery Inventory-55, *GDS* Geriatric Depression Scale, *GHQ* General Health Questionnaire, *HADS* Hospital Anxiety and Depression Scale, *HDRS* Hamilton Depression Rating Scale, *HRQOL* health-related quality of life, *HUI-III* The Health Utilities Index-III, *KAS* Katz Adjustment Scale, *MOQ* Memory Observation Questionnaire, *POMS* Profile of Mood State, *QOL* quality of life, *QOLIE-89, QOLIE-10, QOLIE-31, QOLIE AD-48* Quality of Life in Epilepsy, *SF* seizure free or seizure freedom, *SF-36* The Medical Outcomes Study Short Form, *STAI* State Trait Anxiety Inventory, *VMLT* Verbaler Lern und Merkfähigkeitstest (verbal learning test), *WMS* Wechsler Memory Scale, *WHOQOL-BREF-26* World Health Organization Quality of Life-BREF-26

Appendix 12.2. Summary of Study Characteristics and Results from Noncontrolled Studies of Quality of Life after Epilepsy Surgery in adults

Authors	Surgical procedure	Sample size	Age at onset	Age at surgery	Study age	Outcomes measures	Seizure outcome	Summary of results	Follow-up interval
1. Rose et al. [44]	Temporal lobectomy	47	11.5 years	Not reported	32 years (baseline)	ESI-55 Seizure outcome	44 % SF (Vickrey et al. [7])	Preoperative QOL more predictive of postoperative QOL than seizure outcome Greatest improvement seen in low or medium preoperative QOL scores High preoperative QOL scores did not see the same improvement, but scores remained high postoperatively	Pre-surgery, 1 or 2 years
2. Malmgren et al. [31]	Temporal lobectomy ($n=73$) Extratemporal lobectomy ($n=25$) Other ($n=5$)	103	10.9 years	27.9 years	32.1 years (follow-up)	SF-36 HADS Seizure outcome Single item QOL scale (Aaronson et al., 1992)	46 % SF (no seizures or only auras)	QOL is scored as a continuum in relation to seizure frequency; scores improve with decreased seizure frequency Seizure severity follows the same pattern	Pre-surgery, Average 4 years
3. Selai et al. [32]	Temporal lobectomy ($n=20$) Extratemporal lobectomy ($n=5$)	22	9.6 years	Not reported	32.8 years	QOLAS ESI-55 EQ-5D	100 % >75 % reduction in seizures	QOL scores improved at 1 year follow-up	Pre-surgery, Average 1 year

4. Maganti et al. [42]	Anterior temporal lobectomy	27	25 years	43.8 years	Not reported	QOLIE-31 Seizure outcome Employment	67 % SF (Engle classification)	Postop seizure outcome for US veterans was consistent with outcome seen in general population Better post-surgery seizure outcomes had higher QOL scores Employment outcome was better with good seizure outcome	2–13 years
5. Reid et al. [33]	Anterior temporal lobectomy ($n=32$) Amydalohippocampectomy ($n=16$) Temporal lesionectomy ($n=13$) Extratemporal lesionectomy ($n=3$) Other ($n=3$)	67	11.2 years	Median 29 years	41.4 years	Overall QOL Overall health Impact of epilepsy AEDs Seizure frequency Surgery satisfaction Stigma Mastery Anxiety Self-esteem Depression Affect balance Employment or education HRQOL model (Baker et al. [47])	44.8 % SF	Significantly more SF participants were employed and had a driver's license after surgery SF reported better QOL, psychological and psychosocial outcomes than those with continuous seizures	Average 10.3 years
6. Lowe et al. [39]	Temporal lobectomy	48	Not reported	42.7 years	Not reported	QOLIE-89 Seizure outcome AEDs	80 % SF (Engel classification)	Better seizure outcome had better QOL scores	Average 5.8 years

(continued)

Appendix (continued)

Authors	Surgical procedure	Sample size	Age at onset	Age at surgery	Study age	Outcomes measures	Seizure outcome	Summary of results	Follow-up interval
7. Cankurtaran et al. [38]	Anterior temporal lobectomy	22	10.5 years	30 years	Not reported	WHOQOL-BREF WHO-DAS-II SCID-I BPRS HDRS HARS	Not reported	Improvement seen in social domains of WHO-DAS-II postoperatively All participants were more satisfied with health post-surgery No significant difference found between pre- and postop general evaluation of QOL in WHOQOL-BREF	Pre-surgery, 3 and 6 months
8. Ahmad et al. [40]	Anterior temporal lobectomy w/subpial amygdalohippocampectomy and Lesionectomy (Numbers for each group not specified)	36	Not reported	Not reported	~25 years	QOLIE-31 Seizure outcome	77 % SF (Engel classification)	Improvement shown in all QOL domains in SF group and some domains (seizure worry, overall QOL, emotional wellbeing and social functioning) in not SF group Stronger score gains seen in SF	Pre-surgery and 6 months

9. Langfitt et al. [46]	Temporal lobectomy	138	14.9 years	Not reported	39.5 years (baseline)	QOLIE-89 Seizure control CVLT (verbal memory)	56 % SF at 2 and 5 year 26 % SF at 2 or 5 year	Improved QOL in SF group despite memory decline QOL declined when not SF was accompanied by memory decline and remained stable when there was no memory decline No relationship between cognition and QOL	Pre-surgery, Average 2 and 5 years
10. Tanriverdi et al. [43]	Selective Amygdalohippocampectomy ($n=33$) Cortico-amygdalahippocampectomy ($n=20$) Lesionectomy Temporal lobe ($n=10$)	63	7.1 years	33.8 years	34.4 years	QOLIE-10 Seizure outcome AEDs Employment	70.8 % SF (Engel classification)	Improvement in QOL was seen regardless of seizure outcome after surgery SF had high ratings of QOL than those who continued to have seizures Better QOL when AEDs were reduced or discontinued	Pre-surgery, 6 months, 2 years, and 12 years
11. Buschmann et al. [34]	Extratemporal resection	21	Not reported	Not reported	32.3 years	SHE Seizure outcome BDI Neuropsychological evaluation	52.4 % SF (Engel classification)	QOL improved after surgery regardless of seizure outcome No relationship between QOL and neuropsychological test performance	Pre-surgery and 1 year

(continued)

Appendix (continued)

Authors	Surgical procedure	Sample size	Age at onset	Age at surgery	Study age	Outcomes measures	Seizure outcome	Summary of results	Follow-up interval
12. Cunha and Oliveira [41]	Temporal lobectomy	32	Not reported	Not reported	41.4 years	QOLIE-31 Seizure outcome SCL-90	62.5 % SF (Engel classification)	QOL improved after surgery regardless of seizure outcome. More significant gains seen in SF group than those who continued to have seizures.	Pre-surgery, 1, 3 and 6 months and annually for 1–5 years
13. Elsharkawy et al. [35]	Extratemporal resection	87	13.9 years	30.1 years	37.3 years (follow-up).	QOLIE-31 Seizure outcome AEDs Employment Driving Psychiatric treatment Medical comorbidities	51.7 % SF	Seizure freedom was the most powerful predictor of QOL; SF was associated with higher QOL ratings Medical comorbidities were the second most important predictor of QOL	Average 7.2 years
14. Mohammed et al. [36]	Temporal resection ($n=60$) Extratemporal resection ($n=24$) Hemispherectomy ($n=8$) Callosotomy ($n=6$) More than 1 surgery type ($n=71$)	117	9.1 years	21 years	Not reported	QOLIE-31 Seizure outcome	48 % SF (Engel classification)	The majority reported improvement in quality of life after surgery Postoperative SF was associated with better QOL	Average 26 years

15. Schramm et al. [37]	Hemispherectomy	27	Median 5 years	Median 30 years	Not reported	German version based on ESI-55; 17 item version (Von Lehe et al. [48]) German -Functional status Seizure outcome Morbidity	81 % SF (ILAE classification)	QOL scores improved after surgery.	Median 9.6 years Minimum follow-up 1 year

Abbreviations: *AEDs* antiepileptic drugs, *BDI* Beck Depression Inventory, *CVLT* California Verbal Learning Test, *ESI-55* Epilepsy Surgery Inventory-55, *EQ-5D* EuroQol EQ-5D, *HADS* Hospital Anxiety and Depression Scale, *HARS* Hamilton Anxiety Rating Scale, *HDRS* Hamilton Depression Rating Scale, *HRQOL* health-related quality of life, *QOL* quality of life, *QOLAS* Quality of Life Assessment Schedule, *QOLIE-89, QOLIE-10, QOLIE-31* Quality of Life in Epilepsy, *SCID-I* Structured Clinical Interview for DSM Disorders I, *SF* seizure free or seizure freedom, *SF-36* the Medical Outcomes Study Short Form, *SHE* Subjective Handicap of Epilepsy, *WHO-DAS II* World Health Organization Disability Assessment Schedule, *WHOQOL-BREF-26* World Health Organization Quality of Life-BREF-26

References

1. Wiebe S, Blume WT, Girvin JP, Eliasziw M, Effectiveness and Efficiency of Surgery for Temporal Lobe Epilepsy Study Group. A randomized, controlled trial of surgery for temporal-lobe epilepsy. N Engl J Med. 2001;345:311–8.
2. Engel Jr J, Wiebe S, French J, Sperling M, Williamson P, Spencer D, Gumnit R, Zahn C, Westbrook E, Enos B, Quality Standards Subcommittee of the American Academy of Neurology, American Epilepsy Society, American Association of Neurological Surgeons. Practice parameter: temporal lobe and localized neocortical resections for epilepsy: report of the Quality Standards Subcommittee of the American Academy of Neurology, in association with the American Epilepsy Society and the American Association of Neurological Surgeons. Neurology. 2003;60:538–47.
3. Seiam AH, Dhaliwal H, Wiebe S. Determinants of quality of life after epilepsy surgery: systematic review and evidence summary. Epilepsy Behav. 2011;21:441–5.
4. Taylor RS, Sander JW, Taylor RJ, Baker GA. Predictors of health-related quality of life and costs in adults with epilepsy: a systematic review. Epilepsia. 2011;52:2168–80.
5. Engel Jr J, McDermott MP, Wiebe S, Langfitt JT, Stern JM, Dewar S, Sperling MR, Gardiner I, Erba G, Fried I, Jacobs M, Vinters HV, Mintzer S, Kieburtz K, Early Randomized Surgical Epilepsy Trial (ERSET) Study Group. Early surgical therapy for drug-resistant temporal lobe epilepsy: a randomized trial. JAMA. 2012;307:922–30.
6. Fiest KM, Sajobi TT, Wiebe S. Epilepsy surgery and meaningful improvements in quality of life: results from a randomized controlled trial. Epilepsia. 2014;55:886–92.
7. Vickrey BG, Hays RD, Rausch R, Engel Jr J, Visscher BR, Ary CM, Rogers WH, Brook RH. Outcomes in 248 patients who had diagnostic evaluations for epilepsy surgery. Lancet. 1995;346:1445–9.
8. Kellett MW, Smith DF, Baker GA, Chadwick DW. Quality of life after epilepsy surgery. J Neurol Neurosurg Psychiatry. 1997;63:52–8.
9. Mikati MA, Comair YG, Rahi A. Normalization of quality of life three years after temporal lobectomy: a controlled study. Epilepsia. 2006;47:928–33.
10. Taft C, Sager Magnusson E, Ekstedt G, Malmgren K. Health-related quality of life, mood, and patient satisfaction after epilepsy surgery in Sweden–a prospective controlled observational study. Epilepsia. 2014;55:878–85.
11. McGlone J, Valdivia I, Penner M, Williams J, Sadler RM, Clarke DB. Quality of life and memory after vagus nerve stimulator implantation for epilepsy. Can J Neurol Sci (Le Journal Canadien Des Sciences Neurologiques). 2008;35:287–96.
12. Kim YH, Kim HI. Assessing quality of life for the measurement of outcome after epilepsy surgery. Psychiatry Clin Neurosci. 1995;49:S304–5.
13. Kanchanatawan B, Kasalak R. Quality of life in Thai intractable epileptic patients with and without surgery. J Med Assoc Thai. 2012;95:1232–8.
14. Stavem K, Bjørnaes H, Langmoen IA. Long-term seizures and quality of life after epilepsy surgery compared with matched controls. Neurosurgery. 2008;62:326–34.
15. Bien CG, Schulze-Bonhage A, Soeder BM, Schramm J, Elger CE, Tiemeier H. Assessment of the long-term effects of epilepsy surgery with three different reference groups. Epilepsia. 2006;47:1865–9.
16. Gilliam F, Kuzniecky R, Meador K, Martin R, Sawrie S, Viikinsalo M, Morawetz R, Faught E. Patient-oriented outcome assessment after temporal lobectomy for refractory epilepsy. Neurology. 1999;53:687–94.
17. Choi-Kwon S, Chung CK, Lee SK, Choi J, Han K, Lee EH. Quality of life after epilepsy surgery in Korea. J Clin Neurol. 2008;4:116–22.
18. Engel Jr J. Outcome with respect to epileptic seizures. In: Engel Jr J, editor. Surgical treatment of the epilepsies. New York: Raven Press; 1987. p. 553–71.
19. Wieser HG, Blume WT, Fish D, Goldensohn E, Hufnagel A, King D, Sperling MR, Luders H, Pedley TA, Commission on Neurosurgery of the International League Against Epilepsy

(ILAE). ILAE Commission Report. Proposal for a new classification of outcome with respect to epileptic seizures following epilepsy surgery. Epilepsia. 2001;42:282–6.
20. Markand ON, Salanova V, Whelihan E, Emsley CL. Health-related quality of life outcome in medically refractory epilepsy treated with anterior temporal lobectomy. Epilepsia. 2000;41:749–59.
21. Vickrey B, Perrine K, Hays R, Hermann B, Cramer J, Gordon J, Meador K, Devinsky O. Scoring manual and patient inventory for the quality of life in epilepsy inventory-89 (QOLIE-89). Santa Monica: RAND; 1993.
22. Cramer JA, Perrine K, Devinsky O, Bryant-Comstock L, Meador K, Hermann B. Development and cross-cultural translations of a 31-item quality of life in epilepsy inventory. Epilepsia. 1998;39:81–8.
23. Cramer JA, Perrine K, Devinsky O, Meador K. A brief questionnaire to screen for quality of life in epilepsy: the QOLIE-10. Epilepsia. 1996;37:577–82.
24. Vickrey BG, Hays RD, Graber J, Rausch R, Engel Jr J, Brook RH. A health-related quality of life instrument for patients evaluated for epilepsy surgery. Med Care. 1992;30:299–319.
25. Ware J, Sherbourne C. The SF-36 health status survey: I. Conceptual frame-work and item selection. Med Care. 1992;30:473–83.
26. Skevington SM, Lotfy M, O'Connell KA, Group W. The World Health Organization's WHOQOL-BREF quality of life assessment: psychometric properties and results of the international field trial. A report from the WHOQOL group. Qual Life Res. 2004;13:299–310.
27. Baker G, Jacoby A, Smith D, Dewey M, Johnson A, Chadwick D. Quality of life in epilepsy: the Liverpool initiative. In: Trimble M, Dobson W, editors. Epilepsy and quality of life. New York: Raven Press; 1994. p. 135–50.
28. McLachlan RS, Rose KJ, Derry PA, Bonnar C, Blume WT, Girvin JP. Health-related quality of life and seizure control in temporal lobe epilepsy. Ann Neurol. 1997;41:482–9.
29. Aydemir N, Ozkara C, Canbeyli R, Tekcan A. Changes in quality of life and self-perspective related to surgery in patients with temporal lobe epilepsy. Epilepsy Behav. 2004;5:735–42.
30. Helmstaedter C, Kurthen M, Lux S, Reuber M, Elger CE. Chronic epilepsy and cognition: a longitudinal study in temporal lobe epilepsy. Ann Neurol. 2003;54:425–32.
31. Malmgren K, Sullivan M, Ekstedt G, Kullberg G, Kumlien E. Health-related quality of life after epilepsy surgery: a Swedish multicenter study. Epilepsia. 1997;38:830–8.
32. Selai CE, Trimble MR, Rossor MN, Harvey RJ. Effectiveness of rivastigmine in Alzheimer's disease. Patients' view on quality of life should be assessed. BMJ. 1999;319:641–2.
33. Reid K, Herbert A, Baker GA. Epilepsy surgery: patient-perceived long-term costs and benefits. Epilepsy Behav. 2004;5:81–7.
34. Buschmann F, Wagner K, Metternich B, Biethahn S, Zentner J, Schulze-Bonhage A. The impact of extratemporal epilepsy surgery on quality of life. Epilepsy Behav. 2009;15:166–9.
35. Elsharkawy AE, May T, Thorbecke R, Ebner A. Predictors of quality of life after resective extratemporal epilepsy surgery in adults in long-term follow-up. Seizure. 2009;18:498–503.
36. Mohammed HS, Kaufman CB, Limbrick DD, Steger-May K, Grubb Jr RL, Rothman SM, Weisenberg JL, Munro R, Smyth MD. Impact of epilepsy surgery on seizure control and quality of life: a 26-year follow-up study. Epilepsia. 2012;53:712–20.
37. Schramm J, Delev D, Wagner J, Elger CE, von Lehe M. Seizure outcome, functional outcome, and quality of life after hemispherectomy in adults. Acta Neurochir (Wien). 2012;154:1603–12.
38. Cankurtaran ES, Ulug B, Saygi S, Tiryaki A, Akalan N. Psychiatric morbidity, quality of life, and disability in mesial temporal lobe epilepsy patients before and after anterior temporal lobectomy. Epilepsy Behav. 2005;7:116–22.
39. Lowe AJ, David E, Kilpatrick CJ, Matkovic Z, Cook MJ, Kaye A, O'Brien TJ. Epilepsy surgery for pathologically proven hippocampal sclerosis provides long-term seizure control and improved quality of life. Epilepsia. 2004;45:237–42.
40. Ahmad FU, Tripathi M, Padma MV, Gaikwad S, Gupta A, Bal CS, Sarkar C, Gupta S, Wadhawan AN, Sharma BS, Chandra PS. Health-related quality of life using QOLIE-31: before and after epilepsy surgery a prospective study at a tertiary care center. Neurol India. 2007;55:343–8.

41. Cunha I, Oliveira J. Quality of life after surgery for temporal lobe epilepsy: a 5-year follow-up. Epilepsy Behav. 2010;17:506–10.
42. Maganti R, Rutecki P, Bell B, Woodard A, Jones JC, Ramirez L, Iskandar B. Epilepsy surgery outcome among US veterans. Epilepsy Behav. 2003;4:723–8.
43. Tanriverdi T, Poulin N, Olivier A. Life 12 years after temporal lobe epilepsy surgery: a long-term, prospective clinical study. Seizure. 2008;17:339–49.
44. Rose KJ, Derry PA, Wiebe S, McLachian RS. Determinants of health-related quality of life after temporal lobe epilepsy surgery. Qual Life Res. 1996;5:395–402.
45. O'Donoghue MF, Duncan JS, Sander JW. The subjective handicap of epilepsy. A new approach to measuring treatment outcome. Brain. 1998;121(Pt 2):317–43.
46. Langfitt JT, Westerveld M, Hamberger MJ, Walczak TS, Cicchetti DV, Berg AT, Vickrey BG, Barr WB, Sperling MR, Masur D, Spencer SS. Worsening of quality of life after epilepsy surgery: effect of seizures and memory decline. Neurology. 2007;68:1988–94.
47. Baker GA, Smith DF, Dewey M, Jacoby A, Chadwick DW. The initial development of a health-related quality of life model as an outcome measure in epilepsy. Epilepsy Res. 1993;16:65–81.
48. von Lehe M, Lutz M, Kral T, Schramm J, Elger CE, Clusmann H. Correlation of health-related quality of life after surgery for mesial temporal lobe epilepsy with two seizure outcome scales. Epilepsy Behav. 2006;9:73–82.

Chapter 13
Quality of Life and Psychosocial Outcomes in Children Following Epilepsy Surgery

Mary Lou Smith and Klajdi Puka

Abstract Quality of life (QOL) and psychosocial functioning of children diminishes with the onset of seizures. The adult outcomes of patients show some improvements with good seizure control but impairments in some areas remain. Epilepsy surgery in childhood has the potential to eliminate seizures, which may lead to improvements in QOL and psychosocial functioning. This chapter reviews recent work on the long-term QOL and psychosocial outcomes following epilepsy surgery in childhood. The few studies that have examined these outcomes find overall improvements in QOL, but are not always concordant as to which QOL domains show improvements. Similarly, although improvements are found in overall psychosocial functioning, there is no consensus on which domains improve. Improvements in QOL and psychosocial functioning, when evident, are consistently associated with seizure freedom. More recently, mood and affective symptoms have been found to be integral in ratings of QOL. Further work is needed to identify specific affective symptoms that lead to diminished QOL and psychosocial functioning and to identify other variables that may be involved, such as IQ or memory, and family function.

Keywords Quality of life • Psychosocial • Social • Comorbidities • Education • Mood • Affect • Internalizing disorders • Depression • Anxiety • Emotion • Cognition

Health-related quality of life (QOL) has become a key outcome in the medical and surgical treatment of people with epilepsy [1–4]. Measurement of QOL is a recommended aspect of clinical trials for medications, devices, surgery, and other

M.L. Smith, PhD (✉)
Department of Psychology, The University of Toronto, Toronto, ON, Canada

Neurosciences and Mental Health Program, The Hospital for Sick Children, Toronto, ON, Canada

Department of Psychology, The Hospital for Sick Children, Toronto, ON, Canada
e-mail: Marylou.smith@utoronto.ca

K. Puka, HBSc
Department of Psychology, The Hospital for Sick Children, Toronto, ON, Canada

K. Malmgren et al. (eds.), *Long-Term Outcomes of Epilepsy Surgery in Adults and Children*, DOI 10.1007/978-3-319-17783-0_13

treatments. In recent years, QOL has been increasingly used in the evaluation of the impact of surgery.

Most health researchers have adopted the World Health Organization definition of QOL [5], which has several key components. First, the individual's subjective perception is core to the concept. Second, QOL is a broad construct, encompassing many aspects of life, including physical health, psychological well-being, social function, and independence. Health-related QOL has been seen as most relevant to understanding the impact of epilepsy and its treatment on the individual. In this context, researchers have taken a multidimensional approach, examining the impact of epilepsy on domains such as the patient's physical, psychological, social, and cognitive function. QOL questionnaires are not synonymous with diagnostic instruments that measure symptoms or deficits [1], but rather examine the individual's perception of the influence of their epilepsy on function.

What Is the QOL and Psychosocial Function of Children and Adolescents with Epilepsy?

It has become increasingly recognized that epilepsy is a disorder beyond just seizures. This recognition has been reinforced by the documentation of the comorbidities of epilepsy; children with epilepsy (CWE) have an increased risk of cognitive, academic, behavioral, psychiatric, and social disorders, some of which may be present at, or predate, the time of seizure onset [6, 7]. It is also known that epilepsy of childhood onset is associated with an elevated risk of comorbid disorders that lasts well into adulthood, and these disorders may remain even if seizures remit or are well controlled by medication [8–11]. The presence of what can be an unpredictable disease course, the impact of seizures, medication side effects, and the stigma of epilepsy can in addition pose compromise to QOL. It has been demonstrated that children with epilepsy have poorer QOL than children with other chronic illnesses [12–14], and that the decreased QOL is evident at seizure onset [14].

Both youth with epilepsy and their parents have provided compelling evidence of the impact of epilepsy on QOL. When patients and parents were asked to list their concerns about living with or caring for their children with epilepsy, a wide variety of issues common to both parents and children were raised [15]. Their main concerns are medication side effects, cognitive and academic struggles, safety, the effect of the seizures on the brain, physical and mental development, the unpredictability of seizures and social problems. Parents revealed worries about their children's future with respect to health, self-esteem, and social prospects. The children also indicated a strong hatred for seizures and dislike of hospital visits.

A small number of studies have used individual or group interviews of children and teens to explore their experiences of epilepsy and its impact on QOL. Elliott et al. [16] used open-ended questions to elicit responses within four domains of QOL: physical, psychological (emotional/behavioral), social, and cognitive/academic. In the physical domain, the youth reported excessive fatigue that made it difficult for them to be involved in academic and social endeavors. The majority described periods of intense emotional distress related to their sense of the unpredictability of their seizures and the resultant sense of loss of control over their bodies. They also identified worry about and fear of seizures, sadness and depression, and anger and frustration, the latter related to the seizures, medications, and the extent of parental monitoring. A major concern expressed by the group was their sense of social isolation, imposed by internal factors such as lack of self-confidence and feeling of being different from their peers, and by external factors such as teasing, exclusionary behavior by peers, and restriction of activities and monitoring by parents. The majority of the participants reported cognitive problems, mainly poor memory and difficulties learning in school; these difficulties were compounded by the feeling of being physically and mentally unable to learn. The overarching theme arising from this study was that the youth viewed epilepsy as a barrier to normality.

A qualitative study with focus groups of adolescents revealed that teens have a number of concerns related to identity formation [17]. In this realm, they identified the following key issues: peer acceptance, development of autonomy, school-related issues, worries about the future, and incorporating epilepsy into their sense of self (both its negative and positive consequences). The adolescents also raised a number of epilepsy-related topics, involving medication, the fear of and experience of seizures, their own and others' knowledge of epilepsy and their sense of uncertainty regarding having seizures in the future. Similar methodology with 7–12-year-old children also revealed major concerns about the social impact of epilepsy, and about the direct effects of epilepsy such as the impact of seizures, medications, and the possibility of persistence of epilepsy in the future [18]. An international survey revealed a number of issues common to children, teenagers, and their parents, the most notable of which were worries about independence and future prospects for employment [19].

QOL Outcomes

Long-Term QOL Outcomes Without Surgery

To set the context for understanding the changes in QOL that may occur after epilepsy surgery, in this section we review studies on evolution of QOL over time in individuals (with childhood-onset epilepsy) who have not had surgery. A diagnosis of epilepsy in childhood often results in frequent doctor visits, the intake of countless medications, and limitations to daily activities imposed by the condition and by parents. As well, the fear of having epileptic seizures and enduring the associated stigma can be emotionally burdensome. Such a diagnosis may cause drastic and sudden changes to the individual's life leading to a lowered QOL, which may recover with time as seizure control improves and as the individual learns to cope with daily limitations and accepts the diagnosis. The findings of Speechley et al. [20] are indicative of this developmental course: although patients had significantly lower scores compared to the normative population on most QOL domains postdiagnosis, scores improved rapidly during the first 6 months and then gradually plateaued over the 2-year follow-up period. At 2 years follow-up, subscale scores were more similar to the population norms. Postdiagnosis and at 2 years follow-up, the largest difference between the patients and the normative population was on the emotional impact on parents scale. The presence of cognitive problems, more AEDs, poor family functioning, and increased family demands were predictive of poorer QOL at the 2-year follow-up. Of note was the finding that epilepsy-specific variables such as seizure severity or frequency were not found to be predictive [20, 21].

In the long term, 9 years after initial diagnosis, Baca et al. [22, 23] found significantly better QOL scores for seizure-free patients relative to patients with active seizures. However, no differences were found between patients who were seizure-free for at least 1 year compared to those seizure-free for at least 5 years, suggesting that the course of QOL improvement once seizure freedom is attained is not linear but plateaus with time. This finding is mirrored in adult surgical cohorts [24]. Additionally, chronic comorbidities such as psychiatric disorders, particularly internalizing disorder, were associated with worse QOL in most domains reported by the parent and patient. The presence of a neurodevelopmental spectrum disorder was significantly associated with worse parental ratings of QOL. These findings suggest that poor QOL may be driven by factors beyond epilepsy and seizure factors, a conclusion supported by the generally better outcome of patients with uncomplicated epilepsy, or epilepsy not associated with any other neurological impairments [25, 26].

Similarly, Sillanpaa et al. [27] followed 92 patients, of which 81 % were in remission (seizure-free for the past 5 years), for >30 years, finding that patients in remission and off AEDs had better scores than patients in remission who continued to take AEDs and patients who were not in remission. No significant differences were found between patients and healthy controls in terms of any QOL domains or the total score.

These studies illustrate that although children experience significantly lower QOL following an epilepsy diagnosis, improvements are evident over time, particularly in the first few months following diagnosis, as the patient and parent come to terms with the condition, learn coping strategies, form support networks, and gain improvements in seizure control. Unfortunately, it seems that QOL does not continue to increase linearly following diagnosis or once seizure freedom is attained and begins to plateau with time. Nonetheless, patients with uncomplicated epilepsy and patients who are seizure-free or in remission tend to show similar QOL as the normative population. Cohort studies of children with epilepsy find that long-term outcomes are more similar to the normative population but adverse effects persist particularly associated with psychiatric and neurological comorbidities, AED use, and continued seizures. Although QOL outcomes improve in some patients, it is important to note that adverse effects are persistent even in patients who entered adulthood seizure- and medication-free, suggesting that interrupted neurological and social/emotional development continue to have adverse effects well into adulthood.

Long-Term QOL Outcomes Following Epilepsy Surgery

The majority of long-term follow-up studies that have assessed QOL outcomes following pediatric epilepsy surgery have variable follow-up periods due, in part, to the difficulty associated with following large cohorts of patients over many years. Moreover, several studies do not analyze patients with shorter and longer follow-up periods separately. Many studies do not include a nonsurgical epilepsy control group, which is essential in long-term follow-up studies to identify the effects of surgery, as opposed to the natural progression of the disorder or development of the child. This point is especially important as long-term follow-up studies of pediatric epilepsy patients who do not undergo surgery show improvements in several areas. Hence, without a comparison group improvements may be erroneously attributed to surgery. An additional confound is the lack of preoperative assessment that is characteristic of almost all long-term follow-up studies, without which it cannot be determined whether the patient improved, deteriorated, or experienced no change following surgery. Nonetheless, the research conducted thus far assessing the long-term QOL outcomes following pediatric epilepsy surgery is generally concordant and overall shows promising outcomes for patients. We will first review studies that combine short- and long-term outcomes and then review studies that restrict the follow-up period to a minimum of 2 years.

Studies Combining Short- and Long-Term Follow-Up

Mikati et al. [28] compared QOL outcomes of 19 surgical patients at least 1 year after surgery (mean: 3.84, SD: 2.26 years), 19 nonsurgical epilepsy patients and 19 healthy controls. In comparison to nonsurgical patients, surgical patients had significantly better scores in the QOL behavioral domain and The Hague Side Effects Scale [29]; in contrast, the total QOL score and all other QOL domains were not significantly different. In comparison to healthy controls, surgical and nonsurgical patients scored significantly lower in total QOL score, general health, and physical domain; however, when the surgical seizure-free patients (79 %) were examined separately, they were found to score similarly to healthy controls in all domains. Moreover, better QOL was associated with higher IQ, fewer side effects of medications, and lower severity of seizures. Similarly, Gilliam et al. [30] reported scores similar to the normative population on some, but not all, QOL domains in a group of 33 patients who underwent pediatric epilepsy surgery 6 months to 7 years prior (mean: 2.7 years).

More recently, Gagliardi et al. [31] followed 13 patients with temporal lobe epilepsy (TLE) from pre- to postsurgery (7 months to 10 years later; mean 3.8 years). QOL was measured using a semi-structured questionnaire examining various aspects of QOL. At follow-up, all patients reported very good seizure control and improved QOL scores in general health, medication effects, and environmental influences scales. Physical issues, emotional behavior, cognition, social functioning, and schooling remained unchanged at follow-up. However, almost all patients showed significantly improved QOL total scores.

Roth et al. [32] examined outcomes of 39 patients with tuberous sclerosis complex 3 months to 12 years after surgery (mean: 3.2 years), in terms of seizure control, language, social development/interaction, school performance, independence with daily activities, family QOL, and time spent on epilepsy therapy. Rating their child's current condition compared to before surgery, moderate or major improvements in each outcome category were reported by 46–85 % (mean 65 %) of parents; deterioration was observed in one patient who did not achieve seizure freedom. Additionally, seizure freedom (71.8 %) was significantly associated with higher scores in each category, with the exception of language.

Determining the length of seizure freedom that is associated with improvements in QOL is difficult to extrapolate based on studies that do not restrict the follow-up period. The large range of follow-up periods postsurgery adds variability that ought to be controlled if one is to determine the long-term QOL outcomes of pediatric epilepsy surgery. Despite limitations of sample size and lack of nonsurgical controls, these studies are among the few that have examined QOL in the long-term and provide valuable clues regarding prognosis.

Studies Restricting Follow-Up to Two or More Years

Keene et al. [33] studied 64 surgical patients, at least 2 years after surgery (mean 7.6 years, SD 3.8 years) with the Quality of Life in Epilepsy questionnaire (QOLIE-31; [34]). Patients seizure-free for more than 2 years (55 %) scored significantly better on all domains (see Table 13.1). Those with greater than 50 % reduction in seizures (83 % of the sample) had better outcomes than those who had no significant improvement in the seizure worry, overall QOL, cognitive function, and social function scales.

Although other long-term outcome studies find overall improvements, improvements are not evident across all domains. Elliott et al. [35] studied young adults (ages 18–30) who had undergone epilepsy surgery in childhood a minimum of 2 years before (mean: 8.86, SD: 4.93). They found that surgical seizure-free patients had better QOL in most, but not all, domains of the QOLIE-31 relative to surgical patients with active seizures, and a nonsurgical epilepsy comparison group (see Table 13.1). Additionally, surgical seizure-free patients had better scores relative to nonsurgical patients with active seizures in the QOLIE-31 seizure worry scale and the SHE (Subjective Handicap of Epilepsy Scale) [36] physical scale. Number of AEDs was also significantly predictive of QOLIE-31 medication effects, and sex was significantly predictive of higher scores for males in the QOLIE-31 energy-fatigue and the SHE physical effects subscales. Similarly, Puka and Smith [37] found that 4–11 years (mean 6.93 years) after pediatric epilepsy surgery, or baseline evaluation for nonsurgical patients, seizure-free patients (51 %), regardless of surgical status, showed significantly better scores in most QOL domains (see Table 13.1). Additionally, surgical patients, independent of seizure status, showed significantly better scores in the seizure worry and medication effects subscales. AED use was independently associated with lower scores on the social functioning subscale;

Table 13.1 Summary of QOL results of studies restricting follow-up period to at least 2 years

	Keene et al. [33]	Elliot et al. [35]	Puka and Smith [37]
QOLIE-31/QOLCE			
Total score	A	A	A
QOL item	–	n.s	A
Cognitive function	A	A	n.s
Energy/fatigue	A	n.s	n.s
Social functioning	A	A[a]	A
Emotional functioning	A	n.s	n.s
Seizure worry	A	B	A, C
Medication effects	A	n.s	C
Health perception	–	–	A
SHE			
Self-perception	–	A	–
Physical	–	B	–
Life satisfaction	–	n.s	–

A Seizure-free patients scored significantly better than patients with continued seizures; regardless of surgical or nonsurgical status
B Surgical seizure-free patients scored significantly better than nonsurgical patients with continued seizures
C Surgical patients scored significantly better than nonsurgical patients
n.s not significant
– Domain was not measured
[a]Reported by Lach et al. [38]

other variables – number of years of follow-up and IQ – were not significantly predictive of any QOL domain.

Overall, studies of long-term QOL outcomes following pediatric epilepsy surgery find significant improvements associated with seizure freedom in most QOL domains, although there is variability as to which domains do improve. Of the long-term follow-up studies, few have restricted the follow-up period to at least 2 years; an important factor as QOL may increase rapidly during the first 6 months to 2 years following surgery and plateau with time [20, 24]. Additionally, few studies have compared surgical and nonsurgical patients, and only one has compared pre- and postoperative ratings of QOL. In evaluating the long-term QOL outcomes following pediatric epilepsy surgery, future studies should address these gaps and evaluate key variables that may lead to improved QOL (See Appendix).

What Influences QOL Outcome in Addition to Seizure Control?

Comprehensive models of QOL in childhood epilepsy have been proposed, largely out of recognition that seizure control alone does not completely explain the experience of QOL [12, 20, 21, 39]. These models address the impact of a number of variables, such as those associated with seizures (e.g., duration of epilepsy, age of onset, medication), child variables (e.g., behavior, cognition, psychosocial function), family variables (e.g., family function, stress, maternal anxiety/depression), and community variables (school, availability of social support, the health system). To date, none of the studies on outcome after epilepsy surgery have utilized such a comprehensive model. Although studies have consistently examined at least a subset of the seizure-related variables, only a few have examined the impact of the other categories of variables, specifically the impact of patient affective symptoms. This variable is particularly important, as research has shown that young adults who have undergone surgery in childhood continue to experience psychological distress, even in those who are seizure-free [40]. Significant associations with mood and affective symptoms with QOL have also been demonstrated in the literature on surgery in adulthood [41–44].

The study by Elliott et al. [35] was the first among pediatric long-term outcome studies to incorporate patients' mood, as measured by the Profile of Mood States [45], which assesses anxiety, depression, anger, energy, and confusion. Mood was significantly and independently predictive of 8 out of the 10 QOL subscales examined (QOLIE-31 total score, overall QOL rating, cognitive function, energy/fatigue, emotional functioning, and the SHE self-perception, physical and life satisfaction scales). More recently, Puka and Smith [37] examined the relationship between QOL and affective symptoms, as measured by the internalizing behavior summary score of the Adult- and Child- Behaviour Checklist [46, 47]. A mediation analysis was utilized to determine whether the commonly reported association between seizure freedom and QOL is determined by a third variable, the presence of affective symptoms, such that seizure freedom does not directly affect QOL but it leads to an improvement in affective symptoms which in turn leads to an improvement in QOL ratings. A mediating effect of affective symptoms was significant for all subscales examined: overall QOL, QOL item, cognitive functioning, energy/fatigue, and emotional functioning, social functioning, and health perception. Such findings emphasize the integral role of affective symptoms on QOL in patients with childhood-onset epilepsy.

Psychosocial Outcomes

Due to the high rate of comorbidities, children with epilepsy may experience challenges in a number of domains of psychosocial function, including emotional and behavioral disorders, compromised social behaviors and experiences, and limitations on their educational and vocational opportunities. Many of these topics are discussed in depth in other chapters in this book; thus, our discussion here concentrates mainly on the social realm.

Long-Term Psychosocial Outcomes Without Surgery

Patients with pediatric-onset epilepsy show residual social difficulties in adulthood that remain despite good seizure outcomes. Following a Japanese cohort of 148 patients with childhood-onset epilepsy over 6–37.5 years (mean 19 years), Wakamoto et al. [48] found lower rates of marriage, education, and employment, despite the fact that 63 % of patients were in remission. However, when examining patients with normal intelligence, the education and employment differences were no longer significant. Similarly, a group of patients from Finland followed for >30 years had worse social and educational outcomes in comparison to healthy controls, and patients not in remission were at high risk of having lower socioeconomic status [8, 27, 49]. Patients were also less likely to be married, to live with someone, or to have children. However, patients with "epilepsy-only" had better outcomes in each measure relative to patients with epilepsy and other disabilities, although they were more likely than controls to feel lonely and to have lower perceived control over their lives. Additionally, "epilepsy-only" patients taking multiple AEDs reported lower life satisfaction and poorer health relative to controls. Other studies of long-term psychosocial outcomes reveal similar results [50, 51]. It is also important to note that these adverse social situations remained even in patients who entered adulthood seizure- and medication-free.

Given the persistence of social problems among individuals with childhood-onset epilepsy, an important question is whether surgery and associated seizure outcomes have an impact on social outcomes. To date, there has been little research to address this question.

Long-Term Psychosocial Outcomes Following Surgery

Hum et al. [52] found that 1.5–3.4 years (mean 2.4 years) following surgery, youth with persistent seizures did not report an improvement in their social function, whereas mixed results were found among seizure-free patients. Those who reported improvements commented on the contribution of their decreased fear of having seizures, their perception of feeling normal and increased autonomy (less parental monitoring). Those with continued peer difficulties reported on the lingering stigma and discrimination associated with epilepsy. Similarly, Park et al. [53] found that social adaptation, assessed by the number of intimate friends, was significantly associated with seizure control and school performance 1–5.3 years (mean 3.2) years postsurgery.

Lach et al. [38] utilized various subscales of the QOLIE-31 and SHE to examine the psychosocial outcomes of 71 surgical patients and a control group of 31 nonsurgical patients with active seizures, a minimum of 2 years (mean: 8.86, SD: 4.93) following surgery. General social well-being was found to be significantly better in surgical seizure-free patients compared with patients with active seizures. Additionally, surgical seizure-free patients were less likely to report the perception that their epilepsy posed a handicap in social and personal functioning, and had better scores pertaining to work and activities. The groups did not differ in the number of friends they had, the number of times they had contact with friends on a weekly basis, how well they knew their neighbors, or in their principal activity (i.e., student, employed or unemployed). However, the surgical seizure-free patients were more likely to be involved in a romantic relationship, to have taken a recent extended trip with friends, and to belong to community clubs or organizations.

Keene et al. [54] also found that at least 2 years after surgery (mean 7.6 years, SD 3.8 years) better social outcomes were associated with a greater than 50 % reduction in seizure frequency; such patients were more likely to have stable relationships, be financially independent, and have a higher level of education. This relationship was only significant when patients under the age of 18 ($n = 20$) were excluded from the analysis. Interestingly, correlating the social outcome of financial independence, level of employment, and marital/relationship status with ratings of improved QOL (reported in [33]) did not yield significant results, suggesting that patients' reports of improved QOL may not translate to improved social and socioeconomic status.

Similar to the long term QOL outcomes, overall social functioning improves following pediatric epilepsy surgery. When evident, improvements in social functioning have been associated with seizure freedom or reduction. However, improvements are not seen in all domains even in seizure-free patients and different studies find different areas that improve and areas that remain diminished in the long term. Where social functioning remains diminished, lingering stigma and discrimination have been reported. It is also important to note, that the few studies that have examined long-term social outcomes have not explored the relationship between social outcomes and various family variables (e.g., family function, stress) and child variables (e.g., affective symptoms).

Conclusions and Future Directions

This chapter reveals that QOL and psychosocial function improve in individuals who obtain seizure freedom after epilepsy surgery in childhood. Given that improvements have been associated with seizure freedom in individuals who have not undergone surgery, surgical status itself appears to have little effect on QOL and psychosocial outcomes. The QOL and psychosocial domains that improve in the long-term remain unclear, reflecting the complex nature of such outcomes.

A number of questions await further investigation. Research shows that the QOL trajectories after seizure onset vary, and this situation is likely to be the case after surgery as well. Such trajectories have not yet been explored. To date, few studies have systematically examined long-term outcomes, and the influence of time since surgery, age at surgery, and age at follow-up. The influence of other variables (such as child and family variables), shown or hypothesized to be related to QOL outcomes, await research in pediatric surgical samples. We do know that perception of QOL after surgery is highly influenced by mood or affective state. It is of the utmost importance to not only treat epileptic seizures as early as possible to but to provide support with the social and emotional challenges that arise during childhood, adolescence, and with the transition into adulthood. Strong social support and coping strategies to overcome epilepsy-specific and emotional difficulties may be essential in attaining improved psychosocial and QOL outcomes into adulthood.

Appendix. Summary of Long-Term (≥2 years) Studies of Quality of Life and Psychosocial Outcomes in Children After Epilepsy Surgery

Author, year	Study design	Participants† (children) *N*	Surgical *N*	Males	Age (yr) at surgery (min-max)	% life (yr) with epilepsy	Prognostic indicators studied	Intervention	Seizure outcome measure	Seizure-free *N*	Follow-up (min-max/ years)
Keene et al. [33]	CS	64 (20)	64	39	12.2 (4.8)**	NS	a,b	T-EXT	B	35	7.6 (3.8)** 2 - NS
Keene et al. [54]	CS	64 (20)	64	39	12.2 (4.8)**	NS	a	T-EXT	E	35	7.6 (3.8)** 2 - NS
Lach et al. [38]	CS	102 (0)	71	41	13.5 (3.71)** 0.5–18.4	67(23)**	a,c,e,g,l	T-EXT	A	38‡	8.8 (4.9)** 2–22
Elliot et al. [35]	CS	98 (0)	69	37	13.5 (3.71)** 0.5–18.4	66(24)**	a,c,d,f,h,i,j,m	T-EXT	A	38‡	8.8 (4.9)** 2–22
Puka and Smith [37]	CS	109 (34)	71	68	13.2 (4.3)** 4.25–18.83	58(28)**	a,d,j,k,n	T-EXT	A	Surgical: 40 Controls: 16	6.9 (2.2)** 4–11

CS cross-sectional, *NS* not specified, *T* temporal, *EXT* extratemporal, *A* seizure free > 1 year, *B* seizure free > 2 years, *E* Engel classification, *a* seizure status, *b* type of surgical procedure (temporal resection, extratemporal resection, or hemispherectomy), *c* age of seizure onset, *d* years since surgery/follow-up, *e* proportion of life with epilepsy, *f* duration of epilepsy, *g* age at surgery, *h* current age, *i* sex, *j* AED use, *k* IQ, *l* emotional well-being, *m* mood state, *n* affective symptoms, *yr* years, † All patients were children at baseline or time of surgery-number in parentheses refers to those aged 18 years or less at time of follow-up, ‡ Inclusion criteria for nonsurgical group was active epilepsy, ** Mean (SD)

References

1. Cramer JA. Principles of health-related quality of life: assessment in clinical trials. Epilepsia. 2002;43(9):1084–95.
2. Speechley KN. What if quality of life better expressed outcomes for epilepsy? In: Arts WF, Arzimanoglou A, Brouwer OF, Camfield C, Camfield P, editors. Outcomes of childhood epilepsies. Montrouge: John Libbey Eurotext; 2013. p. 253–62.
3. Perry MS, Duchowny M. Surgical versus medical treatment for refractory epilepsy: outcomes beyond seizure control. Epilepsia. 2013;54(12):2060–70.
4. Thurman DJ, Beghi E, Begley CE, Berg AT, Buchhalter JR, Ding D, et al. Standards for epidemiologic studies and surveillance of epilepsy. Epilepsia. 2011;52 Suppl 7:2–26.
5. World Health Organization. WHOQOL: measuring quality of life. Geneva: World Health Organization; 1997.
6. Baum KT, Byars AW, deGrauw TJ, Johnson CS, Perkins SM, Dunn DW, et al. Temperament, family environment, and behavior problems in children with new-onset seizures. Epilepsy Behav. 2007;10(2):319–27.
7. Fastenau PS, Johnson CS, Perkins SM, Byars AW, deGrauw TJ, Austin JK, et al. Neuropsychological status at seizure onset in children: risk factors for early cognitive deficits. Neurology. 2009;73(7):526–34.
8. Sillanpaa M, Jalava M, Kaleva O, Shinnar S. Long-term prognosis of seizures with onset in childhood. N Engl J Med. 1998;338(24):1715–22.
9. Camfield C, Camfield P. Twenty years after childhood-onset symptomatic generalized epilepsy the social outcome is usually dependency or death: a population-based study. Dev Med Child Neurol. 2008;50(11):859–63.
10. Camfield CS, Camfield PR. Juvenile myoclonic epilepsy 25 years after seizure onset: a population-based study. Neurology. 2009;73(13):1041–5.
11. Camfield P, Camfield C. Idiopathic generalized epilepsy with generalized tonic-clonic seizures (IGE-GTC): a population-based cohort with >20 year follow up for medical and social outcome. Epilepsy Behav. 2010;18(1–2):61–3.
12. Austin JK, Smith MS, Risinger MW, McNelis AM. Childhood epilepsy and asthma: comparison of quality of life. Epilepsia. 1994;35(3):608–15.
13. Wang J, Wang Y, Wang LB, Xu H, Zhang XL. A comparison of quality of life in adolescents with epilepsy or asthma using the Short-Form Health Survey (SF-36). Epilepsy Res. 2012;101(1–2):157–65.
14. Taylor J, Jacoby A, Baker GA, Marson AG. Self-reported and parent-reported quality of life of children and adolescents with new-onset epilepsy. Epilepsia. 2011;52(8):1489–98.
15. Arunkumar G, Wyllie E, Kotagal P, Ong HT, Gilliam F. Parent- and patient-validated content for pediatric epilepsy quality-of-life assessment. Epilepsia. 2000;41(11):1474–84.
16. Elliott IM, Lach L, Smith ML. I just want to be normal: a qualitative study exploring how children and adolescents view the impact of intractable epilepsy on their quality of life. Epilepsy Behav. 2005;7(4):664–78.
17. McEwan MJ, Espie CA, Metcalfe J, Brodie MJ, Wilson MT. Quality of life and psychosocial development in adolescents with epilepsy: a qualitative investigation using focus group methods. Seizure. 2004;13(1):15–31.
18. Moffat C, Dorris L, Connor L, Espie CA. The impact of childhood epilepsy on quality of life: a qualitative investigation using focus group methods to obtain children's perspectives on living with epilepsy. Epilepsy Behav. 2009;14(1):179–89.
19. Baker GA, Hargis E, Hsih MM, Mounfield H, Arzimanoglou A, Glauser T, et al. Perceived impact of epilepsy in teenagers and young adults: an international survey. Epilepsy Behav. 2008;12(3):395–401.
20. Speechley KN, Ferro MA, Camfield CS, Huang W, Levin SD, Smith ML, et al. Quality of life in children with new-onset epilepsy: a 2-year prospective cohort study. Neurology. 2012;79(15):1548–55.

21. Ferro MA, Camfield CS, Levin SD, Smith ML, Wiebe S, Zou G, et al. Trajectories of health-related quality of life in children with epilepsy: a cohort study. Epilepsia. 2013;54(11):1889–97.
22. Baca CB, Vickrey BG, Caplan R, Vassar SD, Berg AT. Psychiatric and medical comorbidity and quality of life outcomes in childhood-onset epilepsy. Pediatrics. 2011;128(6):e1532–43.
23. Baca CB, Vickrey BG, Vassar SD, Berg AT. Seizure recency and quality of life in adolescents with childhood-onset epilepsy. Epilepsy Behav. 2012;23(1):47–51.
24. Spencer SS, Berg AT, Vickrey BG, Sperling MR, Bazil CW, Haut S, et al. Health-related quality of life over time since resective epilepsy surgery. Ann Neurol. 2007;62(4):327–34.
25. Raty LK, Larsson BMW. Quality of life in young adults with uncomplicated epilepsy. Epilepsy Behav. 2007;10(1):142–7.
26. Stevanovic D. Health-related quality of life in adolescents with well-controlled epilepsy. Epilepsy Behav. 2007;10(4):571–5.
27. Sillanpaa M, Haataja L, Shinnar S. Perceived impact of childhood-onset epilepsy on quality of life as an adult. Epilepsia. 2004;45(8):971–7.
28. Mikati MA, Ataya N, Ferzli J, Kurdi R, El-Banna D, Rahi A, et al. Quality of life after surgery for intractable partial epilepsy in children: a cohort study with controls. Epilepsy Res. 2010;90(3):207–13.
29. Carpay HA, Arts WF, Vermeulen J, Stroink H, Brouwer OF, Peters AC, et al. Parent-completed scales for measuring seizure severity and severity of side-effects of antiepileptic drugs in childhood epilepsy: development and psychometric analysis. Epilepsy Res. 1996;24(3):173–81.
30. Gilliam F, Wyllie E, Kashden J, Faught E, Kotagal P, Bebin M, et al. Epilepsy surgery outcome: comprehensive assessment in children. Neurology. 1997;48(5):1368–74.
31. Gagliardi IC, Guimaraes CA, Souza EA, Schmutzler KM, Guerreiro MM. Quality of life and epilepsy surgery in childhood and adolescence. Arq Neuropsiquiatr. 2011;69(1):23–6.
32. Roth J, Olasunkanmi A, MacAllister WS, Weil E, Uy CC, Devinsky O, et al. Quality of life following epilepsy surgery for children with tuberous sclerosis complex. Epilepsy Behav. 2011;20(3):561–5.
33. Keene DL, Higgins MJ, Ventureyra EC. Outcome and life prospects after surgical management of medically intractable epilepsy in patients under 18 years of age. Childs Nerv Syst. 1997;13(10):530–5.
34. Vickrey BG, Perrine KR, Hays RD, Hermann BP, Cramer JA, Meador KJ, et al. Quality of life in epilepsy: QOLIE-31 (version 1) scoring manual. Santa Monica: RAND; 1993.
35. Elliott I, Kadis DS, Lach L, Olds J, McCleary L, Whiting S, et al. Quality of life in young adults who underwent resective surgery for epilepsy in childhood. Epilepsia. 2012;53(9):1577–86.
36. O'Donoghue MF, Goodridge DM, Redhead K, Sander JW, Duncan JS. Assessing the psychosocial consequences of epilepsy: a community-based study. Br J Gen Pract. 1999;49(440):211–4.
37. Puka K, Smith ML. Predictors of long-term quality of life after pediatric epilepsy surgery. Epilepsia. 2015.
38. Lach LM, Elliott I, Giecko T, Olds J, Snyder T, McCleary L, et al. Patient-reported outcome of pediatric epilepsy surgery: social inclusion or exclusion as young adults? Epilepsia. 2010;51(10):2089–97.
39. Lach LM, Ronen GM, Rosenbaum PL, Cunningham C, Boyle MH, Bowman S, et al. Health-related quality of life in youth with epilepsy: theoretical model for clinicians and researchers. Part I: the role of epilepsy and co-morbidity. Qual Life Res. 2006;15(7):1161–71.
40. Smith ML, Kelly K, Kadis DS, Elliott IM, Olds J, Whiting S, et al. Self-reported symptoms of psychological well-being in young adults who underwent resective epilepsy surgery in childhood. Epilepsia. 2011;52(5):891–9.
41. Hamid H, Blackmon K, Cong X, Dziura J, Atlas LY, Vickrey BG, et al. Mood, anxiety, and incomplete seizure control affect quality of life after epilepsy surgery. Neurology. 2014;82(10):887–94.

42. Johnson EK, Jones JE, Seidenberg M, Hermann BP. The relative impact of anxiety, depression, and clinical seizure features on health-related quality of life in epilepsy. Epilepsia. 2004;45(5):544–50.
43. Park SP, Song HS, Hwang YH, Lee HW, Suh CK, Kwon SH. Differential effects of seizure control and affective symptoms on quality of life in people with epilepsy. Epilepsy Behav. 2010;18(4):455–9.
44. Tracy JI, Dechant V, Sperling MR, Cho R, Glosser D. The association of mood with quality of life ratings in epilepsy. Neurology. 2007;68(14):1101–7.
45. McNair D, Lorr M, Droppleman L. POMS: profile of mood states. San Diego: EdiTS/Educational and Industrial Testing Service; 1992.
46. Achenbach TM, Rescorla LA. Manual for the ASEBA adult forms & profiles. Burlington: University of Vermont, Research Center for Children, Youth & Families; 2003.
47. Achenbach TM, Rescorla LA. Manual for the ASEBA school-age forms & profiles. Burlington: University of Vermont, Research Center for Children, Youth & Families; 2001.
48. Wakamoto H, Nagao H, Hayashi M, Morimoto T. Long-term medical, educational, and social prognoses of childhood-onset epilepsy: a population-based study in a rural district of Japan. Brain Dev. 2000;22(4):246–55.
49. Jalava M, Sillanpaa M, Camfield C, Camfield P. Social adjustment and competence 35 years after onset of childhood epilepsy: a prospective controlled study. Epilepsia. 1997;38(6):708–15.
50. Jonsson P, Jonsson B, Eeg-Olofsson O. Psychological and social outcome of epilepsy in well-functioning children and adolescents. A 10-year follow-up study. Eur J Paediatr Neurol. 2014;18(3):381–90.
51. Schneider-von Podewils F, Gasse C, Geithner J, Wang ZI, Bombach P, Berneiser J, et al. Clinical predictors of the long-term social outcome and quality of life in juvenile myoclonic epilepsy: 20–65 years of follow-up. Epilepsia. 2014;55(2):322–30.
52. Hum KM, Smith ML, Lach L, Elliott IM. Self-perceptions of social function 2 years after pediatric epilepsy surgery. Epilepsy Behav. 2010;17(3):354–9.
53. Park CK, Kim SK, Wang KC, Hwang YS, Kim KJ, Chae JH, et al. Surgical outcome and prognostic factors of pediatric epilepsy caused by cortical dysplasia. Childs Nerv Syst. 2006;22(6):586–92.
54. Keene DL, Loy-English I, Ventureyra EC. Long-term socioeconomic outcome following surgical intervention in the treatment of refractory epilepsy in childhood and adolescence. Childs Nerv Syst. 1998;14(8):362–5.

Chapter 14
Subjective Experiences of Epilepsy Surgery in Adults

Kristina Malmgren, Anneli Ozanne, and Sarah J. Wilson

Abstract This chapter reviews the limited literature on patients' subjective expectations and experiences of epilepsy surgery. Patients with drug-resistant epilepsy have widespread fears and misconceptions about epilepsy surgery and often see it as a "last resort." Their expectations of epilepsy surgery include driving, employment, greater independence, and a better social life, as well as less likely changes such as improved memory and cognition. Patients with more practical expectations have been shown to be more likely to consider surgery a success. Certain gender and racial differences have also emerged in a few studies. Adjustment to life after surgery, especially the need to discard the sick role for those who become seizure-free, has been shown to take several years.

Studies of patient-perceived memory changes after temporal lobe resection (TLR) fail to show significant relationships between subjective and objective postoperative memory function. Perceived sexual changes after TLR include improvement in sexuality in those seizure-free but also hypersexuality in some. Patients' perceptions of recurrence of seizures after epilepsy surgery are dominated by psychological issues (perceived loss of self-control, reduced self-confidence, day-to-day stress, and altered expectations for the future) but are also related to the presence of seizure improvement. While the majority of patients report satisfaction after epilepsy surgery, how this should be interpreted is not entirely clear, with a focus on dissatisfaction potentially providing more information.

K. Malmgren, MD, PhD (✉)
Department of Clinical Neuroscience and Rehabilitation, Institute of Neuroscience and Physiology, Sahlgrenska Academy, Gothenburg University, Gothenburg, Sweden

Department of Neurology, Sahlgrenska University Hospital, Gothenburg, Sweden
e-mail: Kristina.malmgren@neuro.gu.se

A. Ozanne, PhD
Institute of Health Care Sciences, The Sahlgrenska Academy, University of Gothenburg, Gothenburg, Sweden

S.J. Wilson, PhD
Melbourne School of Psychological Sciences, The University of Melbourne, Melbourne, VIC, Australia

Comprehensive Epilepsy Program, Austin Health, Melbourne, VIC, Australia

K. Malmgren et al. (eds.), *Long-Term Outcomes of Epilepsy Surgery in Adults and Children*, DOI 10.1007/978-3-319-17783-0_14

There are as yet no published studies of patient experiences with a follow-up of more than 2 years. In one recent preliminary report with a mean follow-up of 13 years, long-term perceptions of the impact of epilepsy surgery in principle equaled the perceptions at the 2-year follow-up. Further studies of patients' long-term experiences after epilepsy surgery are needed.

Keywords Patient experiences • Epilepsy surgery • Long-term outcomes • Qualitative study

Introduction

Assessments of outcomes after epilepsy surgery include many aspects, as exemplified in this volume. Apart from medical outcomes concerning seizures, complications, and cognition, the last decades have seen an increasing amount of patient-related outcome measures such as psychosocial outcomes, health-related quality of life, and mood. However, a surprisingly small number of studies focus on patients' subjective expectations and own narratives of their experiences after surgery compared to the literature in other domains.

This chapter will focus on these issues and is therefore mostly limited to qualitative studies, which deal with patient descriptions obtained via interviews and focus groups, with the exception of a few very relevant questionnaire-based studies. In those studies that have employed a mixed-methods approach (combining qualitative and quantitative methods), the focus will be on the qualitative data. A broad range of databases were searched to identify relevant studies, including Pubmed, CINAHL, PsychINFO, and Scopus.

Perceptions About Epilepsy Surgery in Patients with Drug-Resistant Epilepsy

In the last decade, several qualitative studies have explored perceptions about epilepsy surgery in patients with drug-resistant epilepsy. Using focus groups, one study identified that many patients with intractable epilepsy had a negative attitude towards epilepsy surgery. Patients also felt that their health care providers portrayed epilepsy surgery negatively [1]. In a questionnaire-based study, brain surgery was rated as having a mean dangerousness of 8.3 (on a scale of 1–10) by 94 patients with no history of neurosurgery. In addition, 51 % of these patients would not consider surgical treatment even if it were guaranteed to stop their seizures without causing deficits [2]. In a multicenter questionnaire study of 228 patients attending epilepsy clinics across Italy, widespread fears and misconceptions about epilepsy surgery were disclosed [3].

In a recent study from Canada, in which a brief questionnaire was administered to consecutive adults with focal epilepsy seen in an epilepsy clinic, 55.4 % of the 107 participants (response rate: 83 %) perceived epilepsy surgery to be "very or moderately dangerous" and 61 % agreed with the statement "Brain surgery should be considered a last resort." Sixty percent incorrectly identified the risk of overall serious side effects from epilepsy surgery to be over 10 %. By contrast, over half of the patients had not heard of sudden unexpected death in epilepsy [4].

Choi and colleagues conducted focus groups with patients who had undergone epilepsy surgery in order to develop a patient decision aid for temporal lobe resection (TLR). On reflecting on their own experiences prior to surgery, patients described limited availability of individualized information on the Internet and had a desire for more detailed descriptions of what it would be like to live with the possible negative consequences of surgery. Once patients had received more thorough information, they felt more willing to accept the possibility of experiencing negative outcomes [5].

Patient Expectations and Hopes

In a study of the expectations of 70 presurgical candidates, a rating scale with 20 descriptive terms covering personality, cognitive, and emotional dimensions was used. Patients rated themselves at the time of presurgical investigation and were also asked to rate how they believed they would be if the surgery was successful. The analysis showed that patients were expecting significant positive changes in many dimensions postoperatively, such as having an improved memory, and being more skillful and clever. The authors recommended that such implicit assumptions should be identified and addressed preoperatively, so that candidates can make truly informed decisions about surgery [6].

Taylor and colleagues emphasized the importance of the surgical team undertaking a preoperative interview with patients and their families to derive a list of agreed-upon aims of epilepsy surgery [7]. In a further study using in-depth interviews, the aims of 69 patients and carers were analyzed, identifying five commonly endorsed aims: desire for work, driving, independence, socializing, and freedom from drugs [8]. Using a standardized, in-depth, semi-structured clinical interview, Wilson and colleagues explored the spontaneously generated reasons of 60 patients for seeking surgery. Seventy-two percent reported seizure freedom, followed by driving (45 %), the development of new activities (38 %), and employment opportunities (35 %), with less emphasis on expectations of a psychosocial nature [9]. In a US multicenter cohort study of 389 adults undergoing resective epilepsy surgery, potential gender differences in expectations were explored using a list of 12 items based on the literature and clinical experience. Men and women both ranked anticipated changes in driving and memory as most important. Women rated driving, physical activity limitations, and economic worries as less important, and fatigue and pregnancy concerns as more important than men [10]. In another study from the same group, racial differences in expectations were explored using open-ended questions, allowing expectation themes to be rank-ordered. Among 391 respondents, the two most frequently endorsed expectations were driving (62 %) and job/school (43 %). Nonwhites were found to endorse job/school and cognition more frequently and driving less frequently than whites [11].

A recent study by Patton and colleagues explored the use of "hope language" in epilepsy surgery candidates. Thirty-eight adult patients completed a semi-structured interview 1 day prior to surgery, with transcripts coded thematically using standard qualitative analysis. Ninety-two percent of participants used the word "hope" or one of its derivatives. In 25 participants, hope was used to express optimism associated with the term, whereas in 27 participants, hope inversely expressed forms of dread, tempered expectations, and uncertainty about surgery. The investigators recommended that health care professionals should clarify use of the word "hope" when assessing patient beliefs, goals, and understanding of surgery [12].

Patient-Perceived Impact of Epilepsy Surgery

Short-Term Outcome After Surgery

In a follow-up study by Wilson and colleagues [13], medical and psychosocial factors independently contributing to perceived surgical success were examined. Patient perceptions of the impact of surgery were related to their preoperative expectations. Seizure outcome made the largest independent contribution, but post-operative affect and preoperative expectations made additional unique and significant contributions to perceived success. Twenty-six patients (43 %) clearly identified the operation as a success at a 6-month review. Patients emphasizing practical expectations prior to surgery (i.e., driving, employment, activities) were more likely to consider the operation a success than those who expected it to enhance personal independence, family, or social relationships. A predictive model of perceived surgical success emerged, which highlighted the multidimensionality of outcome, including the importance of discarding sick role behaviors associated with chronic epilepsy after surgery [13] (Fig. 14.1).

Longitudinal Assessment up to Twenty-Four Months

In a longitudinal study by Wilson and colleagues [14], 90 in-depth, semi-structured clinical interviews were conducted with the patient and family, with the aim of exploring the longitudinal course of postoperative adjustment. In particular, they mapped the incidence of symptoms of "the burden of normality" over a period of 2 years, examining symptom occurrence relative to seizure outcome. These

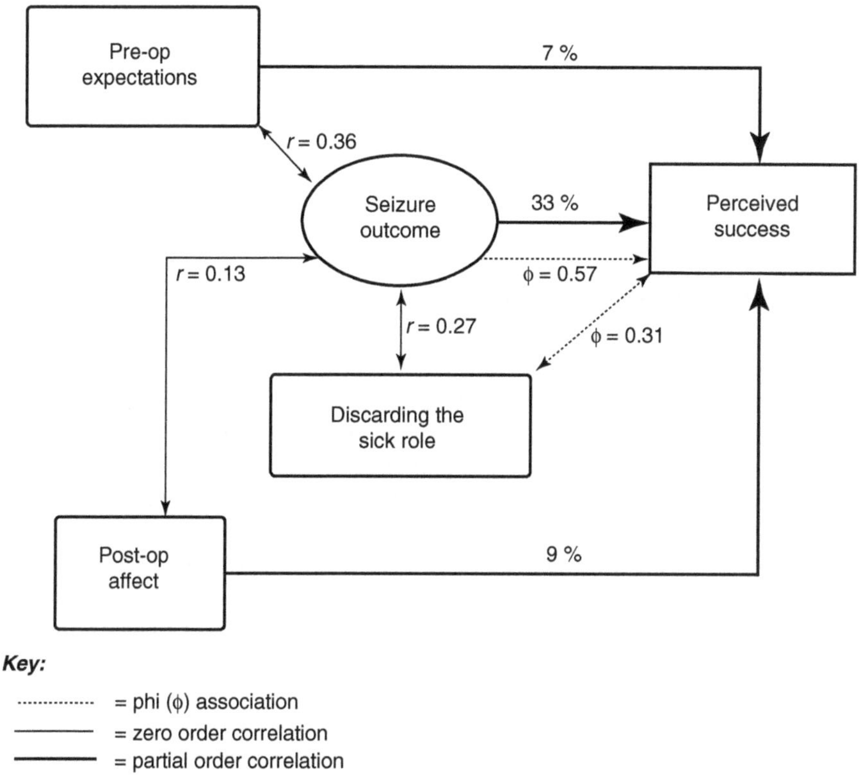

Fig. 14.1 Multidimensional model of surgical outcome showing the independent contributions of seizure outcome, preoperative expectations, and postoperative mood to patient perceptions of surgical success. Note that the patient's ability to discard sick role behaviors also contributes to perceived success but is dependent on being rendered seizure-free (Reprinted from [13], Figure 2 with permission from Elsevier)

symptoms comprise changes commonly reported by patients and families after surgery as they adapt to living without epilepsy [15]. Psychologically, patients often describe feeling and thinking differently about themselves (e.g., having greater self-confidence), including a sense of being "cured" or "transformed" now they no longer have seizures. This may be accompanied by an increase in expectations that patients place on themselves to be "normal" or well, and a desire to catch-up on missed opportunities or time lost due to the effects of chronic epilepsy. It can also lead to significant changes in family roles, particularly as the patient moves towards greater personal independence and new vocational and social activities. Alternatively, some patients may avoid taking on new roles and experience a sense of loss of their epilepsy and some of the benefits it provided.

In total, Wilson and colleagues [14] showed that 66 % of patients reported symptoms of the burden of normality at some time within the first 2 years of surgery. At the 24-month review, patients who had been seizure-free or experienced auras only were significantly more likely to report symptoms compared to patients who had experienced seizures, supporting the notion that the burden of normality arises from a process of adjustment as the patient learns to become well. It has also been shown to be greater in patients with seizure onset before or during adolescence, with these patients reporting greater changes in their self-identity, which can ultimately have positive effects for health-related quality of life [16].

Long-Term Outcome After Surgery

In Sweden, Taft and colleagues recently reported the results of a 2-year outcome study of a national sample of 96 patients assessed before and after epilepsy surgery using health-related quality of life questionnaires, and satisfaction with surgery rated on a 7-point Likert scale [17]. Eighty of these patients (83 %) also answered open-ended questions at baseline, 77 (96 %) at 2 years, and 54 (67.5 %) at a mean long-term follow-up of 13 years after surgery (range 10–16 years) [18]. Preoperative questions tapped patients' hopes and worries concerning epilepsy surgery, and questions at the follow-ups focused on whether surgery had led to benefit and/or harm. Data were analyzed by qualitative content analysis. Preoperatively, patients expressed both expectations (seizure freedom, less medication, a richer social life, better self-confidence) and fears of surgery (continued seizures, complications). Interestingly, the results from the long-term follow-up were mostly consistent with the 2-year follow-up, providing limited support for a long-term reprioritization effect in quality-of-life domains [19]. In particular, patients reported increased independence, a new life, and better self-confidence. Eighty-seven percent reported positive experiences at the 2-year follow-up and 94 % at the long-term follow-up. Some patients, however, also or only had negative experiences of surgery: they felt that life had changed for the worse through psychological problems and or physical complications (25 % after two years, and 19 % at the long-term follow-up). Some seizure-free patients reported difficulties "finding oneself" consistent with the burden of normality [15].

Subjective Experiences of Memory Change After Epilepsy Surgery

Several studies have explored the relationship between objective memory change after TLR and patient report of memory change. In one study of 65 patients undergoing TLR, the prevalence of significant subjective memory decline 1 year after surgery ranged from 3 to 7 %, whereas the prevalence of significant objective memory decline ranged from 26 to 55 % [20]. In another study of 290 patients followed 1 year after TLR, no significant relationships were found between subjective ratings of postoperative memory function and objective indices of change [21].

A meta-analysis of subjective memory complaints derived from 465 TLR patients and 171 informants suggests that following TLR, most patients do not report changes in their memory function. As a result, the authors recommended that a comprehensive discussion of surgical risks and benefits should incorporate both patient impressions and objective memory outcomes [22].

Patient-Perceived Sexual Change After TLR

Christianson and colleagues investigated changes in sexuality and life satisfaction through a cross-sectional survey and obtained answers from 53/91 operated, 15/15 nonoperated patients with drug-resistant epilepsy, and 50/200 healthy controls. Specific questions regarding sexuality revealed a lower sex drive among epilepsy patients compared to controls. In most cases, there were no differences between the operated and the nonoperated patients, although the seizure-free group rated a higher level of life satisfaction and sexuality than the non-seizure-free group [23].

Another study reported 7 patients out of a series of 60, who spontaneously reported hypersexuality after unilateral TLR. All of the patients had significant difficulties with postoperative psychosocial adjustment that preceded the onset of hypersexuality, leading the researchers to conclude that hypersexuality following TLR most likely represents a complex interaction of biological and psychosocial factors [24]. In a study exploring the relationship between the amygdala and sexual drive, 21/45 patients reported a sexual increase after TLR, 14 did not describe any sexual change, and 10 reported a sexual decrease [25].

In a recent survey of 50 married males before and after TLR and 50 healthy controls, self-perceived sexual desire and satisfaction were low in patients compared to controls. Although the majority of the sexual domains improved after TLR, even after a median duration of 5 years, the sexual status of the patients did not match that of controls. Patients who were seizure-free and either AED-free or on monotherapy at the last follow-up, reported a better sexual outcome [26].

Patient Experiences of Seizure Recurrence

There is limited understanding of a patient's experience of the recurrence of seizures after surgery. One in-depth interview study of 15 patients, on average 6 years after surgery, identified key themes using content analysis of patient spontaneous reports of the experience of seizure recurrence. The results showed a prominence of psychological issues over medical concerns. The four most frequently expressed themes were perceived success of surgery, medication, acceptance of seizure recurrence, and personal independence. Despite seizure recurrence, patient sentiments were not universally negative. There was heterogeneity of views, with some reporting ambivalence and others a sense of satisfaction with outcome. Patients with substantial seizure improvement (9/9) were significantly more likely to report positive subthemes of surgical success than patients with no substantial seizure improvement (1/6) [27].

A recent review of the broader literature on suboptimal results after medical interventions (including epilepsy surgery) identified 22 qualitative studies of patients experiencing a range of suboptimal outcomes. In order of frequency, the most common patient experiences included altered social dynamics and stigma, unmet expectations, negative emotions, use of coping strategies, hope and optimism, perceived failure of the treating team, psychiatric symptoms, and control issues. The authors concluded that knowledge of common patient experiences can assist in the delivery of patient follow-up and rehabilitation services tailored to differing outcomes after epilepsy surgery [28].

Family Experiences

Several of the qualitative studies described above include assessment of family experiences. In one in-depth interview study focusing on six families before and 6–8 months after epilepsy surgery, the concept of "sudden health" was described. The findings indicated that families were organized in two primary ways (nesting and crisis) to deal with the epilepsy and the aftermath of surgery. The patient's "sudden health" postsurgery had differing effects on these two types of families that depended on their organizational style, emotional communication, and developmental dynamics [29].

Patient Satisfaction

Since most patient satisfaction surveys in health care settings show high rates of satisfaction, the interpretation of satisfaction as the outcome of an active evaluation has been increasingly called into question. In a study using unstructured in-depth interviews with users of mental health services, many expressions of "satisfaction" were shown to hide a variety of reported negative experiences. The authors concluded that "dissatisfaction" rates may be a more useful indicator of a minimum level of negative experience and, therefore, of potential use in benchmarking exercises [30]. Consistent with this, in a study of the predictors of satisfaction, a lack of unmet expectations was shown to be a powerful predictor of satisfaction at all time-points [31].

A systematic review of eight studies published up to June 2009 focused on patient satisfaction with all types of epilepsy surgery [32]. Satisfaction was assessed using one or more global questions from which four themes emerged: (1) satisfied or dissatisfied, (2) perceived success or failure, (3) overall positive or negative impact, and (4) willingness to repeat surgery or regretting surgery. Overall, 71 % of patients were satisfied; 64 % considered surgery a success; it had a positive effect for 78 %; and 87 % would repeat surgery. Seizure freedom was the most common predictor of epilepsy surgery satisfaction, whereas the presence of postoperative neurologic deficits predicted dissatisfaction. In a recent prospective study of a representative national sample of 96 Swedish patients before and 2 years after epilepsy surgery, 80 % were satisfied with having had surgery and 86 % considered that they had benefited, whereas 20 % thought that surgery caused some harm [17].

Conclusions and Future Directions

The literature on patients' subjective expectations and experiences of epilepsy surgery is limited and most longitudinal studies are limited to follow-ups of 6 months to 2 years (see Appendix). The aspects studied range from preoperative expectations (hopes as well as fears) to how social and psychological changes influence patient perceptions of the success of epilepsy surgery. Since most patients who undergo epilepsy surgery have had epilepsy half of their lives, it is conceivable that it takes several years until their life situation has stabilized. There are, however, as yet no published studies with a longer perspective than 2 years. There is one recent preliminary report with a mean follow-up of 13 years, in which the long-term perceptions of the impact of epilepsy surgery in principle equaled the perceptions at the 2-year follow-up. Patients' long-term subjective experiences of the effects of epilepsy surgery across different domains of life need further study in order to provide epilepsy surgery candidates with realistic counseling, and to consider the need for postoperative rehabilitation efforts.

Appendix. Summary of Studies on Subjective Experiences in Adults After Epilepsy Surgery

Author, year	Study design	Sample size (m/f)	Mean age at surgery (years)	Mean age at seizure onset	Surgical procedure	Seizure outcome (N)	Summary of results	Follow-up interval
Baird et al. 2002 [24]	RE, case reports	7 (2/5)	35	9	TLR	5 seizure-free, 1 with auras, 1 with auras, CPS, GTCS	Hypersexuality following TLR more likely to occur in patients with psychosocial difficulties and contralateral temporal lobe abnormalities	Presurgery and 3 weeks to 9 months after surgery
Baird et al. 2004 [25]	PR, RE, quantitative and qualitative	Patients: 45 (22/23) Controls: 46 (22/24)	36	NR	TLR	NR	21 patients reported sexual increase, 14 no change, 10 sexual decrease	Presurgery and follow-ups for a minimum of 2 years
Baxendale and Thompson 1996 [6]	PR, quantitative	Presurgical group: 70 (33/37) Postsurgical group: 32 (13/19)	Mean preop 31.8	11.7	TLR	1 year postop: Seizure-free or only auras 68.7 %, rare seizures 18.7 %, no worthwhile improvement 12.6 %	Expectations before surgery: be happier, more in control, more hopeful, independent, and interested in life. Seizure-free patients more in control, trends to feeling happier, more hopeful and friendly	Presurgery and 1 year after surgery
Baxendale and Thompson 2005 [21]	PR, quantitative	290 (sex not reported)	Age at study entry or surgery 31.7	11.3	TLR	1 year postop 65.5 % seizure-free	Almost 1/3 experienced deterioration in verbal learning. Significant improvements were better in the right TLR group than in the left TLR group	Presurgery, 6 and 12 months after surgery

Christianson et al. 1995 [23]	PR, quantitative	118 (63/55)	Mean age at interview 37.6	NR	TLR, XTLR	All nonoperated had seizures, 59 % of operated were seizure-free	Lower sexual drive in epilepsy patients than controls. Higher satisfaction among seizure-free operated than those not seizure-free	Postsurgery cross-sectional follow-up time NR
Ozanne et al. 2014 [18]	PR, qualitative longitudinal	80 (42/38)	NR	NR	NR	44/77 seizure-free at 2 years follow-up and 37/54 at long-term follow-up	Hope before surgery: reduction of seizures and medication, richer social life, better self-confidence. Afraid of surgery, continued seizures and complications. Mostly equal results at short- and long-term follow-up. Patients experienced increased independence, a few experienced that life had changed to the worse	Presurgery, 2 years after surgery and 13 years after surgery (range 10–16 years)
Ramesha et al. 2012 [26]	PR, quantitative	50 patients 50 controls (only men)	Pat: 39.8 Controls: 41.3	Median 12 (3–22 yrs)	TLR	Seizure-free: 39 (78 %)	Poor sexual satisfaction after surgery compared with controls	Presurgery and 5 years after surgery (range 1–13 years)
Sawrie et al. 1999 [20]	PR, quantitative	65 operated patients (27/38), 39 controls (20/19)	Surgery group: 34.6 Control group: 36.6	Average epilepsy duration: 22.1 Control group: 17.1	TLR	NR	No significant relation between subjective and objective memory change in operated patents	Baseline and 1 year after randomization

(continued)

Appendix (continued)

Author, year	Study design	Sample size (m/f)	Mean age at surgery (years)	Mean age at seizure onset	Surgical procedure	Seizure outcome (N)	Summary of results	Follow-up interval
Seaburn and Erba 2003 [29]	PR, qualitative	6 patients with their families (2/4)	Mean age at the interview: 39.6 (patients)	15.8	TLR	All seizure-free or greatly reduced seizure frequency	The families were organized in two ways to deal with the disease and the aftermath of surgery. The families' organizational style, emotional communication process, and developmental dynamics affect how "sudden health" will affect them	Presurgery and 6–8 months after surgery
Shirbin et al. 2009 [27]	PR, qualitative and quantitative	15 (6/9)	35.8 (11)	14.4 (12)	TLR, XTLR	All had seizures: 9 were substantially improved	The most frequently expressed themes were perceived success of surgery, medication, acceptance of seizure recurrence, and personal independence	≥12 months since surgery
Williams et al. 2009 [22]	PR, quantitative	64	NR	NR	TLR	NR	Most patients reported no change or improvement in memory after surgery. 7.8% reported deterioration	8.8 months before and 1 year after surgery

Wilson et al. 2010 [16]	PR, quantitative	57 (30/27)	Mean age at interview: 35	Infancy 12 Childhood 14 Adolescent 17 Adult 14	TLR, XTLR	Seizure-free at 1 month: 47 3 months: 41 12 months: 36	Patients with high neuroticism and low extraversion predisposed to greater depression after surgery. Over 70% with high neuroticism reported disrupted family dynamics and difficulties adjusting to seizure freedom	Presurgery, 1, 3, and 12 months after surgery
Wilson et al. 2001 [14]	PR, quantitative, qualitative	90 (38/52)	Mean age at interview: 32.7	11.1	TLR	18 months follow-up: Seizure-free: 47 Auras only: 13 CPS and/or GTCS: 30	66% reported symptoms within the first 2 years of surgery. Symptoms often emerged by the 3-month review and were frequently seen also after 2 years	7–10 days postsurgery 1, 3, 6, 12, 24 month after surgery
Wilson et al. 1999 [13]	PR, quantitative	50 (21/29)	NR	10.6	TLR	NR	Independent effects included patients' preoperative expectations, their postoperative seizure outcome, and affective state. The importance of discarding sick role behaviors associated with chronic epilepsy, after surgery was also highlighted	Presurgery and 6 months after surgery

(continued)

Appendix (continued)

Author, year	Study design	Sample size (m/f)	Mean age at surgery (years)	Mean age at seizure onset	Surgical procedure	Seizure outcome (N)	Summary of results	Follow-up interval
Wilson et al. 1998 [9]	PR, qualitative	60 (23/37)	Mean age at interview: 31.0	10.6	TLR	31/50 seizure-free or auras only. 19/50 CPS and/or GTCS	Patients who perceived surgery as successful endorsed "practical" expectations as driving, employment, activities preoperatively, rather than psychological or social expectations	Presurgery and 6 months after surgery

RE retrospective, *PR* prospective, *NR* not reported, *TLR* temporal, *XTLR* extratemporal, *SD* standard deviation, *CPS* complex partial, *GTCS* generalized tonic-clonic seizures

References

1. Swarztrauber K, Dewar S, Engel Jr J. Patient attitudes about treatments for intractable epilepsy. Epilepsy Behav. 2003;4(1):19–25.
2. Prus N, Grant AC. Patient beliefs about epilepsy and brain surgery in a multicultural urban population. Epilepsy Behav. 2010;17(1):46–9.
3. Erba G, Messina P, Pupillo E, Beghi E. Acceptance of epilepsy surgery among adults with epilepsy–what do patients think? Epilepsy Behav. 2012;24(3):352–8.
4. Hrazdil C, Roberts JI, Wiebe S, Sauro K, Vautour M, Hanson A, et al. Patient perceptions and barriers to epilepsy surgery: evaluation in a large health region. Epilepsy Behav. 2013;28(1):52–65.
5. Choi H, Pargeon K, Bausell R, Wong JB, Mendiratta A, Bakken S. Temporal lobe epilepsy surgery: what do patients want to know? Epilepsy Behav. 2011;22(3):479–82.
6. Baxendale SA, Thompson PJ. "If I didn't have epilepsy …": patient expectations of epilepsy surgery. J Epilepsy. 1996;9(4):274–81.
7. Taylor DC, Neville BG, Cross JH. New measures of outcome needed for the surgical treatment of epilepsy. Epilepsia. 1997;38(6):625–30.
8. Taylor DC, McMacKin D, Staunton H, Delanty N, Phillips J. Patients' aims for epilepsy surgery: desires beyond seizure freedom. Epilepsia. 2001;42(5):629–33.
9. Wilson SJ, Saling MM, Kincade P, Bladin PF. Patient expectations of temporal lobe surgery. Epilepsia. 1998;39(2):167–74.
10. Bower CM, Hays RD, Devinsky O, Spencer SS, Sperling MR, Haut S, et al. Expectations prior to epilepsy surgery: an exploratory comparison of men and women. Seizure J Br Epilepsy Assoc. 2009;18(3):228–31.
11. Baca CB, Cheng EM, Spencer SS, Vassar S, Vickrey BG. Racial differences in patient expectations prior to resective epilepsy surgery. Epilepsy Behav. 2009;15(4):452–5.
12. Patton DJ, Busch RM, Yee KM, Kubu CS, Gonzalez-Martinez J, Ford PJ. Hope language in patients undergoing epilepsy surgery. Epilepsy Behav. 2013;29(1):90–5.
13. Wilson SJ, Saling MM, Lawrence J, Bladin PF. Outcome of temporal lobectomy: expectations and the prediction of perceived success. Epilepsy Res. 1999;36(1):1–14.
14. Wilson SJ, Bladin PF, Saling MM, McIntosh AM, Lawrence JA. The longitudinal course of adjustment after seizure surgery. Seizure J Br Epilepsy Assoc. 2001;10(3):165–72.
15. Wilson S, Bladin P, Saling M. The "burden of normality": concepts of adjustment after surgery for seizures. J Neurol Neurosurg Psychiatry. 2001;70(5):649–56.
16. Wilson SJ, Wrench JM, McIntosh AM, Bladin PF, Berkovic SF. Profiles of psychosocial outcome after epilepsy surgery: the role of personality. Epilepsia. 2010;51(7):1133–8.
17. Taft C, Sager Magnusson E, Ekstedt G, Malmgren K. Health-related quality of life, mood, and patient satisfaction after epilepsy surgery in Sweden–a prospective controlled observational study. Epilepsia. 2014;55(6):878–85.
18. Ozanne A, Graneheim UH, Ekstedt G, Malmgren K. Patient experiences of epilepsy surgery – a longitudinal qualitative study. Epilepsia. 2014;55:174.
19. Sajobi TT, Fiest KM, Wiebe S. Changes in quality of life after epilepsy surgery: the role of reprioritization response shift. Epilepsia. 2014;55(9):1331–8.
20. Sawrie SM, Martin RC, Kuzniecky R, Faught E, Morawetz R, Jamil F, et al. Subjective versus objective memory change after temporal lobe epilepsy surgery. Neurology. 1999;53(7):1511–7.
21. Baxendale S, Thompson P. Defining meaningful postoperative change in epilepsy surgery patients: measuring the unmeasurable? Epilepsy Behav. 2005;6(2):207–11.
22. Williams J, Martin M, McGlone J. The patient's experience of memory change after elective temporal lobe resection. Can J Neurol Sci Le J Can Des Sci Neurol. 2009;36 Suppl 2:S46–50.
23. Christianson SA, Silfvenius H, Saisa J, Nilsson M. Life satisfaction and sexuality in patients operated for epilepsy. Acta Neurol Scand. 1995;92(1):1–6.

24. Baird AD, Wilson SJ, Bladin PF, Saling MM, Reutens DC. Hypersexuality after temporal lobe resection. Epilepsy Behav. 2002;3(2):173–81.
25. Baird AD, Wilson SJ, Bladin PF, Saling MM, Reutens DC. The amygdala and sexual drive: insights from temporal lobe epilepsy surgery. Ann Neurol. 2004;55(1):87–96.
26. Ramesha KN, Radhakrishnan A, Jiayaspathi A, Padickaparambal S, Alexander A, Unnikrishnan JP, et al. Sexual desire and satisfaction after resective surgery in patients with mesial temporal lobe epilepsy with hippocampal sclerosis. Epilepsy Behav. 2012;25(3):374–80.
27. Shirbin CA, McIntosh AM, Wilson SJ. The experience of seizures after epilepsy surgery. Epilepsy Behav. 2009;16(1):82–5.
28. Fernando DK, McIntosh AM, Bladin PF, Wilson SJ. Common experiences of patients following suboptimal treatment outcomes: implications for epilepsy surgery. Epilepsy Behav. 2014;33:144–51.
29. Seaburn DB, Erba G. The family experience of "sudden health": the case of intractable epilepsy. Fam Process. 2003;42(4):453–67.
30. Williams B, Coyle J, Healy D. The meaning of patient satisfaction: an explanation of high reported levels. Soc Sci Med (1982). 1998;47(9):1351–9.
31. Jackson JL, Chamberlin J, Kroenke K. Predictors of patient satisfaction. Soc Sci Med (1982). 2001;52(4):609–20.
32. Macrodimitris S, Sherman EM, Williams TS, Bigras C, Wiebe S. Measuring patient satisfaction following epilepsy surgery. Epilepsia. 2011;52(8):1409–17.

Chapter 15
Subjective Experiences of Children and Parents After Epilepsy Surgery

Siobhan Hannan

Abstract There are few studies examining the child and parent experience of epilepsy surgery, in the shorter or longer term. From the studies available, achievement of seizure freedom is associated with a higher degree of patient satisfaction while ongoing postoperative neurological deficit and/or associated psychosocial and behavioral concerns are associated with lower satisfaction. The small number of studies may reflect challenges with measuring this construct. A systematic evaluation of patient satisfaction, however, should be considered as an additional component when evaluating the efficacy of epilepsy surgery.

Studies considering outcomes in terms of neurological and cognitive, psychiatric and behavioral outcomes, health-related quality of life, and psychosocial outcomes are discussed in other chapters.

Keywords Pediatric epilepsy surgery • Child and parent subjective experience • Patient satisfaction • Health outcomes

Satisfaction with epilepsy surgery can be broadly defined as the child and parent's evaluation of the process of undergoing epilepsy surgery and its associated outcomes [1]. The child and parent's subjective or personal experience of surgery are influenced by a number of factors including seizure freedom, neurological and cognitive sequelae, psychiatric and behavioral outcomes, health-related quality of life, and psychosocial outcomes. There are few pediatric studies examining patient satisfaction alone.

A study reviewing surgical outcomes and parental satisfaction in 48 children with encephalopathy who underwent epilepsy surgery included a telephone interview with parents to review functional outcomes and parental satisfaction 1 year after surgery [2]. No information is provided as to whether the telephone interview consisted of open-ended or closed survey questions. Twenty-seven out of thirty-one

S. Hannan, RN, RSCN, MSc, INP
Paediatric Neurology, Chelsea and Westminster Hospital NHS Foundation Trust, London, UK
e-mail: siobhan.hannan@chelwest.nhs.uk

K. Malmgren et al. (eds.), *Long-Term Outcomes of Epilepsy Surgery in Adults and Children*, DOI 10.1007/978-3-319-17783-0_15

parents (87.1 %) reported overall satisfaction with surgery. All parents (100 %) whose children became seizure-free were reportedly satisfied with the surgery. Of the 18 children who were not seizure-free 14 (77.8 %) were satisfied, due to improvement in alertness, hyperactivity, concentration, facial expression, and responsiveness. The satisfaction rate was 83.3 % in parents whose children underwent resective surgery and 92.3 % in those who had palliative surgery.

Iwasaki et al. examined the benefit of corpus callosotomy in terms of parental satisfaction and seizure outcome and found improvements in frequency, intensity, and duration of seizures were correlated with the level of parental satisfaction [3]. The study included 16 children with early childhood onset epilepsy who underwent one-stage total corpus callosotomy. Length of follow-up ranged from 6 to 45 months (median 24 months). The survey consisted of eight open-ended and two closed (yes/no) questions. In the open-ended questions, specific behavioral changes were described by ten parents; eight with positive, one with neutral, and one with negative comments. Satisfaction was attributed to seizure improvement by eight parents, to the behavioral improvement by five and to both by two parents. The highest level of satisfaction was only reported in patients who achieved seizure freedom from all seizures or drop attacks.

An uncontrolled case series of 13 children demonstrated postoperative reductions in the severity and impact of emotional and behavioral symptoms, following epilepsy surgery, during follow-up of up to eight and a half years [4]. This study also included qualitative data on parental experience via a telephone interview 7.5–8.5 years after surgery. The interview consisted of a series of 16 closed (yes/no) and open-ended questions relating to seizure frequency, overall well-being following surgery, the child's behavior and psychosocial functioning, whether parents regretted surgery or felt it had been successful, and whether parental aims of surgery documented prior to surgery had been met. Documented parental goals for surgery were seizure freedom or a reduction in seizures, with secondary aims for an improvement in developmental progress and/or improvement in behavior and quality of life. Presurgical goals were met in 8 out of 13 subjects and partially met in a further 5 out of 13 subjects. Overall, no parents expressed regrets about their child undergoing surgery and most (70 %) expressed satisfaction with the outcomes for their child following surgery. The biggest predictor of parental satisfaction was seizure freedom, while ongoing prosocial behaviors (conduct disorder, inattention, and hyperactivity; emotional symptoms) was associated with parental dissatisfaction.

Keene et al. conducted a telephone satisfaction survey of 63 patients who had undergone an earlier resection before 18 years of age; mean length of follow-up 7.6 years [5]. The survey consisted of a series of open-ended questions. When asked what if any positive benefits or negative effects they had experienced since surgery, almost 80 % reported some positive effects, 59 % no significant negative effect, and 16 % some negative effects. When asked to rate, on a scale of 0–9, their satisfaction as a result of having had surgery, 52 % reported high satisfaction (6–9); 30 % were indifferent (5); and 17 % were dissatisfied (0–4). The biggest predictor of satisfaction was seizure outcome, with strong positive correlation found between seizure control and degree of satisfaction and between perceived postsurgical neurological deficits and dissatisfaction.

Engelhart et al. reviewed how adolescents and their caregivers looked back on epilepsy surgery performed early in life [6]. The study cohort consisted of 111 participants; 53 children and parents, 3 children only and 55 parents only. The length of follow-up was between 1 and 10 years. The questionnaire asked three principle questions: "Would you do it again?" "With the benefit of hindsight, would you opt again for epilepsy surgery?" "What is the main motive behind your response to the former question?" and "How do you now evaluate the surgical outcome?" The questions were framed as a series of open-ended, multiple-choice and "yes," "no," or "not applicable" questions. Data were processed separately for children seizure-free and those in whom seizures recurred. Of the 56 participating children, 46 (82 %) were seizure-free. Almost all (93 % of the seizure-free children and nine out of ten children with seizures in the previous year) responded "definitely yes" or "probably yes," and one with seizure recurrence responded they would definitely not re-opt for surgery. Three seizure- free children were unsure whether they would opt again for surgery. Among the parents whose children were seizure-free, three (96 %) would definitely or probably re-opt for surgery, whereas 23 (85 %) of those whose children experienced seizures felt the same. Three parents of seizure-free children and two parents with current seizures were unsure whether they would re-opt for surgery and two children with current seizures said they would probably not opt again for surgery. The biggest predictor of satisfaction was seizure outcome, with strong positive correlation found between seizure freedom and a change in "well-being" and degree of satisfaction and between perceived postsurgical recurrence of seizures and neurological deficits and dissatisfaction.

In all of these studies a higher degree of patient satisfaction was consistently associated with overall seizure freedom, while lower satisfaction was associated with ongoing postoperative neurological deficit and psychosocial or behavioral concerns. There are, however, many limitations to these studies including, the heterogeneous nature of patients and lack of uniformity in questionnaires.

Epilepsy surgery has been shown to be an effective treatment for improving seizure control [7, 8]. Studies have also demonstrated cognitive, psychiatric, behavioral, quality of life, and psychosocial improvements as outcomes of surgery [9, 10]. Less attention has been directed toward the subjective experience of children and parents following surgery. Patient satisfaction is a significant aspect of collaborative models of patient-centered health care. Measuring patient satisfaction has an important role in informing the planning, delivery, and evaluation of care [11, 12]. Satisfaction measures provide patient input regarding the effectiveness of medical treatment, have been shown to influence an individual's health-related decision making, and are important indicators of how well treatment has met patient expectations [13, 14]. Patient level of satisfaction with received health care services has also been shown to predict treatment success, compliance, and appropriate use of services [15, 16].

Subjective data enable clinicians to measure whether parental goals of surgery obtained preoperatively are met in the longer term. This approach is a method of maintaining quality control and recording the overall performance of epilepsy surgery programs [17]. From a health-economics perspective, patient satisfaction is also considered an important outcome variable when evaluating treatment effectiveness, and may guide funding decisions regarding health care delivery [18, 19].

The small number of studies on parent and child satisfaction with epilepsy surgery may reflect challenges with measuring this construct [1]. Research examining treatment outcomes demonstrates patient satisfaction is a multidimensional construct incorporating patient-related variables such as treatment expectations, age, gender, and treatment-related variables such as procedure-type; clinician providing treatment, which are accounted for in its assessment [20–23]. In addition, the patient perspective can be measured in many different formats with different methods of data collection and methods of question administration such as the use of closed yes/no or open-ended responses and each of these assessment methods may influence the quality and type of information obtained [1].

Macrodimitris et al. [1] have proposed preliminary guiding principles for measuring satisfaction after epilepsy surgery. Principles suggested include using a specified theoretical model or framework of patient satisfaction, definition of satisfaction, description of possible predictors of postsurgical satisfaction, inclusion of different dimensions of satisfaction, and establishing a specific response format (Table 15.1). The development of a validated tool for measuring child and parent experience and satisfaction would enable a methodical approach to collection of data.

In summary, there are few studies examining the child and parent subjective experience of epilepsy surgery (see Appendix for a summary of the studies discussed in this chapter). Seizure freedom is associated with a higher degree of patient satisfaction while ongoing postoperative neurological deficit and behavioral concerns are associated with lower satisfaction. The small number of studies on parent and child satisfaction with epilepsy surgery may reflect challenges with measuring this construct. Development of a validated tool for measuring child and parent experience and satisfaction after epilepsy surgery may facilitate the systematic evaluation of patient satisfaction as an additional component of its efficacy – an important aspect of collaborative models of patient-centered health care.

Table 15.1 Proposed guiding principles for measuring satisfaction after epilepsy surgery

Use and specify a theoretical model or framework of patient satisfaction to guide the assessment of satisfaction with epilepsy surgery (e.g., a model from the general medical literature, or derived specifically for epilepsy surgery)
Define satisfaction specifically (e.g., satisfaction with epilepsy surgery can be broadly defined as the patient's evaluation [whether positive or negative] of the entire process of undergoing epilepsy surgery and its associated outcomes)
Describe possible predictors of postsurgical satisfaction and if possible assess their impact on satisfaction. These include: Patient characteristics (e.g., age, age at surgery, gender)
Type of surgery (e.g., dominant hemisphere, temporal vs. extratemporal)
Seizure outcome: Presence or occurrence of risk factors (e.g., unrealistic expectations, postoperative neurological deficit, mood disorders), Protective factors (e.g., established plans for postsurgical adjustment; employment)
Include different dimensions of satisfaction, such as (1) how satisfied are you with surgery overall? (2) do you perceive surgery to be a success? (3) do you perceive surgery to be a failure? (4) was the overall impact of surgery positive? or whether questions such as "would you have surgery again in the same circumstances?" are appropriate given the research or clinical question
Establish a specific response format. Ideally, this will be a Likert scale with more than 3 but <10 response options, and provide the scale and wording of response options. If dichotomous analyses (e.g., Yes/No Satisfied/Not satisfied) are done based on responses with >2 response options or gradations, e.g., Likert-type responses), specify the cutoff used for determining what constitutes a negative and a positive response Assess satisfaction longitudinally (e.g., at repeated time points including after 24 months postsurgery)

Table from Macrodimitris et al. [1]. Courtesy of John Wiley & Sons, Inc.

Appendix. Summary of Studies on Subjective Experience of Children and Parents After Epilepsy Surgery

Author, year	Study design	Participants (children)	Males	Age at surgery (min-max/y)	Duration of epilepsy (min-max/y)	Prognostic indicators studied	Intervention	Outcome measures	Good outcome (*N*)	Follow-up (min-max/ mos)
Engelhart, 2013 [6]	RE	56	23	1–17 yr	NS	c,d,f,	T-EXT	O	46	12–120
Hannan, 2009 [4]	PR	13	4	5–17 yr	NS	c,d,f,g,i,k,l	T-EXTs	E	11	90–102
Iwasaki, 2013 [3]	RE	16	NS	1–24 yr	NS	I, m, x	EXT	E	10	6–45
Keene1998 [5]	RE	63	34	NS	NS	c,d,g,i	T-EXT	O	50	78–91
Park, 2013 [2]	RE	48	27	1–16 yr	NS	c,d,f,g,k,l,m	EXT	E	42	12–31

Ref reference, *RE* retrospective, *PR* prospective, *CO* retrospective and prospective combined, *NS* not specified, *T* temporal, *EXT* extratemporal, *A* seizure-free >1 year, *E* Engel classification, *O* other definitions (see text for explanation), *a* febrile seizures, *b* CNS infections, *c* mesial temporal sclerosis, *d* neuromigration defects, *e* vascular diseases, *f* tumor, *g* abnormal MRI, *h* intracranial monitoring, *i* extent of resection, *j* side of resection, *k* EEG/MRI concordance, *l* interictal seizures, *m* postoperative discharges, *x* other variables not studied (mental retardation; unilateral ictal ECoG; subdural ictal EEG; underlying pathology by PET, quantitative MRI, MRI hippocampal volumetry), *yr* year, *mos* months.

References

1. Macrodimitris S, Sherman EM, Williams TS, Bigras C, Wiebe S. Measuring patient satisfaction following epilepsy surgery. Epilepsia. 2011;52(8):1409–17. doi:10.1111/j.1528-1167.2011.03160.
2. Park SY, Kwon HE, Kang HC, Lee JS, Kim DS, Kim HD. Epilepsy surgery in pediatric intractable epilepsy with destructive encephalopathy. J Epilepsy Res. 2013;3(2):48–53.
3. Iwasaki M, Uematsu M, Nakayama T, Hino-Fukuyo N, Sato Y, Kobayashi T, Haginoya K, Osawa S, Jin K, Nakasato N, Tominaga T. Parental satisfaction and seizure outcome after corpus callosotomy in patients with infantile or early childhood epilepsy. Seizure. 2013;22:303–5.
4. Hannan S, Cross JH, Scott RC, Harkness W, Heyman I. The effects of epilepsy surgery on emotions, behavior and psychosocial impairment in children and adolescents with drug resistant epilepsy: a prospective study. Epilepsy Behav. 2009;15 (3):318–24. doi:10.1016/j.yebeh.2009.04.007.
5. Keene D, Loy-English I, Ventureyra E. Patient satisfaction with surgical treatment of refractory epilepsy done in childhood and early adolescence. Childs Nerv Syst. 1998;14:30–2.
6. Engelhart M, van Schooneveld M, Jennekens-Schinkel A, van Nieuwenhuizen O. With the benefit of hindsight: would you opt again for epilepsy surgery performed in childhood? Eur J Paediatr Neurol. 2013;17(5):462–70.
7. Duchowny M, Jayakar P, Resnick T, Harvey AS, Alvarez L, Dean P. Epilepsy surgery in the first three years of life. Epilepsia. 1998;39:737–43.
8. Engel J Jr. Outcome with respect to epileptic seizures. In: Engel J Jr, Van Ness PC, Rasmussen TB, Ojemann LM, editors. Surgical treatment of the epilepsies, 2nd ed. New York: Raven Press Ltd; 1993, p. 609–34.
9. Wyllie E, Comair YG, Kotagal P, Bulacio J, Bingaman W, Ruggieri P. Seizure outcome after epilepsy surgery in children and adolescents. Ann Neurol. 1998;44:740–8.
10. Smith ML, Elliott IM, Lach L. Cognitive, psychosocial, and family function one year after pediatric epilepsy surgery. Epilepsia. 2004;45:650–6.
11. Golin C, Dimatteo MR, Gelberg L. The role of patient participation in the doctor visit. Implications for adherence to diabetes care. Diabetes Care. 1996;19:1153–64.
12. Katz J. Patient preferences and health disparities. JAMA. 2001;286:1506–9.
13. Atkinson M, Sinha A, Hass S, Colman S, Kumar R, Brod M, Rowland C. Validation of a general measure of treatment satisfaction, the Treatment Satisfaction Questionnaire for Medication (TSQM), using a national panel study of chronic disease. Health Qual Life Outcomes. 2004;2:1–13.
14. Taylor T. Understanding the choices that patients make. J Am Board Fam Pract. 2000;13:124–33.
15. McCracken L, Klock A, Mingay D, Asbury J, Sinclair D. Assessment of satisfaction with treatment for chronic pain. J Pain Symptom Manage. 1997;14:292–9.
16. Albrecht G, Hoogstraten J. Satisfaction as a determinant of compliance. Community Dent Oral Epidemiol. 1998;26:139–46.
17. Taylor DC, Neville BRG, Cross JH. New measures of outcome needed for the surgical treatment of epilepsy. Epilepsia. 1997;38:625–30.
18. Eriksen L. Patient satisfaction with nursing care: concept clarification. J Nurs Meas. 1995;3:59–76.
19. Turnbull J, Luther K. Patient satisfaction report paves way to improved care. QRC Advis. 1996;13:1–7.
20. Hall J, Dornan M. Patient sociodemographic characteristics as predictors of satisfaction with medical care: a meta-analysis. Soc Sci Med. 1990;30:7.
21. Fontana A, Rosenheck R. A model of patients' satisfaction with treatment for posttraumatic stress disorder. Adm Policy Ment Health. 2001;28:475–89.
22. Nguyen Thi P, Briancon S, Empereur F, Guillemin F. Factors determining inpatient satisfaction with care. Soc Sci Med. 2002;54:493–504.
23. Revicki DA. Patient assessment of treatment satisfaction: methods and practical issues. Gut. 2004;53 Suppl 4:40–4.

Chapter 16
Informed Consent for Epilepsy Surgery

Ying Meng and George M. Ibrahim

Abstract Informed consent is a critical ethical tenet that is required in order to safeguard patient dignity and autonomy during medical treatment. This chapter explores both the universal and unique challenges involved in obtaining informed consent for epilepsy surgery. We emphasize that patients with epilepsy represent a vulnerable patient population due to the effects of the disease on capacity, agency, and identity. Individuals may be highly motivated to undergo established and experimental surgical procedures due to the medical and psychosocial burden of the illness. Moreover, unique challenges to informed consent may arise in the conduct of pediatric epilepsy surgery and in the context of surgical innovation. An approach to informed consent with discussion of commonly encountered ethical challenges is presented with a view towards facilitating the provision of patient-centered care.

Keywords Assent • Capacity • Consent • Childhood epilepsy • Conflict of interest • Ethics • Epilepsy surgery • Informed consent • Surgical innovation • Therapeutic misconception

---

Conflicts of Interest The authors have no conflicts of interest to declare.

Y. Meng, BASc, MD
Division of Neurosurgery, Department of Surgery, Toronto Western Hospital, University of Toronto, Toronto, ON, USA

G.M. Ibrahim, MD, PhD (✉)
Division of Neurosurgery, Department of Surgery, University of Toronto, Toronto, ON, USA

Institute of Medical Science, University of Toronto, Toronto, ON, USA

Division of Neurosurgery, The Hospital for Sick Children, 555 University Avenue, Toronto, ON, M5G 1Z8, USA
e-mail: georgem.ibrahim@utoronto.ca

K. Malmgren et al. (eds.), *Long-Term Outcomes of Epilepsy Surgery in Adults and Children*, DOI 10.1007/978-3-319-17783-0_16

Introduction

With growing awareness of the benefits of surgical treatment over continued medical therapy, there is increasing acceptance among clinicians and patients alike of surgical intervention for medically intractable epilepsy [1, 2]. Resective surgical treatments result in a greater likelihood of seizure freedom, compared to ongoing medical treatment in subgroups of patients with localization-related epilepsy [3]. Patients without an obvious epilepsy focus may also benefit from palliative strategies aimed at modulating neural circuitry to reduce seizure burden and improve quality of life (see Chaps. 12 and 13). In addition to the need for high-quality evidence in guiding appropriate treatment strategies, the enthusiasm to treat patients with intractable epilepsy surgically must be tempered by pragmatism and ethical principles.

Although many of the ethical concepts pertaining to the conduct of epilepsy surgery are common to other medical procedures, there are also important considerations that are unique to patients with intractable epilepsy. First, epilepsy, as an intrinsic disorder of brain function, may affect an individual's capacity, agency, and identity. Second, patients with epilepsy comprise a vulnerable patient population, who may be highly motivated to undergo surgical intervention due to the medical and psychosocial morbidities associated with the disease. Finally, established and experimental surgical strategies, which aim to resect, disconnect, or modulate the brain's circuitry, may be associated with considerable and often irreversible iatrogenic injury, which must be balanced against an uncertain likelihood of seizure freedom.

While clinicians may encounter multifaceted and complex ethical dilemmas during the care of patients with epilepsy, this chapter will exclusively explore the specific challenge of informed consent. The evidence guiding the decision to proceed with surgical treatment must be understood and presented within the context of the patient's subjective experience with epilepsy through the informed consent process. Informed consent is a dynamic, bidirectional process, which is modified by various factors, including whether the treatment is established or experimental or whether the intervention is life-saving or elective. In this chapter, we first introduce a general approach to informed consent. Subsequently, we discuss challenges in obtaining informed consent from patients with epilepsy undergoing resective and palliative procedures. Finally, we explore difficulties that may be encountered in pediatric patients and those undergoing experimental surgical treatments. Illustrative cases are presented throughout to highlight commonly encountered ethical challenges.

General Approach to Informed Consent

Medical bioethics is guided by four pillars: respect for autonomy, beneficence, nonmaleficence, and justice. Informed consent is integral to the respect for patient autonomy, the inalienable right to self-determination to make decisions without undue influence or coercion [4]. The requirements of informed consent are (a) full disclosure, (b) lack of undue influence, and (c) a capable patient.

The concept of full disclosure often refers to discussion of common and material risks, as explanation of all possible risks is often not feasible [5]. As defined in the case of *Canterbury v Spence*, a risk is said to be material "*when a reasonable person in what the physician knows or should know to be the patient's position would be likely to attach significance to the risk or cluster of risks in determining whether or not to undergo the proposed therapy*" [6]. A general approach is to consider what a reasonable person would want to know to make a sound judgment under those circumstances. The requirement of capacity relates to whether an individual understands and appreciates the procedure, its purpose, and associated risks. Finally, the decision to proceed with treatment must be free of coercion from any external party, a concept that becomes paramount especially when approaching patients for involvement in clinical research.

Informed consent is critical to the success of the therapeutic doctor-patient relationship, which is typically asymmetric with greater vulnerability on the side of the patient [7]. Within the framework of this relationship, the requirement of physicians to speak truthfully to patients regarding surgical treatments, alternatives, risks, and benefits is self-evident. Practically speaking, however, informed consent may be affected by cultural, social, and personal considerations [7]. A "relational" view of autonomy has been proposed, whereby the patient's internal moderating factors are taken into account during this discussion [8, 9]. One example of this is withholding information from patients who do not wish to hear all the risks of the procedure. Informed consent may therefore be viewed as a bidirectional process, which evaluates and addresses the patient's position and contextualizes material risks to his/her life circumstances.

Informed Consent for Resective Surgery in Eloquent Cortex

Illustrative Case 1 A 19-year-old male presents with intractable localization-related epilepsy originating from the left central region. Invasive monitoring reveals a peri-Rolandic seizure-onset zone. The medical team meets with the patient to discuss the procedure.

Risks and Benefits: Contextualization of Harm During Informed Consent

As exemplified by Illustrative Case 1, one challenge in obtaining informed consent from patients with epilepsy is the discussion of risks and benefits, given that epilepsy surgery may lead to a predictable iatrogenic injury, which is justified by the possibility of seizure freedom [10]. The perception that the risks of surgery are too great to justify its utility is one factor responsible for the low rates of patient referral for potentially curative surgical treatments [2, 11]. The lack of consideration of surgical treatments may in turn lead to unnecessary patient suffering and disability.

The conflict between beneficence (providing an opportunity to achieve seizure freedom) versus nonmaleficence (avoiding interventions that may result in a disability) can be mitigated by identifying a hierarchy of need satisfaction during the informed consent discussion [12]. Such an approach demands recognition of the patient's unique experience with the illness.

Contemporary deontologist Frances Kamm defines a principle of "permissible harm" whereby an intervention with significant expectant harmful (i.e., resections near or within eloquent brain regions) is justified if it is an effect or aspect of the greater good. The definition of harm is therefore a contextually significant judgment and must encompass the risks of not treating epilepsy. That is to say, the patient's subjective experience with epilepsy must inform the discussion of risks and benefits during the informed consent process. A patient with frequent, disabling seizures may be more willing to accept the risk of an iatrogenic neurological deficit compared to a patient with rare, nondisabling events. However, it is extremely difficult to quantify likely success. Moreover, whether a particular complication is an acceptable risk is individual to each patient. For example, resection of motor area in the presence of existent hemineglect may be acceptable, but resection of the distal hand regions in an otherwise normal individual cannot be quantified and would seem unacceptable. This triage of the need satisfaction is critical to the informed consent discussion, and to guiding the implementation of surgical strategies in circumstances where risks are high or involve foreseeable iatrogenic injuries.

Informed Consent for Palliative Procedures

Illustrative Case 2 A 21-year-old female with an 18-year history of intractable, nonlocalization-related epilepsy and severe cognitive impairment presents with over 50 seizures per day, of which a substantial proportion are drop attacks causing frequent injury. The multidisciplinary team discusses the benefits of a palliative surgical procedure, such as corpus callosotomy.

Capacity

Capacity, as a sociolegal construct, is variable across different jurisdictions, yet is comprised of two essential elements: the ability to "understand" and "appreciate" risks [13]. The ability to understand risks describes a person's capacity to comprehend and retain information. Conversely, appreciation of risk entails the attachment of personal meaning to factual information during the decision-making process. Assessing a patient's capacity to consent to treatment may be a particular challenge in epilepsy surgery, given that the underlying disorder may alter his/her agency.

As exemplified by Illustrative Case 2, cognitive deficits are common comorbidities in epilepsy [14], which may render a patient incapable of providing informed consent to undergo a surgical procedure.

Capacity is domain specific and thus must be evaluated independently for different decisions. For instance, a patient's level of cognitive deficit may preclude him/her from making financial decisions yet he/she may be capable of consenting to medical treatment. Moreover, when assessing a patient's capacity, clinicians must be mindful of their ability to retain information and gauge their risk perception. Patients often underestimate the risks of medical procedures [15], and those with neurological illnesses specifically are known to poorly retain information in a manner directly related to the disease severity [16]. During the informed consent process, clinicians should have an appreciation of the degree to which epilepsy interferes with cognition. In fact, the intersection of neurological illness and cognition is gaining increasing prominence in the study of medical bioethics. Although beyond the scope of this chapter, the burgeoning field of "neuroethics" specifically addresses the unique ethical challenges encountered in the context of disorders of the brain, which is the seat of identity and substrate of agency and capacity.

Goals of Treatment: Quality of Life and Double Jeopardy

During the informed consent process, the goals of surgery must also be clearly outlined. Case 2 illustrates a situation where seizure freedom is not an expected outcome from surgery, but patient may derive substantial improvement in their quality of life with decreased seizure frequency and consequent injury. Reluctance to consider a palliative procedure for such groups of patients may subject them to a "double jeopardy" [17] whereby they first suffer as a result of their illness and second due to the low priority given to improve their quality of life. Substitute decision-makers may also choose to provide consent to palliative treatments if reduced seizure frequency may facilitate better care for the patients [10]. As with resective surgical procedures, the patient's (and the patient's caregivers') subjective experience with epilepsy must be captured during the informed consent process and guide treatment decisions.

Informed Consent in the Pediatric Patient

Illustrative Case 3 An 11-year-old girl presents with a temporal ganglioglioma and intractable epilepsy. The parents are hesitant about proceeding with surgical treatment as they would prefer the child to make her own decision regarding treatment when she is older. The surgical team meets with the patient and family to discuss options.

Pediatric Capacity and Assent

During particular stages of their development, children are described as egocentric, lacking the ability to understand differing beliefs and opinions, and generalizing subjective experience as societal norm. Views of children as prerational and premoral have been discredited by an increasing body of work establishing their maturity and understanding of illness. Experience is increasingly recognized as a more important predictor of competence than age or ability [18]. Assent, a lesser standard of acquiescence to treatment, is typically therefore obtained from children [19].

As described in Illustrative Case 3, surrogate decision-makers, namely parents, often provide consent (with the child's assent) for treatment. While autonomy, the ethical tenet of self-determination, is central to informed consent, in the case of the child, the idea of his/her best interest is often invoked. This is because children may have never been adequately mature to declare their treatment preferences [20]. The informed consent discussion in these cases, therefore, appeal to the protection of the child's welfare, rather than his//her right to self-determination.

Informed consent based on this premise may seem intuitive, yet is often difficult to obtain in the setting of epilepsy surgery. In cases of life-threatening illness (i.e., obstructive hydrocephalus due to posterior fossa tumors), the best interest of the child is clearly to undergo surgical treatments. Conversely, the decision to undergo epilepsy surgery is often value-laden and encompasses the patient's subjective experience with the illness (as previously described). The challenge for clinicians during the informed consent process is, therefore, to glean such insights from the child and his/her family and position the benefits and risk of the intervention in the context of the child's experience with epilepsy.

Informed Consent in the Setting of Surgical Innovation

Illustrative Case 4 A 12-year-old boy with a 5-year history of medically intractable, nonlesional epilepsy localized to the right posterior head region undergoes invasive monitoring to approximate the epileptogenic zone. Time-frequency analysis of recordings from implanted subdural electrodes, reveal a region of cortex expression pathological high-frequency oscillations (pHFOs). The region of pHFO expression is larger than the visually defined hypothesis of the epileptogenic zone. The comprehensive surgical team meets with the patient and family to discuss the surgical plan.

Informed Consent in the Research Setting

Medical professionals have an obligation to improve the care provided to future patients, and rigorous interrogation of experimental procedures, for example, through the conduct of randomized clinical trials, is the most effective way to legitimize novel therapeutics. As such, numerous quintessential documents and treatises have been drafted to uphold ethical principles in the enrollment of patients in clinical research (Table 16.1).

The importance of a rigorous informed consent process prior to enrollment of subjects into clinical research is critical, as patient perception of risk may not accurately reflect the true risk of the intervention [21]. In the research setting, the actual risk of intervention may not be entirely known; therefore, choices based on perceived risk may be misguided. Patients with epilepsy, or their families, may also be highly motivated to pursue experimental treatments given the suffering they endure, which may lead them to underestimate the risk and overestimate the benefit of participation in research [22, 23].

Therapeutic Misconception

Obtaining informed consent from patients for undergoing experimental treatments may be complicated by the "therapeutic misconception." Patients demonstrate this phenomenon when they fail to recognize the distinction between the competing

Table 16.1 Selected guidelines on the ethical conduct of clinical research

Year published	Publication	Details
1947	The Nuremberg Code	In response to inhumane experimentation during World War II, a 10-point statement to prevent future abuse of human subjects
Multiple Revisions	The Declaration of Helsinki	Declaration of ethical research practices and basic principles for the conduct of clinical research
Multiple Revisions	The Vancouver Group (The International Committee of Medical Editors)	Consensus guidelines on the reporting and publication of research findings
1978	The Belmont Report	In response to the Tuskegee syphilis study, a report emphasizing respect for persons with particular note on informed consent and assessment of risks
1981	The Common Rule	A guideline describing ethical standards for government-funded research in the United States emphasizing the role of Institutional Review Boards (IRBs)
1996	International Conference on Harmonisation of Technical Requirements for Registration of Pharmaceuticals for Human use "Guidelines for Good Clinical Practice"	Standards for the regulation of clinical trials involving human subjects, emphasizing protection of human rights, safety, efficacy, and conflicts of interest

obligations of clinicians as their primary care givers and clinical investigators [24]. Patients who maintain a therapeutic misconception disregard the disadvantages of participating in clinical research that result from the research process itself [25]. Individuals with epilepsy are particularly susceptible to therapeutic misconception as it has been previously shown that less optimism regarding personal care and hopelessness about future health states increases the probability of manifesting this phenomenon [26].

During the informed consent process, care must be undertaken to avoid therapeutic misconception by clearly outlining the primary purpose of experimental research, which is to produce generalizable knowledge and not to benefit the patients enrolled. The discussion must also clearly outline the differences between the research and clinical care elements of the treatment. In order to mitigate therapeutic misconception, participants should understand the following five dimensions of research: (1) scientific purpose, to benefit future patients; (2) study procedures that are not necessary for patient care; (3) uncertainty, which is greater than standard treatments; (4) adherence to protocol, which is more strict than standard treatments; and (5) clinician as investigators, the dual roles of the treating physician [27].

Regulation of Innovation and Informed Consent

Surgical innovation in the modern era requires regulation and careful oversight of its clinical applications. The extent to which a surgical innovation requires regulation and careful oversight of its application to patient care is directly related to the extent to which it deviates from established practices [28, 29]. The extent of its deviation should also be explicitly stated in the informed consent discussion. For instance, Illustrative Case 4 describes a scenario in which invasive monitoring is performed, but the resection margins may be modified by innovative mapping strategies (i.e., pathological high-frequency oscillations). The modified resection plan may be identical or more or less aggressive than traditional methods of identifying the epileptogenic zone. Such discrepancies should be explained during informed consent and reasoning behind different resection strategies should be explored.

Elaborating on this example, during the informed consent discussion, the localization modalities used should be compared to standards of care or other consensus guidelines. There is extensive heterogeneity and interinstitutional variability in the extent to which different localization strategies are employed to determine the epileptogenic zone and ultimate resection strategy in patients with epilepsy [30]. While no unanimous agreements exist on standards of care, various guidelines are in place. For example, the Pediatric Epilepsy Surgery Subcommission of the International League Against Epilepsy (ILAE) has proposed guidelines for the evaluation of surgical candidates including interictal and video electroencephalography (VEEG), structural imaging with magnetic resonance imaging (MRI) and/or computed tomography (CT), functional imaging with single-photon emission CT (SPECT) or positron emission tomography (PET), and neuropsychological evaluation [31, 32]. The extent of institutional deviation from accepted guidelines should be explored and justified both during preoperative planning and informed consent.

Conclusions

The conduct of epilepsy surgery is replete with ethical challenges that are unique to the condition. The impact of the disease of patient agency and capacity as well as the uncertain likelihood of seizure freedom has important implications for the informed consent process. Further challenges may be encountered when obtaining informed consent for epilepsy surgery in children and in the setting of surgical innovations. This chapter provided a general approach to informed consent and explored common ethical dilemmas that may be encountered by clinicians. Patients with medically intractable epilepsy represent a unique neurological patient population. Awareness of ethical challenges in informed consent is central to providing patient-centered care.

References

1. Ibrahim GM, Rutka JT, Snead OC. Epilepsy surgery in childhood: no longer the treatment of last resort. CMAJ. 2014;186:973–4.
2. Ibrahim GM, Barry BW, Fallah A, 3rd Snead OC, Drake JM, Rutka JT, et al. Inequities in access to pediatric epilepsy surgery: a bioethical framework. Neurosurg Focus. 2012;32(3):E2.
3. Wiebe S, Blume WT, Girvin JP, Eliasziw M, Effectiveness and Efficiency of Surgery for Temporal Lobe Epilepsy Study Group. A randomized, controlled trial of surgery for temporal-lobe epilepsy. N Engl J Med. 2001;345(5):311–8.
4. Etchells E, Sharpe G, Walsh P, Williams JR, Singer PA. Bioethics for clinicians: 1. Consent. CMAJ. 1996;155(2):177–80.
5. Bernstein M. Fully informed consent is impossible in surgical clinical trials. Can J Surg. 2005;48(4):271–2.
6. Canterbury v Spence. 464 F (2nd) 1972:772.
7. Surbone A. Telling the truth to patients with cancer: what is the truth? Lancet Oncol. 2006;7(11):944–50.
8. Donchin A. Understanding autonomy relationally: toward a reconfiguration of bioethical principles. J Med Philos. 2001;26(4):365–86.
9. Sherwin S. A relational approach to autonomy in health-care. In: Sherwin S, Feminist Healthcare Network, editors. The politics of women's health: exploring agency and autonomy. Philadelphia: Temple University Press; 1988. p. 19–44.
10. Ibrahim GM, Fallah A, 3rd Snead OC, Elliott I, Drake JM, Bernstein M, et al. Ethical issues in surgical decision making concerning children with medically intractable epilepsy. Epilepsy Behav. 2011;22(2):154–7.
11. Erba G, Moja L, Beghi E, Messina P, Pupillo E. Barriers toward epilepsy surgery. A survey among practicing neurologists. Epilepsia. 2012;53(1):35–43.
12. Tomasini F. Exploring ethical justification for self-demand amputation. Ethics Med. 2006 Summer;22(2):99–115.

13. Appelbaum PS, Grisso T. Assessing patients' capacities to consent to treatment. N Engl J Med. 1988;319(25):1635–8.
14. Spencer S, Huh L. Outcomes of epilepsy surgery in adults and children. Lancet Neurol. 2008;7(6):525–37.
15. Lidz CW, Appelbaum PS, Grisso T, Renaud M. Therapeutic misconception and the appreciation of risks in clinical trials. Soc Sci Med. 2004;58(9):1689–97.
16. Schaeffer MH, Krantz DS, Wichman A, Masur H, Reed E, Vinicky JK. The impact of disease severity on the informed consent process in clinical research. Am J Med. 1996;100(3):261–8.
17. Harris J. QALYfying the value of life. J Med Ethics. 1987;13(3):117–23.
18. Alderson P, Sutcliffe K, Curtis K. Children's competence to consent to medical treatment. Hastings Cent Rep. 2006;36(6):25–34.
19. Weithorn LA, Campbell SB. The competency of children and adolescents to make informed treatment decisions. Child Dev. 1982;53(6):1589–98.
20. Diekema DS. Parental refusals of medical treatment: the harm principle as threshold for state intervention. Theor Med Bioeth. 2004;25(4):243–64.
21. Perrow C. Normal accidents living with high-risk technologies. Princeton: Princeton University Press; 1999.
22. Penman DT, Holland JC, Bahna GF, Morrow G, Schmale AH, Derogatis LR, et al. Informed consent for investigational chemotherapy: patients' and physicians' perceptions. J Clin Oncol. 1984;2(7):849–55.
23. Joffe S, Cook EF, Cleary PD, Clark JW, Weeks JC. Quality of informed consent in cancer clinical trials: a cross-sectional survey. Lancet. 2001;358(9295):1772–7.
24. Appelbaum PS, Lidz CW, Grisso T. Therapeutic misconception in clinical research: frequency and risk factors. IRB. 2004;26(2):1–8.
25. Appelbaum PS, Roth LH, Lidz CW, Benson P, Winslade W. False hopes and best data: consent to research and the therapeutic misconception. Hastings Cent Rep. 1987;17(2):20–4.
26. Goebel S, von Harscher M, Mehdorn HM. Comorbid mental disorders and psychosocial distress in patients with brain tumours and their spouses in the early treatment phase. Support Care Cancer. 2011;19(11):1797–805.
27. Henderson GE, Churchill LR, Davis AM, Easter MM, Grady C, Joffe S, et al. Clinical trials and medical care: defining the therapeutic misconception. PLoS Med. 2007;4(11):e324.
28. Bernstein M, Bampoe J. Surgical innovation or surgical evolution: an ethical and practical guide to handling novel neurosurgical procedures. J Neurosurg. 2004;100(1):2–7.
29. Ibrahim GM, Fallah A, Snead OC, Drake J, Rutka JT, Bernstein M. The use of high frequency oscillations to guide neocortical resections in children with medically-intractable epilepsy: how do we ethically apply surgical innovations to patient care? Seizure. 2012;21:743–7.
30. Harvey AS, Cross JH, Shinnar S, Mathern BW, ILAE Pediatric Epilepsy Surgery Survey Taskforce. Defining the spectrum of international practice in pediatric epilepsy surgery patients. Epilepsia. 2008;49(1):146–55.
31. Cross JH, Jayakar P, Nordli D, Delalande O, Duchowny M, Wieser HG, et al. Proposed criteria for referral and evaluation of children for epilepsy surgery: recommendations of the subcommission for pediatric epilepsy surgery. Epilepsia. 2006;47(6):952–9.
32. Jayakar P, Gaillard WD, Tripathi M, Libenson MH, Mathern GW, Cross JH, et al. Diagnostic test utilization in evaluation for resective epilepsy surgery in children. Epilepsia. 2014;55(4):507–18.

Chapter 17
Managing Expectations of Epilepsy Surgery

Sallie Baxendale

Abstract Although seizure control is the primary aim of epilepsy surgery, candidates who undergo elective surgery for the relief of medically intractable epilepsy often hope that a successful surgical outcome will result in broader changes in their lives. Some of their expectations may be realistic; others may not, or may even be contraindicated by the outcome literature. The expectation literature in epilepsy surgery is small. The most commonly reported expectations in adults of improved employment opportunities and the ability to drive following surgery are realistic hopes for many surgical candidates, but they should be informed of the actuarial outcome data for these likelihoods. Expectations of improvements in cognitive function and a desire to be free from antiepileptic medications are unrealistic aims for the majority of adult candidates. Implicit assumptions about seizure freedom need to be identified and addressed explicitly, and corrected where necessary, so that the candidate can make a truly informed decision regarding a surgical option. While much of the literature to date has been focused on the decision-making processes of their physicians, little is known about how surgical candidates approach and make this decision. Future research should move towards a more inclusive approach and should guard against paternalistic attitudes in the medical profession. Studies to date have exclusively focused on the expectations of epilepsy surgery candidates who live in resource-rich countries. It is likely that there are very significant cultural influences on expectations of epilepsy surgery in different parts of the world. These have yet to be explored. Elective surgery in a pediatric setting has special ethical and legal considerations, over and above those associated with surgery in adults. While a number of authors have discussed these issues at a theoretical level, the expectations of children and teenagers and their parents have yet to be empirically examined. Further work is also needed to create and evaluate a presurgical counseling schedule to ensure that candidates approach surgery with realistic expectations and a longitudinal perspective on change.

Conflicts of Interest The author has no conflicts of interest to declare.

S. Baxendale, PhD, C.Psychol, AFBPsS
Department of Clinical and Experimental Epilepsy,
National Hospital for Neurology and Neurosurgery, London, UK
e-mail: s.baxendale@ucl.ac.uk

K. Malmgren et al. (eds.), *Long-Term Outcomes of Epilepsy Surgery in Adults and Children*, DOI 10.1007/978-3-319-17783-0_17

Keywords Expectation • Hope • Epilepsy surgery • Informed consent • Preparation • Counseling

Introduction

The decision to proceed with epilepsy surgery is complex. Prospective candidates need to weigh up the chances of being seizure-free or having a significant reduction in seizures against the inherent risks associated with the procedure. The magnitude and severity of these risks vary considerably and range from the small risks of surgical catastrophe such as death, stroke, and permanent neurological deficit, to the more substantial, but still small, risks of postoperative infection [1] or a worsening of seizure control following the surgery [2]. The risks of developing a postoperative visual field deficit can be significant for some candidates and disallows the possibility of obtaining a driving license after surgery, even if they become seizure-free [3].

The risks of cognitive decline following surgery form a different class of surgical risk that prospective candidates must consider. These risks are different for each candidate and depend on their premorbid characteristics and the nature of the proposed surgery (see Chap. 5). However, for some candidates the chances of a clinically significant postoperative decline in memory or language function are high, greater than 50 % [4]. In these cases, postoperative decline in cognitive function should be considered by the prospective candidate as the likely "cost" they will pay for surgery, rather than a possible risk.

Thus, the constellation of outcomes of epilepsy surgery is different for every candidate and depends on the premorbid characteristics of the candidate and the nature of the proposed surgery. It is not possible to precisely predict outcome but it is the duty of the epilepsy surgery team to provide the prospective candidate with as full and accurate information as possible with respect to the risks and costs associated with the procedure. This information should be evidence based and must be continually revised and updated. It should also be placed in a longitudinal framework wherever possible.

The "value" of seizure freedom (or a significant reduction in seizures) lies on the other side of the surgical decision-making scale (see Fig. 17.1). This value can only be determined by the surgical candidate. However, the multidisciplinary surgical team can help to ensure that the candidate is able to "balance" this possibility against the possible risks and costs of the procedure, by exploring the wider expectations the candidate has of becoming seizure-free. Although reduction of seizures is the primary aim of epilepsy surgery, patients who undergo elective temporal lobe surgery for the relief of medically intractable epilepsy often hope that a successful surgical outcome will result in broader changes in their lifestyle. Some of their expectations may be realistic; others may not or may even be contraindicated by the outcome literature.

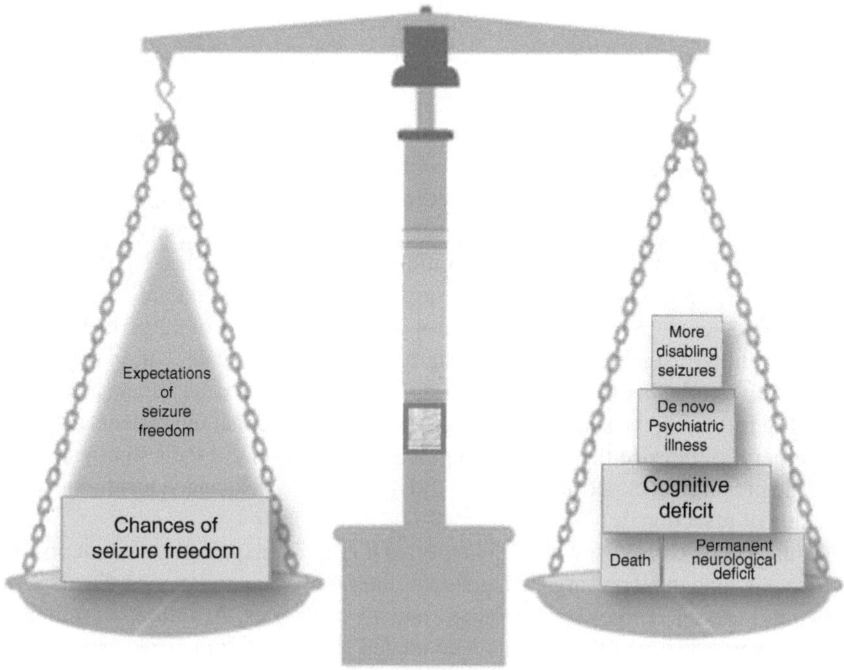

Fig. 17.1 Diagrammatic representation of the risk–benefit ratio that underpins the decision to proceed to epilepsy surgery. The size and weight of the factors on both sides of the scale will depend on individual patient characteristics. An integral part of the presurgical preparation should be an evaluation of the candidate's expectations of seizure freedom to ensure that this component does not have undue weight in the decision-making process

Patients' Expectations of Epilepsy Surgery

A number of studies have examined patient expectations of epilepsy surgery. See Appendix for a summary of these studies. In 1996, my colleague Pam Thompson and I conducted a study in which we asked 70 prospective surgical candidates to rate themselves on 20 descriptive scales covering personality, cognitive, and emotional dimensions [5]. The participants were also asked to rate how they believed they would be if the surgery were successful and their seizures ceased. As a group, the candidates were expecting significant positive changes in many dimensions postoperatively. The patients were expecting to be happier, more in control, and more hopeful, independent, and interested in life. They also expected to be more skillful, be of more value, have a better memory, and be more intelligent than their preoperative selves. While not significant at a group level, some individuals reported that they would become more physically attractive following successful surgery. Many of these expectations do not compare with the psychosocial changes that have been associated with temporal lobectomy in the literature or those reported by 32 patients who had been followed up for 1 year postoperatively.

We hypothesized that surgical candidates who had lived at least part of their adult life without seizures would have a more realistic idea of life without seizures than someone who had been medically intractable since childhood, or infancy. The sample was divided into three groups: those with onset of habitual seizures in very early life (before 7 years), those with an onset in childhood (age 8–16 years), and those with an onset in adulthood, (age >17 years). However, these groups did not differ significantly in their preoperative self-ratings on any of the scales. Neither did the pattern of expectations after successful surgery differ between the three groups.

Wheelock et al. [6] examined the presurgical expectations of 32 patients and 17 of their relatives/significant others using a 7-point rating scale. The patients and their relatives together expected "moderate" to "very much better" changes in quality of life following the surgery. Group analyses suggested that the patients expected the surgery to improve their QOL to a greater degree than did their significant others. The presurgical expectation ratings did not differ by sex, age, educational level, and side of resection.

In the same year, Wilson et al. [7] reported a range of expectations about postoperative outcome in 60 presurgical candidates interviewed using a standardized, semi-structured format. These were classified into 11 categories. At follow-up 6 months after the surgery, it was the patients who tended to endorse "practical" expectations (i.e., driving, employment, activities) preoperatively, rather than expectations of a psychological or social nature (i.e., self-change, relationships) who perceived the operation to be a success. In contrast, a perceived lack of success was reported by those who had greater expectations of psychosocial changes preoperatively.

Taylor et al. [8] used open-ended questions as part of a psychiatric interview to assess the aims and ambitions for change of 69 presurgical candidates. They identified 59 categories of response in total but the desires to drive, work, increase independence, socialize, and gain freedom from medication constituted 50 % of all the aims listed. Although an informed witness (parent/spouse/ friend) was also interviewed, their results are not presented separately in the study. Interestingly, very few of participants in this study identified a desire for improvement in cognitive functioning as an aim for epilepsy surgery, in contrast to the findings of later studies.

More recently, researchers working on the seven-center cohort study in the USA examined 389 prospective candidates' endorsements of 12 potential impacts of epilepsy surgery, and have published their results in a series of studies [9, 10]. Participants were given a list of items based on the literature and the researchers' clinical experience (see Appendix) and told "This list includes items other epilepsy patients have felt were important to them and which they hoped to have changed as a result of surgery. Please rate each item on a scale from 1-10, 1 being not important to you, 10 being extremely important to you." The lifting of driving limitations and an improvement in memory problems were listed by both men and women as their top two expectations of epilepsy surgery [9]. Improvements in emotional well-being and in concentration were also listed in the top five aspects of life that the patients expected to change following surgery.

The literature looking at patient expectations of epilepsy surgery is small. Patient expectations have been studied using guided interviews with open-ended questions, semi-structured interviews, and rating scales. The use of rating scales may introduce a confounding variable in expectation studies, highlighting areas that the patients have not thought of, and missing others. It is noteworthy that expectations of cognitive improvement did not feature in the Taylor et al. [8] study that used open-ended questions, but were prominent in the Baxendale and Thompson [5] and seven-center cohort studies [9, 10] that used specific rating scales. The most commonly reported expectations of improved employment opportunities and the ability to drive are realistic hopes for many surgical candidates, but they should be counseled regarding the actuarial outcome data in the literature on these likelihoods (See Chaps. 10 and 12). Although cognitive changes are common following surgery, improvements in function, particularly in the memory domain occur in less than a third of adult surgery candidates [11]. A desire to be free of medication and its side effects is also a common feature in expectation studies. Again this is unrealistic, particularly in the long term where studies suggest that less than 50 % of epilepsy surgery candidates will be seizure-free and off medication a decade or more after surgery [12, 13]. The small literature to date has exclusively focused on the expectations of epilepsy surgery candidates who live in resource-rich countries. It is likely that there are very significant cultural differences attached to patient's expectations of surgery in different parts of the world. These have yet to be explored.

The Surgical Decision-Making Process

Although there is a large literature on decision making in medicine, relatively little attention has been paid to how epilepsy surgery patients approach their decision to consent to surgery. Rather, the literature has focused on how the medical team managing the patient makes the decision to offer surgery to a candidate. These studies range from evaluations of the specific contributions each presurgical investigation may add [14, 15] to online tools to identify candidates who may benefit from the procedure [16]. Akama-Garren et al. [17], proposed a Markov decision model to evaluate the likely outcomes and associated health utilities associated with a left anterior temporal lobectomy versus continuing with medical management. Three scenarios were considered, which varied in terms of presurgical disability and the potential for a significant postoperative decline in verbal memory abilities. Although interesting from a theoretical standpoint, these approaches have very limited clinical utility. The acceptability of a verbal memory deficit and the burden of epilepsy are unique for each patient at specific points in time and can only be judged by the patients themselves. It is noteworthy that very few studies in this field employ prospective surgical candidates as participants; where they do, there tends to be a rather paternalistic approach [18]. For example, Anderson et al. [19] examined the factors that influence patients who decide not to proceed with epilepsy surgery. Despite the fact that patients who declined surgery were less bothered by their epilepsy (even with comparable severity), more anxious about surgery, and less likely to listen to their doctors (and others), the authors concluded that patient attitudes, beliefs, and anxiety serve as barriers to "ideal care." They concluded that their results provided opportunities for education, treatment, and intervention for the patient group.

An alternative explanation might be that the results provide opportunities for education of the medical team. The participants in this study weighed the risk–benefit ratio of epilepsy surgery in a different way to the researchers and had the advantage of living with the burden of the condition.

Choi et al. [20] used focus groups to elicit the information 20 patients had used to make their decisions about temporal lobe surgery. They used both experiential (i.e., learning about other patient's experiences through testimonials) and factual (i.e., individualized statistical information) sources of information. This kind of information can be used in the development of a patient decision aid designed to assist TLE patients in their decision making about epilepsy surgery. However, despite the obvious clinical need, no such tool has been evaluated under rigorous trial controlled conditions to date.

Expectations of Surgery in a Pediatric Setting

Elective surgery in a pediatric setting has special ethical and legal considerations, over and above those associated with surgery in adults. While a number of authors have discussed these issues at a theoretical level [21, 22], empirical studies of the expectations of children and teenagers and their parents have yet to be published. Given the prominent issues of mental capacity and informed consent in the pediatric population, a research priority would be to formally examine the discrepancies between parental and child expectations, particularly in older children and adolescents.

Summary

The limited literature in this field suggests that the routine presurgical preparations that epilepsy surgery candidates undergo are not sufficient to address the unrealistic expectations they may associate with seizure freedom. Implicit assumptions about seizure freedom need to be identified and addressed explicitly, being corrected where necessary so that the candidate can make a truly informed decision regarding a surgical option. At present, the research suggests that many candidates may overestimate the consequences of seizure freedom. Much of the literature to date has been focused on the decision making processes of the clinicians who decide to offer surgical treatment, rather than the patients who decide to accept it. Future research should move towards a more inclusive, individual approach and should guard against paternalistic attitudes in the medical profession. The patient's experience of epilepsy must be evaluated and valued in this process. Further work is needed to create and evaluate a program to ensure that candidates approach surgery with realistic expectations, and a longitudinal perspective on change. This will allow prospective candidates to make an informed decision regarding their treatment options and ease their postoperative course as far as possible.

Appendix. Summary of Studies on Adult Expectations of Epilepsy Surgery

Study authors	Participants	Measures and design	Main findings
Baxendale and Thompson, [5] UK	$N=70$ elective surgery candidates Age range 16–53 47 % Male/53 % Female	Rating scales along a continuum, with opposite adjectives at each end. These included: Bored–Interested, Happy–Sad, In Control–Helpless, Relaxed– Worried, Satisfied–Dissatisfied, Attractive– Unattractive, Hopeful–Despondent, Confident– Lacking Confidence, Stable–Emotional, Worthless– Of Value, Forgetful–Mindful, Calm–Irritable, Caring–Uncaring, Clumsy–Skillful, Dependent– Independent, Active–Inactive, Difficult–Cooperative, Talkative–Withdrawn, Friendly– Unfriendly, and Stupid–Clever. Participants rated their presurgical selves and their future selves if surgery was successful in eliminating seizures	The participants were expecting to be happier, more in control, more hopeful, independent, interested in life, skillful, and be of more value if they were seizure-free. They also expected to have a better memory and be more intelligent than their preoperative selves Expectations were not related to age of onset, gender, or laterality of the proposed surgery
Wheelock et al., [6] USA	$N=72$ presurgical candidates Age range 18–51 years A subset of their significant others	Brief interviews and semi-structured interview designed to elicit information about subjects' expectations for surgery, using 7-point Likert-type rating scales for quality of life	Patient expectations for improvements in overall quality of life ratings were higher than their significant others Expectations were not related to sex, age, educational level, or side of resection

(continued)

Appendix (continued)

Study authors	Participants	Measures and design	Main findings
Wilson et al. [7] Australia	$N=60$ presurgical TLE candidates Age range 14–8 years 38 % Male/62 % Female	Standardized, semi-structured clinical interview 1. What is the main reason you have sought surgical intervention? 2. Do you see the operation as a chance to change your life? 3. Have you made postoperative plans? 4. Do you plan on engaging on any new activities postoperatively?	11 post hoc categories of expectation identified including seizure cessation, driving, employment, family, social, relationships, independence, medication, self-change, general improvement, new activities 45 % expected to drive 38 % expected to develop new activities 35 % expected new employment opportunities
Taylor et al. [8] Republic of Ireland	$N=69$	Psychiatric interview	59 categories of aims for surgery were initially identified, which were later compressed to 26 The five most frequently cited expectations contributing 50 % of all aims listed were: 1. Improvements in employment status 2. Driving 3. Increase independence 4. Gain freedom from supervision 5. Stop taking medication

Seven-Center Cohort Study [9, 10] USA	$N=396$ Multicenter Study	Semi-structured interview: Participants were asked In what ways do you feel limited by your epilepsy? What do you most hope to change as a result of this surgery? Participants were also given a list and told "This list includes items other epilepsy patients have felt were important to them and which they hoped to have changed as a result of surgery. Please rate each item on a scale from 1 to 10, 1 being not at all important to you, 10 being extremely important to you" (1) Driving limitations, (2) limitations in bicycling, swimming, other physical activities, (3) participation in social situations, (4) level of fatigue, (5) emotional well-being, (6) memory problems, (7) language problems, (8) concentration or attention problems, (9) cosmetic (e.g., dermatologic, weight, etc.), (10) economic worries, (11) pregnancy concerns, and (12) having to take epilepsy medications	15 overarching expectation themes were identified with 61 subthemes. Nine of the 15 unique themes were identified by ≥15 % of the sample: driving (62 %), job/school (43 %), independence (29 %), seizure cessation (26 %), social functioning (23 %), quality of life (20 %), medication discontinuance (20 %), physical activities (18 %), and cognition (17 %). Expectations endorsed by less than 15 % of the sample included embarrassment/stigma, emotional, fatigue, general health, family planning, and no limitation/ no expectation Race and gender may influence presurgical expectations

References

1. Tebo CC, Evins AI, Christos PJ, Kwon J, Schwartz TH. Evolution of cranial epilepsy surgery complication rates: a 32-year systematic review and meta-analysis. J Neurosurg. 2014; 120(6):1415–27.
2. Kanchanatawan B, Limothai C, Srikijvilaikul T, Maes M. Clinical predictors of 2-year outcome of resective epilepsy surgery in adults with refractory epilepsy: a cohort study. BMJ Open. 2014;4(4):48–52.
3. Piper RJ, Yoong MM, Kandasamy J, Chin RF. Application of diffusion tensor imaging and tractography of the optic radiation in anterior temporal lobe resection for epilepsy: a systematic review. Clin Neurol Neurosurg. 2014;124:59–65.
4. Baxendale S, Thompson PJ, Sander JW. Neuropsychological outcomes in epilepsy surgery patients with unilateral hippocampal sclerosis and good preoperative memory function. Epilepsia. 2013;54(9):e131–4.
5. Baxendale S, Thompson PJ. "If I Didn't Have Epilepsy …": patient Expectations of Epilepsy Surgery. J Epilepsy. 1996;9:274–81.
6. Wheelock I, Peterson C, Buchtel HA. Presurgery expectations, postsurgery satisfaction, and psychosocial adjustment after epilepsy surgery. Epilepsia. 1998;39(5):487–94.
7. Wilson SJ, Saling MM, Kincade P, Bladin PF. Patient expectations of temporal lobe surgery. Epilepsia. 1998;39(2):167–74.
8. Taylor DC, McMacKin D, Staunton H, Delanty N, Phillips J. Patients' aims for epilepsy surgery: desires beyond seizure freedom. Epilepsia. 2001;42(5):629–33.
9. Bower CM, Hays RD, Devinsky O, Spencer SS, Sperling MR, Haut S, Vassar S, Vickrey BG. Expectations prior to epilepsy surgery: an exploratory comparison of men and women. Seizure. 2009;18(3):228–31.
10. Baca CB, Cheng EM, Spencer SS, Vassar S, Vickrey BG, Multicenter Study of Epilepsy Surgery. Racial differences in patient expectations prior to respective epilepsy surgery. Epilepsy Behav. 2009;15(4):452–5.
11. Baxendale S, Thompson PJ, Duncan JS. Improvements in memory function following anterior temporal lobe resection for epilepsy. Neurology. 2008;71(17):1319–25.
12. de Tisi J, Bell GS, Peacock JL, McEvoy AW, Harkness WF, Sander JW, Duncan JS. The long-term outcome of adult epilepsy surgery, patterns of seizure remission, and relapse: a cohort study. Lancet. 2011;378(9800):1388–95.
13. Asztely F, Ekstedt G, Rydenhag B, Malmgren K. Long term follow-up of the first 70 operated adults in the Goteborg Epilepsy Surgery Series with respect to seizures, psychosocial outcome and use of antiepileptic drugs. J Neurol Neurosurg Psychiatry. 2007;78(6):605–9.
14. Uijl SG, Leijten FS, Arends JB, Parra J, van Huffelen AC, Moons KG. Decision-making in temporal lobe epilepsy surgery: the contribution of basic non-invasive tests. Seizure. 2008;17(4):364–73.
15. Uijl SG, Leijten FS, Parra J, Arends JB, van Huffelen AC, Moons KG. What is the current evidence on decision-making after referral for temporal lobe epilepsy surgery? A review of the literature. Seizure. 2005;14(8):534–40.
16. Jette N, Quan H, Tellez-Zenteno JF, Macrodimitris S, Hader WJ, Sherman EM, Hamiwka LD, Wirrell EC, Burneo JG, Metcalfe A, Faris PD, Hernandez-Ronquillo L, Kwon CS, Kirk A, Wiebe S, CASES Expert Panelists. Development of an online tool to determine appropriateness for an epilepsy surgery evaluation. Neurology. 2012;79(11):1084–93.
17. Akama-Garren EH, Bianchi MT, Leveroni C, Cole AJ, Cash SS, Westover MB. Weighing the value of memory loss in the surgical evaluation of left temporal lobe epilepsy: a decision analysis. Epilepsia. 2014;55(11):1844–53.
18. Goodyear-Smith F, Buetow S. Power issues in the doctor-patient relationship. Health Care Anal. 2001;9(4):449–62.

19. Anderson CT, Noble E, Mani R, Lawler K, Pollard JR. Epilepsy surgery: factors that affect patient decision-making in choosing or deferring a procedure. Epilepsy Res Treat. 2013;2013:309284.
20. Choi H, Pargeon K, Bausell R, Wong JB, Mendiratta A, Bakken S. Temporal lobe epilepsy surgery: what do patients want to know? Epilepsy Behav. 2011;22(3):479–82.
21. Taylor DC. Treating children and adults: whose body is it anyway? Eur Child Adolesc Psychiatry. 1999;8(4):315–9.
22. Taylor DC, Neville BGR, Cross JH. New measures of outcome of the surgical treatment of epilepsy. Epilepsia. 1997;38:625–30.

Chapter 18
Health Economic Analyses of Epilepsy Surgery

Nathalie Jetté and Samuel Wiebe

Abstract We review general health economics and evidence-based medicine concepts as they pertain to epilepsy. A brief analysis of cost of illness studies in epilepsy demonstrates substantial burden of illness, identifies important components (e.g., antiseizure medications, hospitalizations, indirect costs), and assesses factors associated with burden, such as seizure control. A systematic analysis of long-term, comparative economic evaluations in epilepsy shows that such studies are scarce, many are methodologically weak, and reporting of results is highly variable. Most studies focus on patients with temporal lobe epilepsy, few focus on children or on resource-poor countries, and none addresses the very young or very old. Despite methodological caveats, studies consistently demonstrate the cost-effectiveness of epilepsy surgery, which is often more effective and cheaper than the medical treatment alternatives. We present recommendations for future economic analyses of epilepsy surgery.

Keywords Cost analysis • Cost-effectiveness • Cost-utility • Decision analysis • Health economics • Direct costs • Indirect costs • Intangible costs • Quality-adjusted life years • QALY

N. Jetté, MD, MSc (✉) • S. Wiebe, MD, MSc
Department of Clinical Neurosciences, Foothills Medical Centre, University of Calgary, 1403 29 Street NW, Calgary, AB T2N 2 T9, Canada
e-mail: nathalie.jette@albertahealthservices.ca; swiebe@ucalgary.ca

K. Malmgren et al. (eds.), *Long-Term Outcomes of Epilepsy Surgery in Adults and Children*, DOI 10.1007/978-3-319-17783-0_18

Abbreviations

COI	Cost of illness
EA	Economic analysis
GDP	Gross domestic product
HE	Health economics
ICER	Incremental cost-effectiveness ratio
PWE	Person with epilepsy
QALYs	Quality-adjusted life years
UK	United Kingdom
USA	United States of America
USD	United States dollar
WHO	World Health Organization

Introduction

Clinicians caring for people with epilepsy (PWE) are increasingly faced with the reality of costs, outcomes, and cost containment measures on many fronts. This occurs, for example, when clinicians prescribe new or costly interventions, an area where researchers have developed generic models to help clinicians choose the most cost-effective interventions for individual patients [1]. It is also seen when clinicians advocate additional programs and resources for epilepsy, when advising policy makers and administrators on the best and most efficient use of resources, or when assembling cost-conscious clinical practice guidelines [2]. Researchers in the field of epilepsy may also have to justify or explain their work on the basis of translational and economic consequences.

The words *health economics* (HE) may conjure thoughts of financial and monetary aspects pertaining to health. In reality, HE is about deciding how to allocate finite health resources, about outcomes associated with allocative decisions, and about the benefits gained and forgone by a particular choice of use of resources (i.e., opportunity cost). Additionally, although health resources and benefits are usually expressed in monetary terms, there are many important resources and outcomes that are integral elements of HE, and yet are difficult to quantify monetarily (e.g., intangible costs, time, suffering, or well-being).

HE is relevant to clinicians caring for PWE because they need to be aware of the level of health resource use in various groups of patients, and the opportunity cost of epilepsy and its different treatment options [3]. This can help understand the economic burden associated with epilepsy, how this burden compares with other conditions, and the impact of various types of treatment beyond the usual clinical metrics, such as seizures. The manner in which limited resources are allocated in epilepsy care has important consequences at many levels, from health policy makers and health system managers, through health care facilities and health care providers, to individual patients, their families and caregivers. In this chapter, we review some basic concepts of HE and how to interpret studies in this area, and provide a critical summary of the evidence pertaining to long-term costs and outcomes of surgical interventions.

General Concepts

The broad range in scope and methods of different types of economic analyses (EAs) [4] can be conceptualized in a matrix whose two main axes ask whether both costs and outcomes are considered, and whether alternative courses of actions are compared (Fig. 18.1). The most complete EAs examine both costs and consequences in >1 intervention (right lower corner of Fig. 18.1). *Cost of Illness* (COI) studies itemize and sum the costs of a health condition and are generally used to assess burden of illness and determine major cost components. *Cost-minimization* analyses are used to identify the least costly among those interventions that have similar clinical effectiveness. *Cost-effectiveness* analyses compare interventions that use similar clinical outcome metrics (e.g., number of seizure-free patients), but have different levels of effectiveness (e.g., medical vs. surgical therapy). *Cost-utility* evaluations determine the incremental cost per quality-adjusted outcomes – often

		Costs and Consequences Examined?	
		No	**Yes**
		Only Costs	Costs and Outcomes
Two or more alternatives compared?	**No**	(Partial evaluation) ***Cost description***	(Partial evaluation) ***Cost-outcome description***
	Yes	(Partial evaluation) ***Cost analysis***	(Complete evaluation) ***Cost-minimization*** ***Cost-effectiveness*** ***Cost-benefit*** ***Cost-utility***

Fig. 18.1 Different types of economic analyses

quality-adjusted life years (QALYs). In *cost-benefit* studies all inputs (costs) and outputs (outcomes) are expressed in monetary values, allowing for comparison of disparate interventions and outcomes [5].

Users of HE literature in epilepsy can benefit from a systematic approach to critically appraise the validity and applicability of EAs by applying a simple 9-item checklist (Table 18.1) [6]. The viewpoint of the study determines the range of costs and consequences included in an EA, and can be that of the patients, the health care institution, the insurer or health system, and society as a whole. A broad societal perspective, which incorporates the patient's productivity and ability to work, is often recommended. Because subgroups of patients can have vastly different costs and outcomes, these should be adequately explored and reported. Many issues influence cost measurement and valuation; authors should report the physical quantities of resources used, which allows readers to extrapolate results from one setting to another, and they should distinguish between charges and real costs. The types of costs included in the EA determine its scope. A narrow perspective includes only direct costs (i.e., costs directly attributable to epilepsy and its treatment), which can be medical and nonmedical (transportation, home support, etc.). A broader perspective includes also indirect costs (e.g., productivity costs) and intangible costs (e.g., the value of pain and suffering), although the latter are difficult to quantify monetarily. Of particular relevance in long-term EAs is accounting for the lower value of costs or outcomes incurred in the future. This is usually addressed by discounting future events at a rate of 3–5 % to approximate future to present values. In the absence of long-term medical and surgical epilepsy cohorts or randomized trials, long-term EAs resort to models (such as decision analysis and Markov models-Stochastic model to study health outcomes using health states and health transitions iteratively) in which future costs and outcomes are predicted based on assumptions that should be clearly stated and subjected to sensitivity analyses to assess their robustness.

Table 18.1 Checklist to assess the validity and applicability of economic evaluations

Are the results valid?
1. Did the investigators adopt a sufficiently broad viewpoint (patients, treatment options, and outcomes)?
2. Are the results reported separately for relevant patient subgroups?
3. Were costs measured accurately?
4. Did investigators consider the timing of costs and consequences?
What are the results?
5. What are the incremental costs and effects of each strategy?
6. Do incremental costs and effects differ between groups?
7. Was a sensitivity analysis performed to assess impact of different cost assumptions?
Can I apply the results to patient care?
8. Are the treatment benefits worth the risks and costs (including patient values)?
9. Can I expect similar costs in my setting?

Adapted from Drummond et al. [6]

Sensitivity analysis refers to repeating the evaluation using a range of plausible probabilities of outcomes, costs, and value judgments to assess whether the results change substantially. In interpreting the results of EAs, clinicians should look for incremental analyses based on a ratio of the difference between alternatives in costs and outcomes, and often expressed as an Incremental Cost-Effectiveness Ratio (ICER):

$$\text{ICER} = \frac{[C_A - C_B]}{[O_A - O_B]},$$

where C_A and C_B are the costs of alternatives A and B, and O_A and O_B are the outcomes of alternatives A and B. Costs are usually expressed in monetary units, benefits are expressed in clinical units (seizure freedom) or more often in QALYs, and the ICER is often expressed as Cost per QALY.

A final point pertains to what constitutes a cost-effective intervention, that is, the ICER that warrants adoption of an intervention by a health system. Although more relevant to policy makers than to individual clinicians, this is important to consider given the increasing pressure on clinicians for "bedside allocation" (see above). The World Health Organization's (WHO) CHOICE project has published threshold values for intervention cost-effectiveness in the different world regions based on their gross domestic product (GDP) expressed in 2005 International dollars, and adopting quality adjusted life years (QALYs) as the outcome [7]. The cost-effectiveness of interventions is divided into three categories: (1) very cost-effective if the cost per QALY (ICER) is less than the region's GDP per capita, (2) cost-effective if it is between 1 and 3 times the GDP per capita, and (3) not cost-effective if it is >3 times the GDP per capita. The upper threshold for cost-effective interventions ranges from Int$ 5,086 in the poorest African countries, to Int$ 119,849 in affluent North American countries (Fig. 18.2).

The Cost of Epilepsy

Studies of COI in epilepsy are challenging. First, COI studies incorporating measures of direct, indirect, and intangible costs are rare. Most studies focus primarily on direct costs and even when indirect and intangible costs are incorporated, the components included vary among studies. Second, COI studies span a variety of time horizons, geographic regions (health care costs differ substantially between countries) and populations, making comparisons between studies impossible in the absence of reports of physical units of resources used. Finally, most long-term COI studies of epilepsy (i.e., lifetime costs of incidence cohorts) usually provide estimates based on modeling, because prospective studies with rigorous and comprehensive data collection are sparse. Studies consistently show that antiseizure medications and hospital admissions have become the largest component of direct costs (median 31 % and 34 %, respectively) [5], particularly in those with

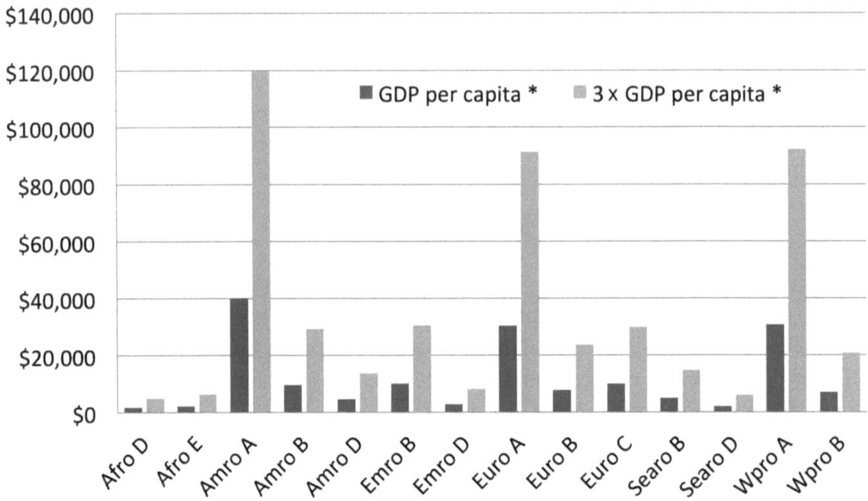

Fig. 18.2 WHO cost-effectiveness thresholds for interventions, expressed as Cost (2005 international $) per QALY *Footnote*: *GDP* gross domestic product; < GDP per capita (very cost-effective); 1–3×GDP per capita (cost-effective); > 3×GDP per capita (not cost-effective). *Afro* African region, *Amro* American region, *Emro* European region, *Euro* European region, *Searo* South East Asia region, *Wpro* Western Pacific region. Suffixes A to E after each region indicate gradation of population health indicators in terms of adult and infant mortality, A = best, E = worst

difficult-to-treat or newly diagnosed epilepsies [8, 9]. Cost estimates vary markedly among studies, as demonstrated in a review of population-based prevalence studies, where the annual per-patient direct costs of epilepsy in Italy and the UK (5 studies) ranged from $803 (USD) to $3,208 (USD) in those with active epilepsy, and it ranged from $126 (USD) to $1,748 (USD) in those with inactive epilepsy [8]. A more recent review also found that the annual direct per-patient costs of prevalent epilepsy in 15 international studies ranged from $55 (USD) in India to $3,065 (USD) in the UK [5].

Although costs of epilepsy vary among studies, direct costs are always higher in the first year after diagnosis (up to four times higher than in subsequent years) [5, 8]. In a systematic review of 22 COI studies in epilepsy worldwide (most from Europe and the USA but also from India, Hong Kong, Oman, Burundi, Chile, and Mexico), every study used a bottom-up approach (using individual patient records) and most only measured direct costs [9]. Antiseizure medications were the main contributor to direct costs, while indirect costs ranged between 12 and 85 % of the total annual costs in the 12 studies that estimated these. Unfortunately, results of bottom-up approach COI studies, although more precise, may not be applicable to population-based cohorts of persons with epilepsy. A systematic review examining predictors of cost and health resource utilization in epilepsy in five studies [10] found no association between demographic factors studied and costs or health resource utilization, while increased seizure frequency and severity along with polytherapy or higher number of AEDs predicted costs.

Epilepsy Surgery Is a Cost-Effective Intervention

In this section, we review long-term EAs of epilepsy surgery, which were identified by searching Embase and Medline on August 1, 2014, using the following strategy: epilepsy AND (economic* or cost or quality-adjusted life years or QALY) AND (surgery or amygdalo-hippocampectomy or amygdalo-hippocampectomy or resection or callosotomy or hemispherectomy or lesionectomy or transection or vagus nerve stimulation or hippocampal stimulation or deep brain stimulation or gamma knife surgery or ablation or subpial transsection). We included studies that examined long-term (5 years or longer) costs and outcomes of epilepsy surgery, and compared epilepsy surgery to another intervention (e.g., medical management). Review articles on the cost of epilepsy and included articles were also hand searched.

Ten articles published between 1995 and 2014 met eligibility criteria (see Appendix) [11–20]. Studies were performed in Canada ($n=3$), the USA ($n=3$), the UK ($n=2$), France ($n=1$), and India ($n=1$). All long-term analyses relied on modeling because there are no actual long-term data. There were only two pediatric studies [11, 14], no studies focused on the elderly, and none addressed palliative surgeries or electrical stimulation aside from two studies examining the cost-effectiveness of vagus nerve stimulation, one of which was a follow-up of the other [12, 13]. Most studies had a health system or insurer viewpoint. Only three studies adopted a societal perspective [15, 17, 19] (although one assumed no productivity changes [15]), and only one study (from France) included intangible costs [19]. All but one study derived long-term estimates of surgical and medical costs from decision analysis modeling [18]. Half of the studies were cost-effectiveness analyses with seizure control as the outcome of interest [14, 17–20], and half were cost-utility analyses [11–13, 15, 16] that calculated QALYs using utility weights derived from the literature, from direct measurement, or by extrapolating from quality of life (not utility) scores. The cost, outcomes, and long-term data sources to generate the models included bottom-up local data, expert opinion, patient surveys, and published studies. Temporal lobe resection was overwhelmingly the commonest surgical procedure considered. Nearly every study used sensitivity analyses, but the variables and results were heterogeneous. Methodological quality was generally poor and the scope tended to be narrow, although more recent studies dealing with resective surgery had substantially improved quality and reporting [11, 19].

Results were reported in a nonstandardized and highly variable manner. In general, seizure freedom was an important factor associated with lower costs after surgery. Every study demonstrated that, in the base model and also in many sensitivity analyses, epilepsy surgery was more effective than medical therapy in the long term (i.e., yielded more QALYs), and it became less costly over time (i.e., surgery dominated medical care). Costs per QALYs for epilepsy surgery were within acceptable ranges when compared to other common interventions and/or treatments [15, 16]. In the USA, the ICER was $15,581 [16] considering only direct costs, and $27,200 considering direct and indirect costs (but assuming no change in productivity). Both of these are below the USA GDP per capita ($40,000) and well within the "very cost-effective" range suggested by WHO thresholds [7]. In general, epilepsy surgery became cheaper than medical therapy anywhere from 7 to 14.4 years after surgery in the base case models, although direct costs dropped rapidly immediately after surgery in seizure-free patients.

In 2002, the International League Against Epilepsy subcommission on the economic burden of epilepsy published methodological recommendations for EAs in epilepsy [21]. It is recommended that studies be carried out in community-based patients with newly diagnosed epilepsy, who would then be followed prospectively, while retrospective and prevalence-based studies should be population-based and use valid case definitions to minimize selection bias. They also suggest capturing a comprehensive set of cost items and to include important direct costs such as antiseizure medications, hospital care, major diagnostic tests, physician visits, treatment of injuries, and antiseizure medication side effects [9, 21]. Recommendations for reporting EAs have also been published and should be adopted in epilepsy surgery studies [22].

Conclusions and Some Recommendations

COI studies in epilepsy highlight the burden of illness and consistently identify the most important cost categories (indirect costs, antiseizure drugs, and hospitalization), and the importance of seizure control. In spite of methodological and reporting limitations, EAs in epilepsy consistently demonstrate that in most situations, epilepsy surgery is cost-effective or dominates (is more effective and less costly) medical treatment over time. However, knowledge gaps in this area exist. Most studies dealt with TLE, most were from North America and Europe, and resource-poor countries were rarely represented. Cost-effectiveness of surgery in the very young, the elderly and for palliative surgical procedures requires further exploration. Prospective long-term studies are nonexistent, and studies using appropriate utility weights and incorporating all aspects of COI (i.e. direct, indirect, and intangible) are scarce.

Some principles to consider in future epilepsy EAs include: (1) clearly defining the population under investigation and only attributing epilepsy-related costs (not comorbidities or clinical trial costs); (2) considering a bottom-up approach aiming for precise and comprehensive estimates of direct, indirect, and intangible costs; (3) being mindful of equity issues arising from inclusion of indirect cost, as children and older adults may appear to have lower costs despite a significant burden of epilepsy; (4) being cautious to extrapolate EA results to different settings as costs may vary substantially; (5) encouraging multicenter studies with standard methodology and reporting to enhance interpretability and applicability of EAs; (6) performing and reporting subgroup analyses, such as age groups, epilepsy syndromes, recent versus chronic epilepsy, and drug-responsive versus drug-resistant epilepsy; (7) performing EAs in non-TLE patients, in palliative procedures and in younger and older patients; (8) accounting for common epilepsy comorbidities both in terms of costs and outcomes.

Appendix. Summary of Characteristics and Results of Long-Term Health Economic Outcome Studies Associated with Epilepsy Surgery

Author, year, country	Study type, methodology, perspective[a]	Study population (data source)	Intervention(s) compared	Main outcome metric (time horizon)	Results
Bowen, 2013 (Canada, Ontario)	Cost-utility HTA with decision (Markov) analysis modeling[b] Perspective: health system/ insurer	Children with drug-resistant epilepsy of all types (Costs: local patients. Outcomes, utilities, long term: literature)	Epilepsy surgery vs. medical management	QALYs (20 years)	Average expected cost per patient, $ (CDN) Surgery: costs: 59,197 QALYs: 11.648 No surgery: costs: 60,985 QALYs: 10.757 ICER: 0.892 (surgery dominates and costs −1,788 over 20 years)
Forbes, 2003 (UK)	Cost-utility Modeling Perspective: not clear – combined from literature	Adults with drug-resistant epilepsy of all types (Costs, outcomes: literature. Utilities: literature and patients using TTO and EQ-5D)	VNS pivotal trials of high vs. low current	QALYs (5 years)	Cost per QALY for VNS implants with battery life of 5 years, NNT=6 for 50 % reduction in seizure frequency (£) VNS:[c] Cost/QALY: (£) 28,849 QALY: 0.285 QALYs gained per successful device
Forbes, 2008 (UK)	Cost-utility Modeling Perspective: not clear – combined from literature	Adults with drug-resistant epilepsy of all types (Update to Forbes 2003 study – all from literature and assumptions)	VNS follow-up data. Control data were historical-assumed	QALYs (6 years)	Cost for VNS implant with battery life of 6 years, NNT=2 for 40–58 % reduction in seizure frequency (£) VNS: costs: (£) 4,423 QALY: 0.285 QALYs gained per successful device

(continued)

Appendix (continued)

Author, year, country	Study type, methodology, perspective[a]	Study population (data source)	Intervention(s) compared	Main outcome metric (time horizon)	Results
Keene, 1999 (Canada, Ontario)	Cost-effectiveness Decision analysis modeling Perspective: health system/ insurer	Children age 5–18 years old with drug-resistant epilepsy (Costs: local patients. Outcomes and long term: literature)	Cortical resection vs. medical management	Seizure outcome (25 years)	Total cost for 64 children over a 25-year period, $ (CDN) Surgery: $9,490,538[d] Medical: $12,378,964 Surgery became less costly than medical therapy after 14 years
King, 1997 (USA)	Cost-utility Decision analysis (Markov) modeling Perspective: societal, but assumed no change in productivity	Adults with drug-resistant TLE (Costs, outcomes: local patients and literature. Utilities: transposed from QOL values in literature – no utilities)	TLE surgery vs. medical management	QALYs CER (lifetime)	Surgery provided average of 1.1 additional QALY compared to continued medical management $ (USD) CER: $27,200/QALY[e]
Langfitt, 1997 (USA, NY)	Cost-utility Decision analysis modeling Perspective: health care provider/insurance	Adults with drug-resistant TLE (Costs: local patients. Outcomes: literature. Utilities: transposed from QOL values in literature – no utilities)	TLE surgery vs. medical management	QALYs CER (lifetime)	CPS free after ATL. $ (USD) CER: $15,581/QALY

Picot, 2004[f] (France)	Cost-effectiveness Decision analysis (Markov) modeling Perspective: societal	Ages 15–60 years old with drug-resistant focal epilepsy (Costs, outcomes: local patients. Long-term: literature)	Epilepsy surgery vs. medical management	Seizure outcome, CER (2 years and lifetime)	ICER = 9,533 € per seizure-free patient at 2 years (€) Surgery became less costly than Medical therapy between 7 and 8 years after surgery
Platt, 2002 (USA)	Cost-effectiveness Decision analysis modeling Perspective: societal	Adults with drug-resistant TLE (Costs, outcomes: literature)	TLE surgery vs. medical management	Seizure outcome Seizure outcome (up to 40 years)	Cost per modeled cohort, $ (USD) Direct costs for surgery lower than medical at 14.4 years Indirect costs became lower for the surgical group 1 year after surgery Direct plus indirect costs became lower for surgical than medical group 7.3 years after surgery
Rao, 2000 (India, Kerala)	Cost-effectiveness Cohort study with descriptive analyses Perspective: Health care payer	119 adults with drug-resistant TLE (Costs, outcomes: local patients. Long term: simple permutation – no modeling)	TLE surgery vs. medical management	Seizure outcome (up to 34 years)	Total direct costs of caring for a TLE patients from age 26 to 60 years old, $ (USD): Medical: 5,000 Surgical: 1,200

(continued)

Appendix (continued)

Author, year, country	Study type, methodology, perspective[a]	Study population (data source)	Intervention(s) compared	Main outcome metric (time horizon)	Results
Wiebe, 1995 (Canada, Ontario)	Cost-effectiveness Decision analysis modeling Perspective: health system/ insurer	100 adults with drug-resistant TLE (Costs, outcomes: local patients and literature)	TLE surgery vs. medical management	Seizure outcome (up to 35 years)	Direct costs, $ (CDN) Year 1 Medical: 856,970 Surgical: 2,775,640 Year: 8.5 Medical = Surgical Year: 35 Medical: 10,741,425 Surgical: 8,117,911

Abbreviations: *ATL* anterior temporal lobectomy, *CDN* Canadian, *CER* cost-effectiveness ratio, *HTA* health technology assessment, *ICER* incremental cost-effectiveness ratio, *MCER* marginal cost-effectiveness ratio, *QALYs* quality-adjusted life years, *TLE* temporal lobe epilepsy, *USD* US dollars

[a]A societal perspective includes indirect costs. Health insurer/system perspective includes only direct costs

[b]A prevalence-based "top-down" health care system budgetary impact model (Markov model) – input variables into the model were seizure status, surgery candidacy evaluation and surgery costs, follow-up costs, utility values, and mortality

[c]Seven models are analyzed and presented in the original study. Only the baseline model results are shown here

[d]10 % of the total surgical program costs occurred within the first year, compared to 1 % of the total medical program costs. By year 14, the costs were the same in both groups, at which point costs for the surgically treated group became less than for the medically treated group

[e]11 models were analyzed and presented in the original study. Only the basic model results are shown here

[f]The only study that assessed direct, indirect, and intangible costs

References

1. Sinclair JC, Cook RJ, Guyatt GH, Pauker SG, Cook DJ. When should an effective treatment be used? Derivation of the threshold number needed to treat and the minimum event rate for treatment. J Clin Epidemiol. 2001;54(3):253–62.
2. Eccles M, Mason J. How to develop cost-conscious guidelines. Health Technol Assess. 2001;5(16):1–69.
3. Ubel PA, Arnold RM. The unbearable rightness of bedside rationing. Physician duties in a climate of cost containment. Arch Intern Med. 1995;155(17):1837–42.
4. Detsky AS, Naglie IG. A clinician's guide to cost-effectiveness analysis. Ann Intern Med. 1990;113(2):147–54.
5. Pillas D, Selai C. Economic aspects of epilepsy and antiepileptic treatment: a review of the literature. Expert Rev Pharmacoecon Outcomes Res. 2005;5(3):327–38.
6. Drummond M, Goeree R, Moayyedi P, Levine M. Economic analysis. In: Guyatt G, Rennie D, Meade MO, Cook DJ, editors. Users' guides to the medical literature a manual for evidence-based clinical practice. 2nd ed. New York: McGraw-Hill; 2002.
7. Table: threshold values for intervention cost-effectiveness by Region. Geneva: World Health Organization; 2005 [cited 2014 August 2014]. Available from: http://www.who.int/choice/costs/CER_levels/en/.
8. Begley CE, Beghi E. The economic cost of epilepsy: a review of the literature. Epilepsia. 2002;43 Suppl 4:3–9.
9. Strzelczyk A, Reese JP, Dodel R, Hamer HM. Cost of epilepsy: a systematic review. Pharmacoeconomics. 2008;26(6):463–76.
10. Taylor RS, Sander JW, Taylor RJ, Baker GA. Predictors of health-related quality of life and costs in adults with epilepsy: a systematic review. Epilepsia. 2011;52(12):2168–80.
11. Bowen JM, Snead OC, Chandra K, Blackhouse G, Goeree R. Epilepsy care in Ontario: an economic analysis of increasing access to epilepsy surgery. Ont Health Technol Assess Ser. 2012;12(18):1–41.
12. Forbes R. Cost-utility of vagus nerve stimulation (VNS) therapy for medically refractory epilepsy – an update. Seizure. 2008;17(4):387–8. Epub 2008/06/28.
13. Forbes RB, Macdonald S, Eljamel S, Roberts RC. Cost-utility analysis of vagus nerve stimulators for adults with medically refractory epilepsy. Seizure. 2003;12(5):249–56.
14. Keene D, Ventureyra EC. Epilepsy surgery for 5- to 18-year old patients with medically refractory epilepsy – is it cost efficient? Childs Nerv Syst. 1999;15(1):52–4; discussion 5.
15. King Jr JT, Sperling MR, Justice AC, O'Connor MJ. A cost-effectiveness analysis of anterior temporal lobectomy for intractable temporal lobe epilepsy. J Neurosurg. 1997;87(1):20–8.
16. Langfitt JT. Cost-effectiveness of anterotemporal lobectomy in medically intractable complex partial epilepsy. Epilepsia. 1997;38(2):154–63.
17. Platt M, Sperling MR. A comparison of surgical and medical costs for refractory epilepsy. Epilepsia. 2002;43 Suppl 4:25–31.
18. Rao MB, Radhakrishnan K. Is epilepsy surgery possible in countries with limited resources? Epilepsia. 2000;41 Suppl 4:S31–4.
19. Picot MC, Neveu D, Kahane P, Crespel A, Gelisse P, Hirsch E, et al. Cost-effectiveness of epilepsy surgery in a cohort of patients with medically intractable partial epilepsy – preliminary results. Rev Neurol (Paris). 2004;160 Spec No 1:5S354–67. Epub 28 08 2004. Evaluation medico-economique de la chirurgie des epilepsies partielles pharmaco-resistantes de l'adulte. Etude cout-efficacite – resultats preliminaires.
20. Wiebe S, Gafni A, Blume WT, Girvin JP. An economic evaluation of surgery for temporal lobe epilepsy. Epilepsy. 1995;8:227–35.
21. Begley CE, Beghi E, Beran RG, Heaney D, Langfitt JT, Pachlatko C, et al. ILAE commission on the burden of epilepsy, subcommission on the economic burden of epilepsy: final report 1998–2001. Epilepsia. 2002;43(6):668–73.
22. Siegel JE, Weinstein MC, Russell LB, Gold MR. Recommendations for reporting cost-effectiveness analyses. JAMA. 1996;276(16):1339–41.

Chapter 19
Long-Term Outcomes of Epilepsy Surgery: Knowledge Gaps and Future Directions

Kristina Malmgren, Sallie Baxendale, J. Helen Cross, and Philippe Ryvlin

Abstract Although epilepsy surgery has long been recognized as an effective treatment for carefully selected adults and children, studies of long-term seizure control are relatively rare and studies of the wider aspects of surgical outcome are even more scarce. In summarizing the literature, many of the chapters in this volume have highlighted what we do not know about epilepsy surgery outcomes rather than what we do. This chapter highlights the gaps in the adult and pediatric literature and discusses the roles that networking, collaboration, and adherence to a basic set of standards may play in addressing the current shortcomings of the literature.

Keywords Networking • Collaboration • Multicenter studies

The chapters in this volume have reviewed the long-term outcomes of epilepsy surgery in both pediatric and adult populations. Although epilepsy surgery has long been recognized as an effective treatment for carefully selected adults and children (see Chapter 1), studies of long-term seizure control are relatively rare and studies of the wider aspects of surgical outcome are even more scarce. In summarizing the literature, many of the chapters in this volume have highlighted what we do not know

K. Malmgren, MD, PhD (✉)
Department of Clinical Neuroscience and Rehabilitation, Institute of Neuroscience and Physiology, Sahlgrenska Academy, Gothenburg University, Gothenburg, Sweden

Department of Neurology, Sahlgrenska University Hospital, Gothenburg, Sweden
e-mail: Kristina.malmgren@neuro.gu.se

S. Baxendale, PhD, C.Psychol, AFBPsS
Department of Clinical and Experimental Epilepsy, National Hospital for Neurology and Neurosurgery, London, UK

J.H. Cross, MB ChB, PhD, FRCP, FRCPCH
Section of Clinical Neuroscience, UCL-Institute of Child Health, Great Ormond Street Hospital & Young Epilepsy, 4/5 Long Yard, WC1N 3LU London, UK

P. Ryvlin, MD, PhD
Department of Clinical Neurosciences, Centre Hospitalo-Universitaire Vaudois, Lausanne, Switzerland

K. Malmgren et al. (eds.), *Long-Term Outcomes of Epilepsy Surgery in Adults and Children*, DOI 10.1007/978-3-319-17783-0_19

about epilepsy surgery outcomes rather than what we do. The literature reviewed in this volume has a direct impact on what we as clinicians should tell potential surgical candidates about the procedure. Unlike some surgeries in other branches of medicine, epilepsy surgery outcomes are dynamic and not fixed at the 1-year follow-up time point. The oft quoted chances of being seizure-free at 1 year (60–70 %) do not tell the whole story. Long-term outcome studies suggest that less than 50 % of adults will remain seizure-free after surgery in the long term (see Chap. 3). The odds of achieving and sustaining seizure freedom are not the same thing. It is imperative that the long-term perspective forms an integral part of presurgical counseling of prospective surgical candidates. Similarly, Chaps. 10, 11, 12, 13, 14, and 15 highlight the wider aspects of surgical outcome that must be addressed in both the examination of preoperative expectations and the maximization of the postoperative opportunities that improved seizure control can bring, but are by no means automatic.

Knowledge Gaps in the Adult Literature

As discussed in Chap. 3, the best longitudinal long-term seizure outcome data in adults concern those who have had temporal lobe resection. There is much less information on the longitudinal course in other patient cohorts. For many resection types, the numbers of patients in single-center long-term studies are limited and for almost all studies there is a lack of controls. Multicenter observational studies following both operated and nonoperated patients are needed in order to obtain more robust data on long-term seizure outcomes.

Similarly, the literature on the long-term changes in cognitive function in people who undergo epilepsy surgery is small and currently limited to series that have undergone temporal lobe resections. Longitudinal studies suggest that the majority of epilepsy surgery candidates have stable memory functions at assessments conducted more than 5 years after surgery, with scores comparable to those they obtained 12–24 months after the operation. However, there is a subset of patients in whom ongoing seizures are associated with progressive memory impairment. Group data obscure individual trajectories of change, which can vary widely. Neuropsychological outcomes must be considered within the context of the individual patients' capacity for decline at the preoperative assessment.

There are no data on the long-term psychiatric outcomes of epilepsy surgery patients. Given the fluctuating nature of psychiatric conditions, longitudinal, routine clinical follow-up of surgical patients is the only way to track individual trajectories in mental health following surgery. In the shorter term, postsurgical depression and/or anxiety disorders are the most frequent psychiatric disorders identified after resective epilepsy surgery. A presurgical psychiatric history has been found to be associated with an increased risk of postsurgical recurrences or exacerbations. In a majority of patients, symptoms are expected to remit by 1 year, though persistent psychopathology has been found in up to 15 % of patients.

Studies on mortality after epilepsy surgery are very heterogeneous in terms of age groups, types of epilepsy and surgery, methods for reporting mortality outcomes, and comparison groups. Even though most studies report lower mortality among those rendered seizure-free versus those with recurrent seizures after surgery, the trend in the same direction was nonsignificant in the two population-based studies. However, in several studies seizure outcome status was assessed at a specific time point after surgery, typically 2 years, whereas follow-up of survival may extend over many decades. Further population-based long-term studies of both seizure outcome and mortality are warranted.

Studies specifically investigating educational and vocational outcomes in adults are also scarce. Seizure freedom is the strongest predictor of improvement in occupational status after surgery, followed by presurgical educational attainment and employment status. The review of the literature in Chap. 10 highlights the need for longer-term longitudinal studies to accurately track individual trajectories of educational and vocational outcomes relative to medically treated patients and healthy controls to determine whether surgery results in significant improvements, or whether outcomes are primarily accounted for by presurgical functioning.

In the majority of the studies of quality of life (QOL) after epilepsy surgery in adults reviewed in Chap. 12, follow-up intervals were no more than 1–2 years. In these short-term studies improvements in QOL do not automatically accompany seizure freedom and there are many nonseizure-related aspects of life that influence QOL. Outcome studies with follow-up periods of 1–2 years are likely to underestimate the benefits of seizure freedom conferred by surgery. Studies with longer-term follow-ups and including comparisons with control groups are needed in order to be able to accurately measure impact in this domain.

The expectation literature in epilepsy surgery is small. Implicit assumptions about seizure freedom need to be identified and addressed explicitly, and corrected where necessary, so that the candidate can make a truly informed decision regarding a surgical option. While much of the literature to date has been focused on the decision-making processes of their physicians, little is known about how surgical candidates approach and make this decision. It is likely that there are very significant cultural influences on expectations of epilepsy surgery in different parts of the world. These have yet to be explored. Further work is also needed to create and evaluate a presurgical counseling schedule to ensure that candidates approach surgery with realistic expectations and a longitudinal perspective on change.

The literature on adults' subjective expectations and experiences of epilepsy surgery is limited and most longitudinal studies have follow-ups of no more than 6 months to 2 years. Since many adult patients who undergo epilepsy surgery have had epilepsy since childhood, it is likely that it will take a number of years for them to adjust to life without seizures. Patients' long-term subjective experiences of the effects of epilepsy surgery across different domains of life need further study in order to provide epilepsy surgery candidates with realistic counseling.

Knowledge Gaps in the Pediatric Literature

The range of candidates coming to epilepsy surgery in childhood is wide. This aside, the primary outcome aim remains seizure freedom. Longitudinal data following children into adulthood remain few. Although outcome in the shorter term may give a degree of indication of the likely longer-term outcome, attrition does occur over time related to pathology and type of procedure, and the psychosocial consequences of this are apparent. Who is at risk of relapse in the longer term remains, however, unclear as groups reported are often mixed, with regard to age, duration of epilepsy, pathology, and type of procedure undertaken. However, it is also not clear whether outcome scales developed for surgery in adults are relevant in children. Further discussion is required as to what would be a relevant measure, and whether this could incorporate a measure relative to the duration of follow-up. Further, data suggest medication should be withdrawn earlier rather than later to determine who will need to remain on AEDs in the longer term. However, whether medication withdrawal may be possible in some individuals in the longer term and how this may relate to other outcome measures also remains unclear.

The rate of cognitive impairment is high in children with early-onset epilepsy. Parents recognize the impact of the epilepsy, and expectations remain high that improvement will be seen. Although limited data suggest this may be true in the longer term, study has only been performed in limited groups. Further longitudinal prospective study is required in a wide range of individuals to be more accurate in our counseling of families prior to surgery, and whether there is an optimal timing to surgery. Psychiatric comorbidity also remains high and although the rate has been determined to be high both pre and postoperatively, there are little data to indicate who may be at risk for the emergence of a psychiatric disorder, specifically in the longer term. Further work is required to determine individual risk factors, and optimize the timing of surgery accordingly. Finally, it is clear that educational and employment outcomes are enhanced by surgery in childhood, more so than surgery in adulthood, but it is unclear as to what degree employment is commensurate with educational achievement.

Quality-of-life trajectories following epilepsy surgery in childhood are yet to be explored. Long-term quality-of-life studies following epilepsy surgery in childhood are required, with determination of the influence of time since surgery, age at surgery, and age at follow-up, as well as other variables such as child and family variables. Perception of overall outcome and consequently QOL after surgery is highly influenced by mood or affective state and consequently it is important for provision of the appropriate support with the transition into adulthood. Strong social support and coping strategies to overcome epilepsy-specific and emotional difficulties may be essential in attaining improved psychosocial and QOL outcomes. Further, subjective experiences are again highly influenced by circumstance as well as affective state. Although they appear highly related to seizure outcome, with the emotional change seen over time through childhood into adulthood, perceptions of outcome may be related to circumstances rather than any relationship to the surgery itself. This aside, the small but existing literature is problematic in interpretation in view of the different methodologies utilized. The development of a validated tool that could be applied more widely would greatly enhance our understanding of this element.

In many of the studies performed to date, outcomes are often reported postoperatively, but without the availability of a control group – namely what would be likely to occur with medical treatment alone? How do the risks and benefits of surgery compare? Elective surgery in a pediatric setting has special ethical and legal considerations, over and above those associated with surgery in adults. While a number of authors have discussed these issues at a theoretical level, the expectations of children and teenagers and their parents have yet to be empirically examined. There is the compelling requirement for further studies evaluating all outcomes longitudinally following surgery in childhood into adulthood, and beyond. Appropriate counseling prior to surgery, and some indication of requirements for follow-up into adulthood could then be given.

Health Economics

The systematic analysis of long-term, comparative economic evaluations in epilepsy summarized in Chap. 18 shows that such studies are scarce, many are methodologically weak, and reporting of results is highly variable. Also, there are no prospective long-term studies. The limited literature suggests that epilepsy surgery is more effective and cheaper than the medical treatment alternatives. In future studies many methodological aspects need to be addressed, for example, multicenter studies with standard methodology and reporting.

Networking, Collaboration, and Raising Standards

The conclusions that can be drawn from many of the studies reviewed in the preceding chapters are limited by methodological shortcomings. Several of these limitations derive from heterogeneous practices, both in terms of clinical activity and methods of outcome assessment. Scientific publications as well as case discussion during international epilepsy surgery meetings and courses, point to a large variation in presurgical protocols among centers. Investigations such as PET, ictal SPECT, MEG, high-density EEG, and fMRI are advocated in some epilepsy surgery programs, but not in others. The type and indications for invasive EEG, as well as the surgical methods and strategy, also greatly vary between centers. While part of this heterogeneity might reflect national or regional differences in access to specific technology or reimbursement, significant variability in presurgical programs is also observed within the same country, reflecting limited effort towards harmonization. This is also reflected in the current practice parameters and guidelines of epilepsy surgery. Accordingly, the 2003 AAN guidelines on epilepsy surgery concluded that "determination of the localizing and prognostic values of specific presurgical diagnostic tests and presurgical evaluation strategies based on the current published literature would be difficult to impossible because of the tremendous variation from center to center in the way these tests are performed and the manner in which data are reported" [1]. It remains difficult to evaluate how the type of presurgical and surgical strategy influences outcome, but one might suspect a link between these strategies and the variability currently observed between series in long-term seizure freedom rates even after the most common resection type in adults, anterior temporal resections. Differences in the selected population and methods used to investigate or report postoperative seizure outcome might also partly explain this variation as discussed in Chap. 3.

Many of the above issues can be addressed in future studies by networking, collaboration, and adherence to a basic set of standards for long-term outcome studies. The multicenter study of epilepsy surgery launched in the early 2000s by seven large US epilepsy surgery centers is one of the pioneering but rare initiatives in the field [2]. More recently, the Director General for Health of the European commission launched a global program aiming at providing harmonization of optimal care for rare or complex diseases in Europe. This program is organized around European Reference Networks for which a legal framework has been adopted by the European Parliament in March 2014. Two pilot Networks of Cooperation were created within that framework, one in the field of pediatric oncology, and the second, E-PILEPSY, focusing on epilepsy surgery. E-PILEPSY offers a web-based approach to the multiple issues raised by the large heterogeneity of practices in the field. Greater access to relevant information on epilepsy surgery will be made available to patients, relatives, primary care physicians, and referring neurologists in all EU languages through a currently developed web site (http://www.e-pilepsy.eu/). Harmonization of practice will be promoted by: (1) the development of regularly updated systematic reviews and guidelines, (2) access to tutorials and software dedicated to EEG and neuroimaging postprocessing as well as neuropsychological evaluation, on a shared IT platform, (3) video-conferences where complex cases will be discussed at the EU scale, (4) a monitored prospectively completed database to follow practices and outcome in each of the participant centers. E-PILEPSY is currently comprised of 28 partners, including the International League Against Epilepsy (ILAE), the World Health Organization (WHO), and the European Epilepsy Monitoring unit Association (EEMA). Its scope is to enlarge in the near future with the view to represent an inclusive initiative for all European-based epilepsy surgery centers willing to share experience in order to progress towards dissemination and harmonization of optimal care.

Conclusions

Epilepsy surgery has a profound impact on the brains of those operated. Patients and parents have hopes for improvements that are not limited to seizure control but pertain to many other areas of life. When planning this volume, we therefore wanted to focus on longer-term outcomes from epilepsy surgery in both adults and children, and to assess many of the different outcome domains that have been identified as important. Our aim was to address outcomes beyond at least a 5-year time period following surgery. However, as many chapters within this volume have made clear, longer-term data are very scarce or completely missing, and so the authors have only been able to summarize studies of shorter follow-ups. We hope that this volume will inspire those working in the field to address these knowledge gaps in collaborating to conduct methodologically sound, prospective long-term outcome studies, which in many cases will need a multicenter design and control groups.

References

1. Engel Jr J, Wiebe S, French J, Sperling M, Williamson P, Spencer D, et al. Practice parameter: temporal lobe and localized neocortical resections for epilepsy. Epilepsia. 2003;44(6): 741–51.
2. Berg AT, Vickrey BG, Langfitt JT, Sperling MR, Walczak TS, Shinnar S, Bazil CW, Pacia SV, Spencer SS, Multicenter Study of Epilepsy Surgery. The multicenter study of epilepsy surgery: recruitment and selection for surgery. Epilepsia. 2003;44(11):1425–33.

Index

K. Malmgren et al. (eds.), *Long-Term Outcomes of Epilepsy Surgery in Adults and Children*, DOI 10.1007/978-3-319-17783-0

F

G

H

I

L

R

S

T

MIX
Papier aus verantwortungsvollen Quellen
Paper from responsible sources
FSC® C105338

If you have any concerns about our products,
you can contact us on
ProductSafety@springernature.com

In case Publisher is established outside the EU,
the EU authorized representative is:
Springer Nature Customer Service Center GmbH
Europaplatz 3, 69115 Heidelberg, Germany

Printed by Libri Plureos GmbH
in Hamburg, Germany